SECOND EDITION

Social and Behavioral Foundations of Public Health

For Graham and Elliot

SECOND EDITION

Social and Behavioral Foundations of Public Health

Edited by
Jeannine Coreil
University of South Florida

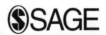

Los Angeles • London • New Delhi • Singapore • Washington DC

For information:

SAGE Publications, Inc.
2455 Teller Road
Thousand Oaks, California 91320
E-mail: order@sagepub.com

SAGE Publications Ltd.
1 Oliver's Yard
55 City Road
London EC1Y 1SP
United Kingdom

SAGE Publications India Pvt. Ltd.
B 1/I 1 Mohan Cooperative Industrial Area
Mathura Road, New Delhi 110 044
India

SAGE Publications Asia-Pacific Pte. Ltd.
33 Pekin Street #02-01
Far East Square
Singapore 048763

Printed in the United States of America

Library of Congress Cataloging-in-Publication Data

Social and behavioral foundations of public health/edited by Jeannine Coreil. — 2nd ed.
    p. cm.
Includes bibliographical references and index.
ISBN 978-1-4129-5704-5 (cloth : alk. paper)

   1. Public health—Social aspects. 2. Public health—Psychological aspects. 3. Social medicine.
I. Coreil, Jeannine. [DNLM: 1. Social Medicine. 2. Public Health. WA 31 S6767 2009]

RA418.C673 2009
362.1—dc22   2008031846

This book is printed on acid-free paper.

10   11   12   13   10   9   8   7   6   5   4   3   2

Acquisitions Editor:	Kassie Graves
Editorial Assistant:	Veronica Novak
Production Editor:	Carla Freeman
Copy Editor:	QuADS Prepress (P) Ltd.
Typesetter:	C&M Digitals (P) Ltd.
Proofreader:	Jenifer Kooiman
Indexer:	Diggs Publication Services
Cover Designer:	Tony Lemos
Marketing Manager:	Carmel Schrire

Contents

Preface

Several considerations guided the development of this second edition of *Social and Behavioral Foundations of Public Health.* Feedback on the first edition from students and colleagues was very helpful. For example, our selection of a schema to depict levels of the social ecology of health model was based on field testing with public health students of several graphical figures found in the literature. Selection of content for the book was influenced by the 10 *core competencies in social and behavioral sciences* identified by the Association of Schools of Public Health (ASPH, 2006) for graduate education in public health. Developed by the ASPH Education Committee during 2004 to 2006 with input from hundreds of professionals and educators in the field, the competencies are part of a comprehensive outline of basic knowledge and skills needed for preparing individuals for the Master of Public Health degree. The competencies are organized by five core discipline-specific domains: epidemiology, biostatistics, social and behavioral sciences, health policy and management, and environmental health sciences. In addition, seven competencies that cut across disciplines were identified: communication and informatics, diversity and culture, leadership, professionalism, program planning, public health biology, and systems thinking. The core competencies for the social and behavioral sciences (SBS) include the following:

1. Identify basic theories, concepts, and models from a range of social and behavioral science disciplines that are used in public health research and practice.

2. Identify the causes of social and behavioral factors that affect the health of individuals and populations.

3. Identify individual, organizational, and community concerns, assets, resources, and deficits for social and behavioral science interventions.

4. Identify critical stakeholders for the planning, implementation, and evaluation of public health programs, policies, and interventions.

5. Describe steps and procedures for the planning, implementation, and evaluation of public health programs, policies, and interventions.

6. Describe the role of community and social factors in both the onset and the solution of public health problems.

7. Describe the merits of social and behavioral science interventions and policies.

8. Apply evidence-based approaches in the development and evaluation of social and behavioral science interventions.

9. Apply ethical principles to public health program planning, implementation, and evaluation.

10. Specify multiple targets and levels of intervention for social and behavioral science programs and/or policies.

All the SBS competencies are addressed in the book, some to a greater degree than others. A few of the book chapters focus on a particular competency, such as the chapters on behavioral and social science theory (Competency No. 1), social epidemiology (No. 2), community-based approaches to health promotion (No. 3), planning health promotion and disease prevention programs (Nos. 4 and 5), and social environment and health (No. 6). Competencies 7 through 10 are addressed in several of the book's chapters.

A number of the cross-cutting competencies are also addressed in the book. In particular, "systems thinking" permeates the entire book because of its social ecological orientation and organization around the social ecology of health model. Systems thinking is defined as "the ability to recognize system level properties that result from dynamic interactions among human and social systems and how they affect the relationships among individuals, groups, organizations, communities and environments" (ASPH, 2006, p. 23). Multilevel systems perspectives are applied to most of the topics in the book, providing diverse examples of the application of this framework in public health. In addition, the "diversity and culture" competency is addressed to a substantial degree, particularly in the chapters on comparative health cultures and on health disparities, diversity, and cultural competence.

The ASPH core competencies will form the basic content for the recently inaugurated Certified in Public Health (CPH) credentialing process (overseen by the newly created National Board of Public Health Examiners). These professional developments, along with the addition of many newly accredited schools and programs for public health education in the United States, reflect the maturation of the field and its increasing relevance for addressing contemporary health problems. The social and behavioral sciences have much to contribute to this process.

While the first edition of this book marked the "coming of age" of the social and behavioral sciences in public health, the second edition reflects the increasing maturity of this interdisciplinary field. Several new chapters have been added, and the content and focus of previous chapters have been expanded, updated, and reorganized to illustrate the relevance of their themes for socio-ecological-systems thinking. "Health Disparities, Diversity, and Cultural Competence" (Chapter 9) takes a critical, reflexive approach to current issues and practices in the diversity arena. Two new chapters—"Planning Health Promotion and Disease Prevention Programs" (Chapter 13) and "Approaches to Policy and Advocacy" (Chapter 16)—expand on the practical applications of the field. The importance of a life-course perspective is highlighted by the addition of chapters on adolescent health and reproductive health, which complement aging and public health. The addition of "Special Topics" chapters on childhood obesity, injury prevention, violence, and occupational health reflects the growing importance of these areas of specialization.

The book is organized into six parts: I. Introduction and Overview; II. Theoretical Foundations; III. Sociocultural Contexts of Health; IV. Special Populations Through the Life Cycle; V. Intervention, Methods and Practice; and VI. Special Topics. Part introductions relate the component chapters to overarching themes addressed in each part. The "Afterword" discusses new directions anticipated in the application of the social and behavioral sciences to public health.

—Jeannine Coreil

REFERENCE

Association of Schools of Public Health. (2006). *Master's Degree in Public Health Core Competency Development Project* (Version 2.3). Washington, DC: ASPH Education Committee. Retrieved May 6, 2008, from www.asph.org/userfiles/version2.3.pdf

Acknowledgments

This book reflects the generous collaboration, assistance, and support of many people. I especially want to thank the 16 authors who accepted the invitation to contribute chapters. Their willingness to make time for writing these chapters and their openness to suggestions for making the chapters fit the goals of the book are much appreciated. My coauthors from the first edition, Carol Bryant and Neil Henderson, provided valuable input in planning the second edition. The editorial staff at Sage, including Margaret Sewell, Kassie Graves, Veronica Novak, Carla Freeman, and Shamila Swamy, were very helpful in moving the project forward and putting the manuscript in order. Several colleagues provided critical feedback on the draft chapters, including Robbie Baer, Ann McElroy, Stephanie Marhefka, Carol Bryant, Kokos Markides, and Carla VandeWeerd. I would also like to thank the following reviewers, who provided valuable suggestions on the organization and content of the book:

Bettina M. Beech
Vanderbilt University

Mary McElroy
Kansas State University

Jan Warren-Findlow
University of North Carolina at Charlotte

Robert M. Huff
California State University, Northridge

Alina Perez
Nova Southeastern University

Vicki L. Tall Chief
University of Oklahoma Health Sciences Center

Kathy Zavela Tyson
University of Northern Colorado

Charlotte Noble saved my sanity through her assistance with formatting and editing the manuscripts, designing the graphics, obtaining reprint permissions, and communicating with the authors. Terri Singer provided last-minute editorial assistance as well. Karen Dyer and Elizabeth Hamilton carefully read the first edition and offered suggestions for making it more student-friendly. Many friends and colleagues gave encouragement and support. I am particularly grateful to my sons, Graham and Elliot, who cheered me on and never tired of hearing about the latest developments. This book is dedicated to them.

PART I

Introduction and Overview

The first three chapters set the stage for the remainder of the book by providing a history and overview of the social and behavioral sciences in public health; by tracing the evolutionary stages of human history and their corresponding disease patterns; and by presenting basic concepts in social epidemiology, the area of inquiry where social science perspectives intersect those of public health.

Chapter 1 reviews the professional development of the field and the emergence of the "new public health" paradigm and introduces the social ecology of health model as the organizing framework of the book. Application of the model to public health problems is illustrated through case studies of eating disorders, HIV/AIDS, and health program planning.

In Chapter 2, the basic principles of population dynamics are presented, and the relationship between disease patterns and population size is discussed. Following is a discussion of demographic, epidemiologic, and health transitions in human history. Building on these principles, the relationship between disease and cultural evolution is described by examining changes in nutrition and health across the stages of foraging groups, settled villages, preindustrial cities, industrial cities, and postindustrial society.

Current issues in social epidemiology are reviewed in Chapter 3, with particular attention to the relationship between health and socioeconomic status, race, and ethnicity. Global inequalities in health are also explored by comparing high-income countries with low- to middle-income countries. The concepts of distal, intermediate, and proximate determinants of health are presented in relation to the Causal Continuum.

CHAPTER

1

Why Study Social and Behavioral Factors in Public Health?

Jeannine Coreil

A lthough the social and behavioral sciences are among the newer disciplines to be integrated into public health, the roots of this integration reach deeper than is often recognized. These roots are explored in the opening History section of this chapter, which overviews the professional development of the interdisciplinary field of social and behavioral sciences applied to public health. In the New Public Health paradigm, sociocultural and psychological factors figure importantly in problem analysis, as illustrated in the case study of the social impact of a natural disaster. Next, the overarching framework for the book, the social ecology of health model, is introduced and described in terms of multiple levels of social-behavioral influence on health problems. The application of the model to understanding and addressing health issues is illustrated through three examples, including eating disorders, HIV/AIDS, and a WIC training program.

HISTORY

Public health has always been concerned with the ways in which social conditions influence the health and well-being of communities and human populations. The disciplines of public health and social science both emerged in the latter part of the 19th century along with the recognition of the needs of the poor and marginalized groups and the association between living conditions and health. However, it was not until the mid-20th century that

Author's Note: Parts of this chapter are reprinted by permission from Coreil, J. (2008). Social Science Contributions to Public Health: Overview. In K. Heggenhougen & S. Quah (Eds.), *International Encyclopedia of Public Health* (Vol. 6., pp. 101–114). Oxford, UK: Oxford University Press.

professionally trained social scientists became actively involved in public health programs, and by the 1980s, accredited schools of public health in the United States were required to provide formal training in the social and behavioral sciences. The most important challenges for improving health in the 21st century involve social, cultural, and behavioral change. Our knowledge about how social and behavioral factors affect health has grown enormously, but effecting the individual and societal changes needed to reach public health goals is no easy task. Political and economic barriers deeply rooted in the social order constrain what is practically feasible. Nevertheless, emerging new approaches to structural change offer possibilities for surmounting these obstacles and producing higher levels of global community health.

Table 1.1 highlights important milestones in the history of social science contributions to public health. In the 19th century, social theorists in Europe called attention to the unequal distribution of infectious disease among the population, with the poor and working classes being the most prone to infection, and cited the unhealthy living conditions of crowded urban slums, inadequate diet, and physically taxing labor as contributing to the poor health of the disadvantaged. Many important figures contributed to a broad discourse that framed public health issues as socially produced—some with an overt political agenda, such as Marx and Engels; others with a more epidemiologic approach, such as Snow, Panum, and Farr; some as activist physicians, such as Villermé and Guérin; and still others, such as Virchow and Durkheim, with a more sociological orientation (Janes, Stall, & Gifford, 1986). Often referred to as 19th century "social medicine," this period is significant for establishing the idea that public health is a social science and that social structures and change generate population-level health effects. Moreover, social reform to improve health is also rooted in the early work of advocates such as Virchow and Chadwick. The late 19th century saw the rise of the Sanitary Movement, with organized efforts to improve standards of hygiene and living and working conditions. However, the turn of the century ushered in the bacteriological era, and attention shifted to the discovery and control of biological pathogens in the early decades of the 20th century.

The growth of social and behavioral science applications in public health was strengthened by the redefinition of health in 1948 within the newly formed World Health Organization (WHO) as "a state of complete physical, mental and social well-being, and not merely the absence of disease or infirmity." Since that time, the WHO and other national and international organizations have affirmed the importance of psychosocial well-being as an integral component of health. This expanded conceptualization of health required the expertise of many disciplines to formulate policies and design programs to improve health conditions around the globe. The scope of health promotion again expanded in 1986 with the adoption of the Ottawa Charter for Health Promotion (WHO, 1995), which identified the fundamental prerequisites for a healthy society, including peace, shelter, education, food, income, a stable ecosystem, sustainable resources, social justice, and equity. This expanded agenda set the stage for an even broader role for social science in public health. The need for comprehensive, multisector approaches to global health promotion was reaffirmed and further outlined in 2005 through the Bangkok Charter for Health Promotion (WHO, 2007).

TABLE 1.1   Important Milestones in the History of Social Sciences in Public Health

Period	Event	Significance
Greco-Roman & Islamic	Organized efforts to protect the health of vulnerable populations	Emergence of social welfare values in society; use of preventive practices for both physical and mental health
19th century	European social theorists define medicine/public health as "social science"	Social determinants identified as fundamental causes of health and illness: political advocacy for social reform
19th century	Snow and Farr in Britain, Panus in Denmark, and others	Use of social science methods for epidemiological investigation
Late 19th century	Sanitary Movement	Organized efforts to improve lifestyle, living and working conditions of urban poor within industrializing nations
1948	WHO defines health to include mental and social well-being	Set stage for addressing psychosocial factors in health and illness
1950s	Anthropological research on community health	Recognition of cultural factors as barriers to public health interventions; first planned culture change projects to improve health
1955	Medical Sociology Section of the American Sociological Association established	Medical sociology attains subdisciplinary status
1958	Publication of the Health Belief Model	Launched the health behavior change paradigm for public health intervention
1964	U.S. Surgeon General's Report on Smoking and Health	Beginning of movement to reduce health behavior risks to public health
1967–1972	Society for Medical Anthropology, organized in 1967, becomes a section of the American Anthropological Association in 1972	Medical anthropology attains subdisciplinary status
1978	Health Psychology Section of American Psychological Association established	The field of health behavior research and intervention is professionally recognized
1978	Alma Ata Conference on Primary Health Care	Set long-term global agenda to develop comprehensive, community-based approaches to promote basic health
1980s	Behavioral and Social Science Council of the U.S. Association of Schools of Public Health established	Formalization of social and behavioral sciences as integral component of public health training programs
1986	Ottawa Charter for Health Promotion	Identified fundamental social prerequisites for ensuring health and well-being
2005	Bangkok Charter for Health Promotion	Reaffirmed social prerequisites and highlighted role of economic development in health promotion

SOURCE: Reprinted by permission from Coreil, J. (2008). Social Science Contributions to Public Health: Overview. In K. Heggenhougen & S. Quah (Eds.), *International Encyclopedia of Public Health* (Vol. 6., pp. 101–114). Oxford, UK: Oxford University Press.

Many observers have noted that the AIDS epidemic, which became global in the 1980s, had a significant impact on the position of social and behavioral research in public health. It was the first modern pandemic that could not be controlled primarily through environmental and technological means, such as sanitation and vaccines. Controlling the spread of HIV required changing social norms and values as well as individual behavior, and social scientists rose to the challenge in large numbers (Benoist & Desclaux, 1995). Anthropologists, sociologists, psychologists, and other social scientists have made important contributions to understanding HIV risk behavior and designing interventions to promote safer sex and reduce transmission from injection drug use. Important conceptual and methodologic advances have accompanied this expanded role.

The 1950s: Seminal Developments

The post–World War II era ushered in a period of tremendous growth and development for the social and behavioral sciences in public health. There were two main thrusts in this groundbreaking era, one focused on health modernization in developing countries and the other on population-based screening for medical conditions. It was an era of great optimism about the potential for social engineering of health development and the application of social science methods to understanding and improving the health of populations (Paul, 1956).

In the international arena, anthropologists began working on projects aimed at improving the health and diet of traditional populations in the 1930s and 1940s (Firth, 1934; Malinowski, 1945; Richards, 1939). Beginning in 1950, a number of anthropologists were appointed to key positions in international health organizations, including the WHO; the Rockefeller Foundation; and the Institute for Inter-American Affairs, the forerunner of the U.S. Agency for International Development (USAID).

> The appointment of anthropologists to institutional posts paralleled the rapid expansion of public health programs worldwide as modern medicine was introduced on a large scale in many areas. The primary role of anthropologists was seen as that of identifying significant cultural barriers to the acceptance of new public health programs. (Coreil, 1990, p. 5)

Many of the important development projects of this era are described in the classic volume edited by Benjamin Paul, *Health, Culture and Community* (1955). These studies defined culture as a barrier to desirable health practice and introduced the role of the social scientist as a culture broker whose expertise can be applied to facilitate directed change. In particular, the focus was on diffusion of health technology to solve problems of "underdevelopment" by overcoming resistance to change grounded in traditional values, institutions, and practices. The conceptualization of culture as a barrier to good health became firmly rooted in social science thinking throughout the latter half of the 20th century, and it persists to the current day in various reformulations, such as "cultural awareness" and "cultural diversity." However, critics have also challenged this perspective as reflecting ethnocentric and neocolonial ideas of progress through culture change (see Chapter 9).

Concurrent to the above developments, the 1950s brought forth in industrialized countries focused attention on mobilizing large numbers of people to take part in various public health campaigns. Here again, officials encountered resistance to citizen participation and turned to social science expertise for solutions. In this case, social psychologists took the lead in developing approaches to analyze the problem and formulate interventions based on emergent models of individual behavior change. The seminal framework that emerged was the health belief model. Drawing on cognitive and behavioral theories of human behavior, the model conceptualized health practices as motivated by value expectancies, or subjective assessments of the personal benefits of particular outcomes and the expectations that certain actions will achieve desired goals (Janz, Champion, & Strecher, 2002). Developed in the context of a campaign to screen the adult U.S. population for tuberculosis (TB) through voluntary chest X rays offered in mobile clinics, the model was advanced to help explain why, despite the availability of free and convenient screening opportunities, participation remained low. The model posits that the decision to take action to protect one's health is determined by four factors: (1) whether people consider themselves susceptible to the condition, (2) whether the condition is perceived as having serious personal consequences, (3) whether a specific action is expected to reduce the risk of getting the condition or the consequences of it, and (4) whether the perceived benefits of the action outweigh the subjective costs or barriers to taking action. This rational cost-benefit model dominated health behavior change programs for several decades, with various elaborations and modifications over time, and set the stage for the development of other cognitive-behavioral models of health practice. Various behavior change models based on principles of motivation and learning theory were elaborated in subsequent decades and came to occupy a central position in health promotion interventions (see Chapter 4).

Maturation of the Field

Social science contributions to public health were bolstered significantly by the development of more sophisticated conceptual models and methods of research and data analysis, including both quantitative and qualitative techniques. The maturation of the field is reflected in the scope and influence of scholarly articles published in the multidisciplinary journal *Social Science & Medicine*, which first appeared in 1966 and currently boasts a large international readership and a high-impact rating among scientific journals. In the 1980s, significant developments occurred through the involvement of social scientists in international health activities related to child survival programs, HIV/AIDS, and tropical diseases. These activities were promoted and funded through intergovernmental agencies such as United Nations Children's Fund (UNICEF), WHO, and TDR (the interagency, collaborative Special Program for Research and Training in Tropical Diseases) as well as through bilateral development agencies such as USAID, the Canadian International Development Agency, and their European counterparts. Established in 1975, TDR in particular has played an important role in advancing social science research on tropical diseases, through programs that train developing country scientists and support research focused on sociocultural factors and health. A noteworthy strength of its programs has been the promotion of gender-focused research.

Shift From Infectious to Chronic Disease

Over the course of the 20th century, the public health enterprise underwent significant transformation as a result of a radical shift in focus from infectious diseases to chronic conditions as the major challenges to population health in industrialized societies. Tied to demographic, environmental, and social change, this transformation, also known as the *epidemiologic transition* (see Chapter 2), required profound alterations in how public health problems were addressed. Chronic conditions such as heart disease, cancer, diabetes, mental illness, and health problems of older persons replaced TB, pneumonia, childhood diarrhea, and other infections as the leading causes of morbidity and mortality in industrial countries (although TB, malaria, and, later, AIDS remained the major killers in developing countries). As chronic diseases and disability became the focus of public health interventions, the role of social and behavioral factors became increasingly important for disease prevention and control. Multilevel models that emphasized the social and political environment reemerged to replace the traditional medical model grounded in the germ theory of disease as well as the traditional public health model emphasizing host-agent-environment interactions. Anthropology, sociology, political science, demography, gerontology, and other social sciences made important contributions to this reframing of public health. With their focus on broad social processes and macrolevel determinants, the social sciences helped redefine the public health agenda as one integrally concerned with policy, economics, social organization, and cultural dynamics across diverse institutions. This shift built on advances in the professional development of these disciplines, theoretical and methodological contributions, and political advocacy on the part of diverse communities (see Chapter 16).

Primary, Secondary, and Tertiary Prevention

One of the ways in which public health is often contrasted with clinical medicine is the degree to which it focuses on *prevention* of disease and disability, while medical practice emphasizes the *treatment* of health problems after they occur. It is commonplace in public health to further differentiate between *primary, secondary, and tertiary prevention.* In primary prevention, the focus is on activities that forestall the development of pathological conditions. For example, preventing the onset of heart disease through healthy lifestyle behavior would fall in this category. Secondary prevention, on the other hand, refers to detection of disease or its precursors at an early stage to take ameliorative action that can thwart full development or enable measures to keep the problem in check. Regular screening for detectable conditions such as hypertension, breast and colorectal cancer, diabetes, and sexually transmitted infections falls in this category. Finally, tertiary prevention includes interventions at later stages of disease to prevent secondary complications, sustain optimal disease management, and ensure the best quality of life. Treatment for hypertension, diabetes, depression, osteoporosis, lymphedema, and other chronic conditions illustrates the third category of prevention. Social and behavioral factors figure importantly in all three types of prevention; however, over the decades, interest has grown particularly in their potential contribution to primary prevention. Health economists have demonstrated that it is far more cost-effective to prevent conditions before they develop than to provide long-term care for chronic conditions. The cost factor is particularly salient as more people live to an advanced age and governments are mandated to ensure the provision of care. There is also the desire for people to live healthy, productive lives for as long as possible.

Of all the public health disciplines, the social and behavioral sciences can make unique contributions to primary prevention. Influencing lifestyle patterns and the social context in which people live is fundamental to prevention of the major health conditions facing society today. It also poses one of the greatest challenges, because the force of macrolevel influences on individual behavior is tremendous. One need only consider the facts of the contemporary way of life—such as sedentary daily routines; people spending many hours of the day in front of computers; increasing reliance on processed and "fast" food; and the tendency toward workaholism, lack of sleep, and chronic stress—to appreciate the obstacles facing such programs. It is a basic tenet of intervention that it is far easier to modify the more proximate determinants of health, such as individual food choices, than it is to alter the intermediate and distal forces that affect those choices. Changing the organization of society and the core components of culture poses an enormous challenge, yet there is growing recognition that only through alteration of the fundamental causes of disease (e.g., inadequate income and access to health care, unemployment, racial and gender discrimination, lack of social support, stressful work settings, failure to provide educational opportunities) can true primary prevention be realized (Link & Phelan, 1995).

Professional Development of the Field

At the close of the 20th century, important conferences and publications marked the maturation of the field and recognition of the significance of "higher-level" analysis of the social and cultural aspects of health. In 1998, the U.S. Centers for Disease Control and Prevention (CDC), in collaboration with the American Psychological Association and other professional social science organizations, sponsored a multidisciplinary conference, Public Health in the 21st Century: Behavioral and Social Science Contributions. Two years later, the National Institutes of Health (NIH) organized an agenda-setting conference, Towards Higher Levels of Analysis: Progress and Promise in Research on Social and Cultural Dimensions of Health (Schneiderman, Speers, Silva, Tomes, & Gentry, 2001). A recurrent theme in these meetings was the recognition that, despite impressive advances in understanding the biological and genetic bases for disease, "Knowledge about biological and genetic markers is important but limited in predicting who gets sick, who seeks treatment for health problems, and who recovers from illness. The social sciences contribute to filling these gaps in our understanding of health" (NIH, 2001, p. 1). These conferences marked a critical juncture in the development of the field—that is, the accumulation of knowledge about the complex interplay of macro- and microlevel influences on health, as well as new technologies for putting into practice strategies for influencing the impact of those factors. Outside the United States, similar events and publications marked this important turning point in the field, such as the volume published by the French Association for Medical Anthropology Applied to Development and Health (AMADES), *Systèmes et politiques de santé: De la santé publique à l'anthropologie* (Hours, 2001); the creation of the WHO Commission on Social Determinants of Health (2005); and the 2007 conference, Social, Cultural and Economic Determinants of Health, held in Portugal.

THE NEW PUBLIC HEALTH

In the 20th century, the field of public health underwent tremendous change and diversification. In the early part of the century, infectious diseases posed the greatest health challenge for people, whether they lived in industrialized countries or developing nations. Control of communicable diseases was the focus of public health practice, through organized efforts such as provision of safe water and sanitation, immunization services, and monitoring and surveillance of disease outbreaks. After 1930, antibiotic therapy became an essential component of infection control, and it remains an important aspect of public health programs that deal with sexually transmitted diseases and other communicable illnesses. In the second half of the century, however, with the emergence of chronic diseases, injury, substance abuse, and other health problems as the focal public health challenges, the dominant paradigm has shifted toward social and behavioral approaches to disease prevention and health promotion. While the more traditional activities of infection control and environmental protection remain important in today's world, much attention and effort are now focused on changing the social conditions that undermine health as well as the behavioral patterns that put people at risk of illness and injury.

Sometimes referred to as the "new public health," this emergent paradigm in public health parallels the reconceptualization of individual health within the field of medicine along similar lines (Frenk, 1993). Whereas in the past, the germ theory of disease dominated medical research and practice, we now view individual health as shaped by complex interacting systems of biological, social, and environmental factors. While tremendous advances in biomedical technology have dramatically improved our ability to treat illness and prolong life through the use of sophisticated diagnostic testing, powerful drugs, and advanced surgery, medicine has increasingly recognized the importance of cultural context, social organization, and lifestyle choices for individual health. Variously labeled "social medicine," "behavioral medicine," and "medical ecology," the new medical model shares with public health a broadened framework for analyzing health problems in terms of complex biosocial systems.

A number of developments contributed to the rise of the social ecology paradigm in medicine and public health (Krieger, 1994). One was the shift in epidemiologic patterns from infectious to chronic diseases noted above. This shift was part of a broader, postindustrial transformation of society, involving changing demographic trends and patterns of morbidity and mortality. People now live longer and healthier lives, and the health problems they do face involve conditions that cannot be "cured" in the traditional sense. The major illnesses affecting industrial populations today, such as heart disease, cancer, and diabetes, can only be controlled through primary prevention or "managed" over the long term to improve quality of life. Prevention and treatment of chronic diseases depends heavily on behavioral practices such as diet, exercise, substance use, and stress reduction. Likewise, behavior and social conditions are the central components of preventive approaches for other leading public health problems such as unintended pregnancy, substance abuse, motor vehicle accidents, and violence. Even with the new and emergent (or resurgent) infectious diseases, such as HIV/AIDS, TB, and sexually transmitted diseases, sociobehavioral factors are widely recognized as critical for their control.

Another important contribution to the social ecology model of public health has been the wealth of scientific discoveries linking biology, behavior, and culture. Nearly all diseases and health conditions are now known to have multifactorial etiologies involving complex interactions of processes located inside and outside people's bodies. We know, for example, that stress is an underlying component of all illness, including both acute infections and chronic disorders, and that physical and psychological stress can affect one's ability to fight disease and restore health. In fact, illness is increasingly viewed as a breakdown in the body's natural defense system, which is highly sensitive to internal emotions and external stressors in the social environment (see Chapter 5). The negative impact of social discord, whether from family relationships, the work setting, or school pressure, can play as important a part in whether someone gets a cold or flu as exposure to specific pathogens. Indeed, some argue that psychosocially mediated immunity is the primary factor in most people's susceptibility to infection (Kaplan, 1991). It is worth noting that only 25 years ago, researchers were just beginning to investigate the relationship between stress and illness; today, the role of stress in health is well documented, and research has spawned a dynamic field of study called psychoneuroimmunology.

Research on stress and health is closely linked to studies of social support—that is, the way in which our connections to other people has a protective effect on well-being. It has been shown, for instance, that people who interact with a large network of friends and family members get sick less often and recover from illness faster than those who do not. Similarly, people who live alone have higher rates of death and suicide than those who live with others (Syme, 1986). These trends illustrate one kind of mechanism through which the social environment can affect health status. The social environment can also influence health through social structural arrangements, which position people at different places in society and mediate access to resources such as education, income, medical services, status, and prestige (Link & Phelan, 1995). Because people occupy different positions in the socioeconomic structure, disease and mortality are not evenly distributed within a population. The field of study that addresses such variation in health risks is known as social epidemiology. Many advances in understanding social risk factors have occurred in recent decades, leading to redefinitions of health as "socially produced" and increased attention to interventions focused on organizational change (Goodman, Steckler, & Kegler, 1997).

We have also learned a great deal about how cultural factors influence health—for example, the ways in which people think about and behave regarding food, the relative value they place on work and leisure, how health and illness are perceived and managed, and the role of ethnic identity in shaping disease patterns. Approaches to studying cultural influence have broadened to encompass notions of gender culture, family culture, organizational culture, and corporate culture, all having important lessons for public health research and practice. In Chapter 2, we take a closer look at disease history in relation to long-term cultural evolution, highlighting the relationship between human subsistence strategies and patterns of disease and injury.

Another development that has enlarged the scope of public health is its expansion into new arenas of social welfare, including primary care services; reproductive health; child and family protection; injury prevention; and the health consequences of natural disasters, war, and political violence, to name but a few. Contemporary public health encompasses an enormous diversity of specialized fields, which in turn draw on the knowledge and perspectives of many disciplines. The social and behavioral sciences have become increasingly relevant in this robust endeavor, contributing new conceptual, methodologic, and policy perspectives to the field. Nowadays it is just as likely to find public health professionals talking about consumer satisfaction, political advocacy, and community empowerment as about more traditional issues such as disease surveillance and government regulation. While the "new public health" has been widely endorsed by diverse disciplines and constituencies within the health arena, it is not without critics (Bunton, Nettleton, & Burrows, 1995; Petersen & Lupton, 1996). The latter apply poststructuralist perspectives to highlight the ever-expanding control public health institutions tend to exert on everyday life, through social constructions, the creation of expert knowledge, moral discourse on behavior, interpersonal relations, and other health "risks."

To illustrate the holistic approach outlined above, the following section presents a case study analyzing the sociocultural and behavioral impact of an acute environmental crisis, the 1989 oil spill in Prince William Sound, Alaska, and subsequent efforts to clean up the area.

CASE STUDY   The *Exxon Valdez* Oil Spill

The grounding of the *Exxon Valdez* oil tanker in 1989 released 11 million gallons of crude oil into a once-pristine environment where Native Alaskans depended heavily on marine resources for their livelihood. A year after the accident, the anthropologist Lawrence Palinkas and colleagues conducted a population-based survey of nearly 600 households in 13 localities (Palinkas, Downs, Petterson, & Russel, 1993). The researchers measured demographic variables, levels of exposure to the spill, impact on social relations within families and the community, changes in traditional subsistence activities, and indicators of mental and physical health. By comparing respondents with high exposure scores and those with less exposure to the effects of the spill and cleanup, a dose-response relationship could be established for different consequences.

The damage from the oil spill, along with the ensuing efforts to clean up the area, set off a chain of events with profound social, cultural, and psychological impacts on the affected communities. Exposure status was significantly associated with degree of reported decline in social relations, including conflicts among family members, neighbors, friends, and coworkers. Not only did the spill dominate daily conversation in the year following the accident, but a large proportion of residents were directly involved in the intensive cleanup efforts, which required a large labor force over several months. The high wages offered to attract workers made it difficult for local communities to retain unskilled employees, and many families were disrupted when one or both parents worked long hours away from home. Only the able-bodied could handle the work, so not everyone benefited from the cleanup operation, causing some resentment among those excluded. Conflicts with outsiders who came for the lucrative work were commonplace. In some villages, more than 40% of respondents reported friendships ending over cleanup disputes, often related to whether one worked on the cleanup or not. Those who worked in the cleanup reported spending less time with friends and less participation in religious activities and festivals and in volunteer activities compared with those less exposed to the spill.

Economic disputes were also rampant, over issues such as equitable distribution of monetary compensation among permit holders and crewmen for lost fishing. Furthermore, involvement in the spill and its aftermath had a dramatic effect on subsistence activities for this population. Hunting, fishing, and harvesting of certain traditional foods had long played an important symbolic role in maintaining native identity, culture, and family solidarity. These activities were drastically curtailed because of environmental pollution from the spill and because so many people were working long hours in the cleanup. Issues of cultural survival were seriously discussed in relation to the disaster (Picou, Gill, & Cohen, 1997).

Finally, in the health arena, high-exposed individuals scored significantly higher than low-exposed persons on measures of psychiatric disorders and physical health status, and they reported higher perceived increases in community levels of substance abuse and domestic violence. Exposure status was associated with generalized anxiety disorder, posttraumatic stress disorder, and depression. It was also linked to higher numbers of physician-verified illness conditions occurring postspill as well as a self-assessed decline in health status. These data were corroborated by documented increases in visits to community clinics for primary care and mental health services throughout the region. Furthermore, the psychosocial impact of the spill differentially affected ethnic groups living in the region. Other studies of the disaster found that Alaska Natives reported higher levels of stress and posttraumatic stress symptoms than did non-Native commercial fishermen (Gill & Picou, 1997; Palinkas, Petterson, Russel, & Downs, 2004). These findings corroborate studies of other disasters in which ethnic groups were affected in different ways (Palinkas, in press), and they underscore the importance of cultural context in understanding the impact of disasters.

The *Exxon Valdez* oil spill illustrates the extensive ways in which environmental disasters can produce direct and indirect social and psychological effects in affected communities. At a more general level, it illustrates the harmful impact of rapid sociocultural change in a case example that is likely to recur in other areas of the world. It allows the examination of the association of processes of sociocultural change and subsequent health and well-being. It would be interesting to investigate the long-term impacts of the Alaskan spill; however, access to affected populations for purposes of research has been severely limited due to litigation issues (L. A. Palinkas, personal communication, November 26, 2007).

SOCIAL ECOLOGY OF HEALTH MODEL

The *Exxon Valdez* case study highlights a variety of social and behavioral factors that are relevant to a holistic analysis of public health problems. These dimensions were presented without reference to a particular organizing framework; however, in the remainder of this volume we will use the social ecology of health model as an organizing framework for understanding health problems and planning interventions.

A number of formulations of the social ecological model have been developed. They all have in common the notion of multilevel systems of mutual influence and interaction, moving from the individual level through linkages to larger social networks including the family, community, social institutions, the state, and global systems. Key concepts include system integration, change, and adaptation over time (Richard, Potvin, Kishchuk, Prlic, & Green, 1996). One formulation of the model that has gained prominence is that developed by McLeroy and colleagues for application to health promotion (McLeroy, Bibeau, Steckler, & Glanz, 1988). This model is organized around five hierarchical levels of influence: (1) intrapersonal factors, (2) interpersonal processes and relations with primary social groups, (3) institutional factors, (4) community factors, and (5) public policy. It has been widely applied to the study of diverse health topics, including physical activity, drug use, adolescent pregnancy, infant feeding, cancer, and heart disease.

The model we are using in this textbook is very similar to that of McLeroy and colleagues (1988) in that it organizes determinants of health according to five hierarchical levels of influence—that is, intrapersonal, interpersonal, organizational, community, and society. Our visual depiction of the model is adapted from Hanson and colleagues' (2005) Injury Iceberg model, with the tip of the iceberg or triangle representing behavior and successive underlying levels representing social contextual and structural factors (see Figure 1.1). Examples of factors influencing health at the intrapersonal level include biological and psychological factors such as genetics, cognition, and personality. At the interpersonal level, we identify home, family, and peer group influences, while the organizational level might include work and school settings, civic associations, and health care organizations. At the level of community, we can identify factors such as ethnicity, social class, social capital, public facilities, and the built environment. The more macrolevel societal factors include policy issues, national ethos and cultural values, infrastructure, economics, and education. Aspects of the physical environment are positioned toward the left side of the pyramid, while social contextual factors are located to the right. Our model also incorporates the notion of proximate, intermediate, and distal determinants of health (see Causal Continuum, Chapter 3), with the more proximate factors located near the tip of the pyramid, the individual level; intermediate factors corresponding with interpersonal and organizational levels; and distal factors corresponding with community and societal influences. This model can be applied to the analysis of many public health problems, as will be illustrated throughout the book.

Although systems strive toward equilibrium, perfect balance is never achieved because systems are open to internal and external changes and thus constantly require adjustment or adaptation. Because all levels of an ecosystem are integrated, change at any level of the system may require adjustment at other levels. The process of adaptation in response to change is one way

FIGURE 1.1   The Social Ecology of Health Model

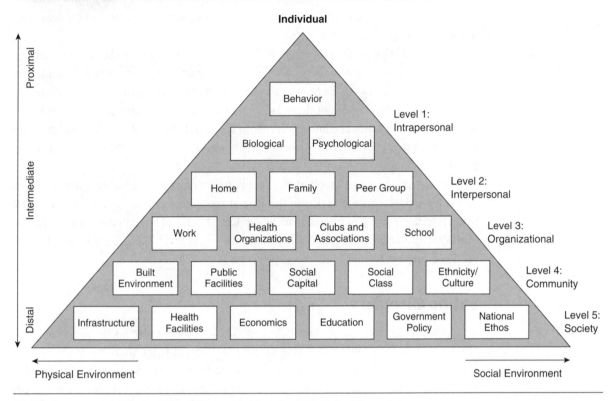

SOURCE: Hanson et al. (2005). *Health Promotion Journal of Australia, 16,* 5–10. Used by permission.

of conceptualizing stress, and again it can occur at different levels, including psychological distress, family dysfunction, community disruption, rapid culture change, and environmental degradation. Sociocultural or environmental change can have repercussions that eventually affect communities, families, and individuals (Ell & Northen, 1991). For example, an economic recession often leads to high unemployment rates; within families, a provider may lose his or her job, leading to loss of medical benefits and reduced income, which affects access to health care. Social support can buffer the negative effects of stress at different levels of the system, such as through close friendships, strong families, community resources, and one's integration with (or alienation from) the larger society.

Although we have emphasized social environmental factors above, because of the subject matter of this book, the social ecology of health model also incorporates aspects of the physical environment. At the household level, we can consider housing conditions and hazards in the home; at the community level we must take into account physical aspects such as the built environment, water quality, air pollution, toxic waste, noise, crowding, and other features; at the societal level, examples of physical environmental concerns might include atmospheric change (e.g., global warming), changes in flora and fauna (e.g., deforestation, vector habitat), climatic stress (e.g., heat waves, cold spells), and natural disasters (floods, tornadoes, hurricanes). The impacts of these biophysical phenomena are always mediated through social system arrangements that shape how humans respond to and manage environmental events.

In public health, we are concerned with changes emanating from the larger social system, including government legislation, regulation, and budgetary matters that directly affect health issues. The health of the economy almost always has social welfare repercussions. We are also concerned with more local-level institutions, such as state politics, community health services, school systems, and law enforcement. The social ecology of health model provides a framework that allows one to locate these disparate public health issues within a coherent organization.

To illustrate the model's application to public health problems, we present three examples. The first provides a brief overview of the general approach, using eating disorders as a case study. Next, the model is more systematically applied at different levels to the chronic epidemic of HIV/AIDS. Finally, a practical application of the model in designing a public health intervention is presented.

Eating Disorders

As a brief illustration of the model's application, we can discuss the different levels of influence on the problem of eating disorders. In recent years, there has been increasing recognition of the seriousness, prevalence, and repercussions of eating disorders in the United States. Although obesity can be considered an eating disorder, we will focus this example on malnutrition related to anorexia and bulimia as it affects adolescent girls. Purging, the use of laxatives, self-induced vomiting, and related unhealthy behaviors have been associated with poor self-esteem in young women, an intrapersonal factor strongly influenced by the social context in which girls live. Familial pressure to excel, peer pressure to maintain an ideal body size, and media images depicting ultrathin fashion models and celebrities all contribute to the tendency of young girls to set unrealistic goals for their physical appearance. Girls who suffer from eating disorders often have a distorted self-image and seek to attain control over their lives through purging and extreme dieting. More distal social structural influences on the problem include gender stereotypes whereby women are valued for their physical beauty and as sex symbols, with the female body being used to sell consumer products. The popular media give lavish attention to topics of weight, weight loss, and dieting, reinforcing the importance accorded to maintaining an ideal body size. The cult of celebrity in American society leads to excessive attention to the thinness or fatness of Hollywood and television stars. Young girls have limited exposure to role models that reflect realistic physical attributes of women.

The HIV/AIDS Epidemic

In the early 1980s, the HIV/AIDS epidemic burst on the international stage signaling alarming and sobering challenges. Here was a highly lethal infection with unclear etiology and transmission, spreading rapidly among disparate social groups and with no effective treatment in sight. In North America and Europe, during the early stages of the epidemic, the disease affected primarily gay men, hemophiliacs, and injection drug users. In 1984, the microbial agent, HIV (human immunodeficiency virus) was identified, along with transmission routes involving sexual practices and contaminated blood, and a test for HIV became available in 1985. Screening of blood supplies eliminated the risk of infection from transfusions, but altering sexual and drug use practices proved to be a much bigger public health challenge. It soon became clear that more than any other major health problem addressed to date, AIDS was a disease in which social and behavioral factors played a dominant role in etiology and control. Primary prevention was the only effective intervention available. Moreover, efforts to curb the epidemic through behavior change (i.e., safer sexual practices) encountered overwhelming obstacles at both individual and societal levels. Of particular interest was the way in which social responses to the disease revealed disturbing patterns of moral condemnation, stigmatization of marginal groups, and questionable ethics in research and medical care.

Before long, the heterosexual transmission pattern dominant in developing countries emerged as a serious problem in the global North as well. However, as noted in the previous section, not everyone in the population was equally at risk; not surprisingly, groups living in poverty at the margins of society were the most affected (with the exception of gay men)—ethnic and racial minorities, sex workers, and people living in high-crime urban neighborhoods. The social epidemiology of AIDS mirrored the health situation of the world's cities.

Applying the social ecology of health model to the HIV/AIDS epidemic underscores the fact that the epidemic served as a lightning rod for a host of psychosocial issues (Rushing, 1995). At the individual level, the illness was charged with intense emotion: fear of diagnosis for its victims, who often could anticipate social rejection and discrimination and an agonizing deterioration ending in death, as well as anxiety among health workers, whose job put them at risk of infection.

The social impact of the epidemic on families, communities, and health care systems was profound. Many people with AIDS were abandoned by their families on account of fear, shame, and economic hardship. The devastating effects included family disintegration, orphaned children, and infants born HIV positive through exposure in utero. In some areas, the magnitude of adults affected seriously diminished the productive workforce. To its credit, the gay community responded positively by organizing for political advocacy and spearheading local educational campaigns. Because the disease involved expensive medical care for multiple conditions over an extended time period, issues of access to care surfaced quickly, highlighting ongoing ethical dilemmas about who should bear the burden of health care costs and how to allocate limited therapeutic resources. Even with the advent of effective drug treatment, which has reduced health care costs, issues of equitable distribution have remained unresolved. Likewise, ethical controversies continue in the realm of research involving subjects from poor countries, which cannot afford the costly new medicines.

At the societal level, the collective moral outrage tended to find a scapegoat in "undesirable" groups that deviated from the norms of the privileged majority. A striking example of such a response was the labeling of Haitians in general as a "risk group" for several years, clearly a reflection of racially based fears of social contamination from foreigners. Most telling was the stark exposure of the deep-seated homophobia triggered by the crisis. Scientific thinking was incredibly suspended as the dogma of "punishment for sin" was espoused from pulpit to podium, and government officials blocked efforts to increase public funding for AIDS research and educate the public about safe sex. The social control functions of illness labeling (see Chapter 7) were clearly operating in many domains during the epidemic. Cultural taboos about sex prevented open discussion of the problem for a long time. The pernicious effects of gender stratification also were evident in the epidemiology of and failure to control the spread of HIV, particularly in poor countries, where women's economic dependence on sexual relations with men placed them at risk of infection.

At the global systems level, the HIV/AIDS epidemic has generated tremendous international collaboration in policy development, research, and treatment. The annual International AIDS Conference, first convened in 1990, has grown into one of the largest assemblies of scientists and professionals in the health field. A more recent offshoot of this meeting, the International AIDS Impact Conference, provides a forum for scholars working in intervention programs and with populations affected by the disease. In recent years, substantial financial support through the Global Fund to Fight AIDS, Tuberculosis and Malaria and President Bush's Emergency Plan for AIDS Relief has enabled noteworthy progress in making effective drugs available to low-income countries.

WIC Training Program

The previous example illustrates how the socioecological model can help identify various factors that affect health problems at different levels. The model also has utility in planning public health programs. The following example describes the application of the ecological model to designing a training program for county health department employees. The focus of the program was training staff involved in the Child Growth Monitoring Project (CGMP) of the New York State WIC (Women, Infants and Children) program. Worldwide, monitoring the growth of infants and children is a fundamental public health activity and is considered an essential component of disease prevention and health promotion in both industrialized and developing countries (de Onis, Wijnhoven, & Onyango, 2003). Children are regularly weighed and measured for height and head circumference to ensure that healthy growth is occurring and to intervene if it falters. In the United States, public sector involvement in child growth monitoring is focused on the Special Supplemental Nutrition Program for Women, Infants and Children, which provides nutrition education and counseling to mothers as well as food supplements and growth monitoring for children. Prior to planning health intervention programs, social and behavioral scientists often conduct formative research to guide program development. In the New York project, researchers used the ecological model to guide formative research "because it offered a concrete framework to account for the reciprocal interaction of behavior and environment" (Newes-Adeyi, Helitzer, Caulfield, & Bronner, 2003, p. 283). The goal was to identify priorities for training WIC staff in plotting and interpreting growth data and implementing nutrition education and counseling for mothers of enrolled children. The researchers focused their data collection efforts on those ecological levels considered potentially amenable to change through training—individual, interpersonal, and organizational. At the individual level, the study found that WIC staff held positive attitudes about the usefulness of growth monitoring in their work but did not include nutritional counseling for caretakers as part of the anthropometric assessment of children. At the interpersonal level, provider-client interaction was found to focus primarily on completion of paperwork for certification of eligibility, with little attention to the client's perspective on the child's growth progress. At the organizational level, the research found that the sequencing of child measurement and caretaker counseling was disjointed, with counseling typically occurring 1 to 2 months after growth assessment. Taken together, the study results showed "gaps in the counseling skills of the WIC providers as well as organizational issues that did not promote the application of comprehensive growth monitoring as advocated in the literature" (Newes-Adeyi et al., 2003, p. 287). Based on these findings, the training program that was developed focused on reinforcing the link between anthropometry and nutritional counseling.

One of the lessons learned in the CGMP study was the recognition on the part of the researchers that the study "could have benefited from utilizing a more comprehensive ecological model in the design of the formative research" (Newes-Adeyi et al., 2003, p. 288). For example, it became evident that a missing piece involved provider-provider relationships in the implementation of a team approach to growth monitoring. There appeared to be less than full support for the team approach, and more information on this aspect would have been helpful. At the community level, lack of information about formal and informal professional networks of WIC staff limited the planners' ability to incorporate strategies for using such networks in the training program. Finally, at the policy level, a better understanding of state-level regulations and policies would have helped in identifying ways to reinforce new strategies for implementing coordinated assessment and counseling.

CONCLUSION

The foundations of social and behavioral science perspectives in public health have roots in 19th-century ideas about the social bases of health. These same ideas continue to have relevance for framing health problems as embedded in complex social environmental contexts. The social ecology of health model provides a framework for understanding the multiple levels of influence on health outcomes. Conceptual and methodologic advances across disciplines have improved research and practice in this field. Application of the model to the examples of eating disorders, HIV/AIDS, and program planning illustrates the kinds of factors that come into play at different levels.

The chapters that follow will explore in greater depth how social, cultural, and behavioral factors influence disease patterns as well as individual and collective responses to ill health. The next chapter takes a historical perspective by examining changes in health conditions across different time periods of human history.

REFERENCES

Benoist, J., & Desclaux, A. (1995). *Sida et anthropologie: Bilan et perspectives.* Paris: Karthala.

Bunton, R., Nettleton, S., & Burrows, R. (1995). *The sociology of health promotion: Critical analyses of consumption, lifestyle and risk.* London: Routledge.

Coreil, J. (1990). The evolution of anthropology in international health. In J. Coreil & D. Mull (Eds.), *Anthropology and primary health care* (pp. 3–27). Boulder, CO: Westview Press.

Coreil, J. (2008). Social science contributions to public health: Overview. In K. Heggenhougen & S. Quah (Eds.), *International encyclopedia of public health* (Vol. 6., pp. 101–114). Oxford, UK: Oxford University Press.

de Onis, M., Wijnhoven, T., & Onyango, A. (2003). Worldwide practices in child growth monitoring. *Journal of Pediatrics, 144*(4), 461–465.

Ell, K., & Northen, H. (1991). *Families and health care.* New York: Gruyter.

Firth, R. (1934). The sociological study of native diet. *Africa, 7,* 401–414.

Frenk, J. (1993). The new public health. *Annual Review of Public Health, 14,* 469–490.

Gill, D. A., & Picou, J. S. (1997). The day the water died: Cultural impacts of the *Exxon Valdez* oil spill. In J. S. Picou, D. A. Gill, & M. J. Cohen (Eds.), *The* Exxon Valdez *disaster: Readings on a modern social problem* (pp. 167–187). Dubuque, IA: Kendall-Hunt.

Goodman, R. M., Steckler, A., & Kegler, M. (1997). Mobilizing organizations for health enhancement: Theories of organizational change. In K. Glanz, F. M. Lewis, & B. K. Rimer (Eds.), *Health behavior and health education: Theory, research and practice* (pp. 287–312). San Francisco: Jossey-Bass.

Hanson, D., Hanson, J., Vardon, P., McFarlane, K., Lloyd, J., Muller, R., et al. (2005). The injury iceberg: An ecological approach to planning sustainable community safety interventions. *Health Promotion Journal of Australia, 16*(1), 5–10.

Hours, B. (Ed.). (2001). *Systèmes et politiques de santé: De la santé publique à l'anthropologie* [Systems and health policies: From public health to anthropology]. Paris: Karthala.

Janes, C. R., Stall, R., & Gifford, S. M. (1986). *Anthropology and epidemiology.* Dordrecht, the Netherlands: Reidel.

Janz, N. K., Champion, V. L., & Strecher, V. J. (2002). The health belief model. In K. Glanz, B. K. Rimer, & F. M. Lewis (Eds.), *Health behavior and health education: Theory, research, and practice* (pp. 45–66). San Francisco: Jossey-Bass.

Kaplan, H. B. (1991). Social psychology of the immune system: A conceptual framework and review of the literature. *Social Science & Medicine, 33*(8), 909–923.

Krieger, N. (1994). Epidemiology and the web of causation: Has anyone seen the spider? *Social Science & Medicine, 39*(7), 887–903.

Link, B. G., & Phelan, J. (1995). Social conditions as fundamental causes of diseases. *Journal of Health and Social Behavior, 35*(Extra issue), 80–94.

Malinowski, B. (1945). *The dynamics of culture change: An inquiry into race relations in Africa.* New Haven, CT: Yale University Press.

McLeroy, K. R., Bibeau, D., Steckler, A., & Glanz, K. (1988). An ecological perspective on health promotion programs. *Health Education Quarterly, 15*(4), 351–377.

National Institutes of Health. (2001). *Toward higher levels of analysis: Progress and promise in research on social and cultural dimensions of health* (Executive Summary, NIH Publication No. 01–5020). Washington, DC: Office of Behavioral and Social Sciences Research.

Newes-Adeyi, G., Helitzer, D. L., Caulfield, L. E., & Bronner, Y. (2003). Theory and practice: Applying the ecological model to formative research for a WIC training program in New York State. *Health Education Research, 15*(3), 283–921.

Palinkas, L. A. (in press). The *Exxon Valdez* oil spill. In Y. Nuria, S. Galea, & F. Norris (Eds.), *Mental health consequences of disasters.* New York: Cambridge University Press.

Palinkas, L. A., Downs, M. A., Petterson, J. S., & Russel, J. (1993). Social, cultural, and psychological impacts of the *Exxon Valdez* oil spill. *Human Organization, 52*(1), 1–13.

Palinkas, L. A., Petterson, J. S., Russel, J. C., & Downs, M. A. (2004). Ethnic differences in symptoms of post-traumatic stress after the *Exxon Valdez* oil spill. *Prehospital and Disaster Medicine, 19*(1), 102–112.

Paul, B. (1955). *Health, culture and community: Case studies of public reactions to health programs.* New York: Russel Sage.

Paul, B. D. (1956). Social science in public health. *American Journal of Public Health, 46*(11), 1390–1396.

Petersen, A., & Lupton, D. (1996). *The new public health: Health and self in the age of risk.* Thousand Oaks, CA: Sage.

Picou, J. S., Gill, D. A, & Cohen, M. J. (Eds.). (1997). *The* Exxon Valdez *disaster: Readings in a modern social problem.* Dubuque, IA: Kendall/Hunt.

Richard, L., Potvin, L., Kishchuk, N., Prlic, H., & Green, L. W. (1996). Assessment of the integration of the ecological approach in health promotion programs. *American Journal of Health Promotion, 10*(4), 318–328.

Richards, A. (1939). *Land, labour and diet in Northern Rhodesia: An economic study of the Bemba tribe.* London: Oxford University Press for the International African Institute.

Rushing, W. A. (1995). *The AIDS epidemic: Social dimensions of an infectious disease.* Boulder, CO: Westview Press.

Schneiderman, N., Speers, M. A., Silva, J. M., Tomes, H. & Gentry, J. H. (2001). *Integrating behavioral and social sciences with public health.* Washington, DC: American Psychological Association.

Syme, L. S. (1986). The social environment and disease prevention. *Advances in Health Education and Promotion, 1*(A), 237–265.

World Health Organization. (1995). *The Ottawa Charter for Health Promotion* (WHO/HPR/HEP/95.1). First presented at the First International Conference on Health Promotion, Ottawa, Ontario, Canada, November 21, 1986.

World Health Organization. (2005). *The Commission on Social Determinants of Health.* Retrieved April 7, 2007, from www.who.int/social_determinants/en

World Health Organization. (2007). *The Bangkok Charter for Health Promotion in a Globalized World.* Retrieved March 22, 2007, from www.who.int/healthpromotion/conferences/6gchp/bangkok_charter/en/index.html

2

Historical Perspectives on Population and Disease

Jeannine Coreil

I n this chapter, we delve into human prehistory to examine the scope of health changes that have affected human populations since ancient times. Our discussion reveals how aspects of human population demography and cultural organization interact to produce distinctive sets of disease challenges. In particular, the discussion focuses on the interrelationship between settlement patterns and subsistence technology—that is, the organized system for procuring food, shelter, and other necessities of life. To lay the groundwork for this discussion, we begin with an overview of the basic principles and processes of population dynamics.

POPULATION DYNAMICS

Demography is the branch of science that investigates the vital statistics of a population, such as births, deaths, marriages, and divorces. It is an important area of research for public health because epidemiologic patterns are closely linked with population parameters and because public health practice is organized around defined populations and their unique health profiles. Needs assessment and program planning in public health rely heavily on standardized demographic indicators. Thus, it is important for public health professionals to understand and evaluate the significance of these various measures.

The demographic indicators most commonly used in public health relate to fertility, mortality, and population growth. Fertility concerns the rate of childbearing in a population and is measured in several ways. *Total fertility* refers to the mean number of children born per woman in a particular population. On average, this figure ranges between 1 and 10. For example, in 2008 the total fertility in the United States was 2.1, and in Niger it was 7.1. The *crude birth rate*, on the other hand, is based on the number of children born in a given year per 1,000 population. This indicator may range from 10 to 50. The indicator often seen in the literature is the *age-adjusted fertility rate,* determined by the number of live births per 1,000 women 15 to 44 years old or some other defined age group. The fertility of certain subgroups of society often receives special attention, such as adolescent childbearing, because of social concerns related to health risks, morality, and human welfare. Also, fertility patterns of different ethnic groups sometimes generate discussion because of the implications for changing demographics and majority-minority group relations.

Mortality rates are usually computed for specific age groups and phases of life. The *crude death* rate, however, refers to the number of deaths in a year per 1,000 people. *Infant mortality rate* (IMR) is one of the most widely used demographic measures in public health because it has come to be recognized as the most sensitive indicator for overall health and quality of life of a population. The IMR is determined by the total number of deaths among infants in the first year of life per 1,000 live births. Over the course of human history, infant mortality has varied considerably, from as high as 500, analogous to a 50% death rate, in the Middle Ages, to less than 10 today in most industrialized countries. Because deaths among adults occur less frequently than among infants and children, the *adult mortality rate,* is calculated using a larger denominator than infant mortality; it is the number of deaths over a year per 100,000 in a population. *Maternal mortality* is a specialized indicator based on reproductive deaths, broadly defined to include those attributable to pregnancy and childbirth as well as contraception and abortion. Like infant mortality, it is calculated in relation to the number of live births to control for fertility (i.e., exposure to maternal mortality risk), and like adult mortality, it uses the 100,000 denominator because of the lower frequency of the event. The indicator is called the *maternal mortality ratio* and is based on the number of deaths among women related to reproductive causes per 100,000 live births. Great disparities exist in maternal mortality between developed and developing countries, where the ratios vary from as low as 5 in Scandinavian countries to more than 500 in sub-Saharan Africa.

The third demographic process of concern to public health is population growth rates, the speed at which groups increase or decrease in size. Overall population growth is a function of the two processes just defined, fertility and mortality, and in addition, migration must be taken into consideration. The basic formula for determining population growth is as follows:

$$P_1 + B - D \pm M = P_2,$$

where

P_1 = population size at Time 1,

B = births,

D = deaths,

M = net migration ("in" minus "out"), and

P_2 = population size at Time 2.

The magnitude of the difference between P_1 and P_2 indicates the absolute increase or decline in a population. If converted to a percentage of P_1, this statistic represents the *population growth rate*, which typically ranges between 0 and 4.0.

The pace of population growth is often described as "slow," "moderate," "rapid," or "explosive." Table 2.1 depicts the population growth rates associated with these labels, along with the corresponding "doubling time" (the number of years it takes for the population to double itself) and examples of countries currently experiencing different rates. Population problems arise when human welfare (any value held by the people concerned) suffers because of the number, composition, distribution, or growth rate of a population. Overpopulation occurs when there are too many people to meet their basic needs, but having too few people, or underpopulation, also can pose problems, such as inadequate numbers to sustain communities. Composition refers to the sociodemographic profile of the group, such as ethnic breakdown and sex ratios. A markedly skewed sex ratio, for example, can affect fertility patterns.

Maldistribution of the population can take a variety of forms, including geographic and social dimensions. For example, regional and urban/rural concentrations can create problems for city planning, water resource management, and health service organization. On the social side, age structure is important for broad human welfare concerns, such as the challenges posed by the increasing elderly population in industrial countries. When we think of population problems, however, rapid population growth rates come to mind first, particularly in poorer countries that still have agrarian economic systems and value large families.

Overpopulation leads to malnutrition, high infant and child mortality, environmental degradation, political tension, and severe strain on social services. It has been linked to famine, disease, and war. Maldistribution of food resources within countries exacerbates precarious food security situations. Additionally, one of the saddest casualties of war is the widespread starvation that often ravages the most vulnerable segments of the embattled

---

TABLE 2.1 Population Growth Rates, Doubling Time, and Representative Countries

Growth Rate	Doubling Time (in Years)	Descriptive Label	Representative Countries
0.0–0.4	140	Slow	Japan, European Union
0.5	130		Netherlands, China
1.0	70	Moderate	United States, Brazil
2.0	35	Rapid	Haiti, Pakistan
3.0	23		Somalia, Uganda
4.0	18	Explosive	Yemen, Afghanistan

SOURCE: United Nations Population Fund (2007).

populations. Refugee camps fill with displaced families, women, children, and elderly uprooted from their homes and weakened by disease and food deprivation. The international community and relief agencies mobilize food and medical aid, but too often such goods become weapons of war themselves, used by military groups to perpetuate the destructive conflicts (Maren, 1997).

But there is another side to population pressure and that is overconsumption and waste, the misuse of resources to the detriment of well-being (Crocker & Linden, 1998). The picture of this malady is widespread obesity, overflowing landfills, and toxic chemicals in breast milk. It is the spoils of postindustrial societies, whose populations produce waste and control global resources vastly out of proportion to their numbers. Ecologists use the term *net primary production* (NPP) to refer to the amount of energy captured by green plants from sunlight and transformed into living tissue. It is the base of all food chains and provides the energy that powers all nature. Human beings, a single species among millions, consume about 40% of land-based NPP. Such "overgrazing" has been linked to global warming, ozone depletion, topsoil degradation, species extinction, and loss of tropical rainforest. Consuming such a huge proportion of the earth's resources, some argue, leaves too little for the natural world to maintain conditions for the long-term well-being of the ecosystem. Furthermore, the 40% NPP is disproportionately consumed by the wealthiest segments of the richest countries; 20% of the world's people consume 82% of global resources, leaving the vast majority of people with far too little (Imhoff et al., 2004). For example, a person living in the United States consumes, on average, more than 500 times the energy used by someone who lives in a poor country such as Ethiopia.

Worldwide population growth reached an all-time peak of 2.0 in 1960, sparking vocal alarm and debate among demographers regarding the maximum number of people the earth can support in a healthy state without degrading the environment (*carrying capacity*). Some doomsday scenarios predicted dire consequences before the end of the 20th century, while more moderate perspectives are tempered by the anticipation of natural and socially engineered population controls. By 1970, global population growth had slowed considerably, quelling fears of imminent catastrophe, but recent increases have renewed concerns about overpopulation. Experts identify the optimal world population growth rate to be 0.5%, yet the current global population is increasing at a rate of 1.5% per year.

What is particularly noteworthy about the demographic history of the human species is the rapid acceleration of population growth rates in recent centuries. As shown in Table 2.2, for thousands of years, human numbers across the globe were quite low, and population size increased very slowly. A significant increase occurred about 10,000 years ago with the Neolithic Revolution, the development of agriculture. Another swell began in the 18th century with the Industrial Revolution and its concomitant urbanization and mass production of goods and services. Now we have entered the postindustrial era, characterized by slower rates of population growth, although many parts of the world have only recently begun the process of industrialization. Sometime near the middle of the 21st century, demographers predict that world population will reach a plateau, then slowly decline. Futurists differ considerably, though, in their visions of how desperate the human welfare situation will become before that point is reached.

Year	Rate (%)
100,000 BP	0.002
10,000 BP	0.05
1800	0.4
1900	0.7
1960	2.2
1970	2.0
1980	1.7
1990	1.5
2000	1.3
2050	0.4

TABLE 2.2 Human Population Growth Rates Through Time

Current Challenges and Approaches to Population Problems

Since 1600, the human population has increased from about 0.5 billion to more than 6 billion. The increase in the last decade of the 20th century exceeds the total population in 1600. Compared with human history prior to World War II, the world's population growth rate is unprecedented. Within the lifetime of some people now alive, the world's population has tripled. If global total fertility drops to the highest projection, 2.5 in the 21st century, by 2050 there will be 12 billion people on earth, and this number will continue to rise. If it falls to 1.7, the lowest prediction, global population will peak at 7.8 billion in 2050 and then begin to decline. Even the latter scenario might give cause for concern, since estimates of the earth's carrying capacity range from fewer than 1 billion to more than 1 trillion people, with most estimates falling between 4 and 16 billion.

Proposals for solutions to the world's population problems confront formidable intellectual and ideological minefields. The various approaches can be grouped into three categories or "schools of thought" (Cohen, 1995). First, the "Bigger Pie School" subscribes to the liberal philosophy that more resources can be produced through improved technology such as the agricultural "green revolution" based on genetically engineered crops and advanced chemical fertilizers. Second, the "Fewer Forks School" seeks to reduce the number of people and/or the expectations of people served, such as through family planning programs and encouraging people to eat lower on the food chain and reduce waste. Third, the "Better Manners School" advocates changing the terms under which people interact both politically and economically and includes solutions based on freer markets, socialism, wealth redistribution, and less corruption.

The biggest source of population growth is what is called *population momentum,* the very high fraction of young people in developing countries who begin having children at an early age. Approaches to counteract population momentum include raising the average age at child-bearing, inducing women to have fewer children, and making contraceptive services more available to adolescents.

The second largest source of increased population is *unwanted fertility.* In developing countries, one birth in four is estimated to be unwanted. In many places, families still desire large numbers of children. Surveys conducted between 1990 and 2001 in 27 countries in Africa, Asia, and Latin America found that desired family sizes everywhere exceeded two children. In sub-Saharan Africa, people wanted nearly six children (INFO Project, 2003). Approaches to reducing fertility, including wanted and unwanted, generally encompass some form of investment in human development, such as improved access to education, enhancing the status of women, and improving the health and survival of children.

DEVELOPMENTAL TRANSITIONS

Demographic and health researchers have described a number of large-scale population changes, or "transitions," that accompany developmental change in human societies. Originally proposed to explain the changes that occur as countries undergo industrialization, much of the focus of these discussions is on contemporary developing countries, with extrapolation to earlier historical periods. Developing societies are undergoing complex transitions in the areas of population trends, disease patterns, and health behavior. These processes have been described, respectively, as demographic, epidemiologic, and health transitions. Each of these will be briefly discussed in turn.

Demographic Transition

History has shown that as societies undergo the shift from rural agricultural economies to urban industrialized ones, population processes follow a predictable course of change, referred to as the *demographic transition* (Notestein, 1983). The pretransition period is characterized by high rates of fertility and mortality, particularly infant and child mortality, producing moderate rates of population growth. During the period of transition, death rates first begin to decrease in response to improvements in living conditions and health care, but there is a lag time during which fertility remains high. This is because the factors favoring large family sizes, such as expectations for high mortality among children, are slow to change. This results in elevated population growth rates, characteristic of many developing countries today and the reason why population growth is sometimes used to define underdevelopment. Over time, fertility decreases in response to falling mortality, producing the low growth rates characteristic of industrialized nations.

Epidemiologic Transition

Along with the demographic changes just described, corresponding changes occur in the pattern of diseases that dominate the health profile of a society. Table 2.3 illustrates common

TABLE 2.3	Illustrative Health Problems of Children and Adults, Pre- and Posttransition	

Age Category	Pretransition	Posttransition
Children	Diarrhea	Congenital defects
	Acute respiratory infection	Growth failure
	Polio, tetanus	Micronutrient deficiency
	Undernutrition	Mental development problems
	Malaria	Injury
	Intestinal helminths	
Adults and elderly	Tuberculosis	Mental disorders
	Malaria	Circulatory disease
	AIDS/STDs	AIDS/STDs
	Parasitic diseases	Cancers
	Injury	Injury
	Maternity problems	Chronic pulmonary disease

SOURCE: Mosley, W. H., Jamison, D. T., & Henderson, D. A. (1990). Reprinted by permission from the *Annual Review of Public Health*, Volume 11 © 1990 by Annual Reviews www.annualreviews.org.

health problems experienced by young and older age groups pre- and posttransition. The pretransition situation is characterized by high rates of infectious diseases, including diarrheal diseases, respiratory infections, and parasitic diseases, which, coupled with poor nutritional status, leads to excess deaths in the younger age groups. As infectious diseases decline, more children survive to adulthood, life expectancy increases, and chronic diseases affecting the older population become the major health problems of a society, as currently seen in posttransition industrialized countries. These processes are referred to as the *epidemiologic transition* (Omran, 1983), and most developing countries are currently in the early stages of this transformation. In both pre- and posttransition societies, HIV/AIDS and injuries are important adult health problems, and in posttransition societies, children are also significantly affected by injuries. The increase in injuries posttransition is largely related to motor vehicle injuries (see Chapter 19).

Health Transition

The concept of the *health transition* is a more recently defined area of study, which seeks to understand the cultural, social, and behavioral determinants of health that underlie the epidemiologic transition (Caldwell, 1993). Health transition research looks beyond changes in material standard of living and medical services to understand the behavioral and sociocultural factors that influence health conditions in all societies, with most work concentrated in poor countries. Some of the important findings to emerge from this work include the far-reaching effects of maternal education on a variety of health activities and the impact of household organization on health-related behavior. The accumulating body of research on health behavior in developing countries would fall within the health transition rubric, although many such studies are not explicitly identified as health transition research.

Shifts in demography and disease patterns do not occur in isolation from other sociocultural changes. The ecosocial approach followed in this volume directs our attention to contextual conditions that both enable and limit the kinds of health problems encountered in a population. In the following section, we take a historical look at the various "stages" and transitions that have characterized human disease history, including what some anthropologists call the "first" demographic transition (Handwerker, 1983), which accompanied the Neolithic Revolution. We examine disease from the perspective of cultural evolution.

DISEASE AND CULTURAL EVOLUTION

Key Concepts

One of the most important concepts in this discussion is human *culture,* the patterned ways of thought and behavior that characterize a social group, which are learned through socialization processes and persist through time. However, like all aspects of dynamic systems, culture is never static. It is constantly changing and evolving at variable rates over time. *Culture change* can be described as long term or short term, depending on the time depth involved. *Long-term culture change* takes place over several generations, centuries, or millennia, such as the shift from one form of subsistence to another. For example, the move from a hunting and gathering livelihood to food-producing subsistence is an example of long-term culture change. *Short-term culture change,* on the other hand, occurs within a single generation or a few years. Examples of short-term culture change include the introduction of automobiles, mass communication, Western medicine, and computer technology within a society. *Cultural evolution* refers to the process of long-term culture change that is slow and developmental, often described in terms of stages, where one form builds on the previously existing phase.

Following Polgar (1964) and Armelagos and Dewey (1978), we organize the following discussion along five constellations of subsistence mode and settlement pattern: (1) foraging groups, (2) settled villages, (3) preindustrial cities, (4) industrial cities, and (5) postindustrial society. The discussion draws on several sources related to historical trends in fertility, health, and nutrition in human populations (Cohen, 1989; Cohen, Malpass, & Klein, 1980; Fabrega, 1997; Stuart-Macadam & Dettwyler, 1995; Ungar & Teaford, 2002, among others). Note that two abbreviations are used to denote time periods: "Before Present (BP)" indicates the number of years prior to the current day, while "Before Common Era (BCE)" replaces the traditional "Before Christ (BC)" designation. It should be noted that there can be overlap between the stages. For example, there may be foraging groups living in the same area as farmers and trading with them, and some groups may engage in both hunting and herding at the same time. Furthermore, many countries have very diverse populations and regional development that encompass traditional subsistence modes as well as urbanization and industrialization.

1. Foraging Groups (3 million BP)

If the time depth of culture history were depicted as a continuous line across a wide surface, it would appear that almost the entire trajectory were taken up with the original human subsistence mode, the foraging group, with only a tiny segment at the end representing all the subsequent phases. The vast preponderance of human history was spent in the hunting and gathering stage, and some would argue that we are "hardwired" to be most adapted socially, biologically, and emotionally to this form of life (see highlight on Evolutionary Medicine below).

Foraging, or hunting and gathering, is a subsistence technology that relies almost totally on human energy and simple tools to collect wild plants and kill free-roaming animals. All pre-human and human groups foraged for food until about 10,000 to 15,000 years ago. Today, less than 1% of human groups rely primarily (more than 75%) on food gathering, hunting, and fishing. The few groups that remain are found in marginal lands not suitable for agriculture in the desert fringes of Australia, Southern Africa, and North America; in the forests of Asia, South America, and Central Africa; and in the frozen wastelands of Siberia and the Arctic. Even these groups have contact with technologically more complex groups, from whom they may obtain food and other supplies. Competition for land and other resources with more complex societies places the technologically simpler foragers at a disadvantage, often with deleterious effects on their way of life and health status.

Foragers live in small groups that move frequently in their search for food; that is, they are nomadic. While there is a good deal of variation in the size of foraging groups, population density rarely exceeds one person per square mile. The exact size of a group and its density is constrained by the resources available and the nomadic lifestyle.

With the exception of a few groups living in extremely harsh regions, such as the Arctic, foraging tribes have enjoyed generally good nutritional status and leisurely work schedules. The !Kung Bushmen, studied in great detail by Richard Lee (1968), offer a good example. Typically, the !Kung woman collects enough food in 2 days to feed her entire family for a week or an average of 240 calories of plant food per hour. The rest of her time is spent cooking, fetching wood, embroidering, dancing, storytelling, resting, and visiting with friends. This steady mix of work and leisure varies little throughout the year. The man's schedule is more uneven. Hunting may occupy an entire week, followed by several leisurely weeks. As with the woman, 2 or 3 days of hunting produce enough food for the entire week. Even the most avid hunter in the tribe studied by Lee worked only 32 hours per week.

Most foragers' diets are high in complex carbohydrates and low in fat, especially saturated fats. The roots, leaves, berries, plant shoots, and the highly nutritious mongongo nut are among a surprising variety of the plant foods the !Kung gather from their desert environment. Meat is consumed less regularly than plant food, contributing 20% to 30% of the diet's calories. Groups living in the Arctic are an exception: They rely almost exclusively on hunting, with animal products contributing as much as 90% of the calories in their diet. Although this diet contains more than enough protein, the entire animal (entrails, organs, stomach contents, etc.) must be consumed to obtain the vitamins and minerals needed to sustain life.

Foragers tend to be lean, robust, and tall and suffer from few nutritional deficiencies. Nutritional surveys of contemporary hunters and gatherers show them to be generally free from severe protein-calorie malnutrition, scurvy, rickets, or vitamin B deficiency diseases. Although malnutrition and starvation are rare, loss of subcutaneous fat during leaner times of the year has been noted, suggesting that the amount of energy available at those times is not optimal. The chronic diseases we see in more modern societies are also rare in these simple societies. The active lifestyle and low fat content of many foragers' diets help protect them from cardiovascular disease. Also, fewer people reach the ages at which these illnesses occur.

In foraging groups, fertility remained low because women breast-fed their infants for extended periods, often until a child reached 4 years of age (Lee, 1980). Frequent nipple stimulation from infant suckling inhibits ovulation in the lactating mother, leading to births spaced several years apart. In some cases, infanticide was practiced when a second child was born too soon after an older sibling. Child spacing was essential in these nomadic groups, where young children had to be carried from one camp to another. Population density remained low, so epidemic infectious diseases were not a serious problem. There was not sufficient concentration of people living in close proximity to one another to maintain a reservoir of new hosts for disease organisms to flourish.

However, life expectancy was low in early human populations because of the hardships of life and the primitive state of medical care. Parasitic diseases were prevalent, and people were exposed to the risks of injury and trauma, animal predation (including insects and snakes), sepsis from wounds, and interpersonal violence (homicide and war). Maternal mortality was very high because prehistoric obstetrical care offered limited help for complications of childbirth. Feeble, handicapped, and sickly members of the group had lower survival chances within the vigorous demands of everyday life.

⊗ **Focus:** Evolutionary Medicine ⊗

An interdisciplinary field of study emerged in the 1990s, which draws heavily on what we know about human biocultural adaptation during the foraging phase of history. *Evolutionary medicine* examines current-day medical problems from the perspective of how ancient patterns of life continue to influence health and illness (Neese & Williams, 1996; Trevathan, Smith, & McKenna, 1999, 2008). Also known as *Darwinian medicine,* the specialty draws on the disciplines of human ecology, physical anthropology, archaeology, genetics, developmental psychology, and the clinical sciences. Evidence is pieced together from ethnographic studies of extant foraging groups, the fossil record, archaeological data, and primate research. The basic principles center on the tenet that culture evolves faster than biology, so physiologically humans are still primarily adapted to a foraging lifestyle. Consequently, certain modern cultural practices conflict with our biological makeup, leading to a variety of health problems.

A wide range of health problems have been examined through the lens of evolutionary medicine. Foremost among these are the role of diet and physical activity in contemporary chronic diseases, the relationship between culture change and reproductive health, child care practices and infant health, environmental factors and respiratory conditions, and the modern-day lifestyle and psychiatric problems.

Worldwide, there is growing concern about the "epidemic" of obesity and its contribution to chronic diseases, including cardiovascular disease, diabetes, and some cancers. Concern is particularly marked in postindustrial societies, where diets are high in fats, carbohydrates, and refined sugar, and sedentary lifestyles limit physical activity at all ages (see Chapter 17). Sometimes referred to as the malnutrition of affluence, the abundance of food in industrialized societies contributes to obesity. Human nutritional requirements are still based on the foods that were consumed during the 5 to 7 million years of hominid evolution. Our evolutionary heritage has programmed the human body to enable people to survive in environments with fluctuating food supplies. Our bodies are equipped with efficient mechanisms for accumulating body fat and excellent defenses against the depletion of these energy stores. These biological mechanisms place people with access to an abundant food supply at risk of gaining excessive amounts of weight (Hill & Peters, 1998).

In addition to obesity as a risk factor for chronic disease, there is evidence that the mismatch between human evolutionary biology and current dietary and physical activity patterns may be linked to the "metabolic syndrome" implicated in the etiology of coronary heart disease and diabetes. Characterized by abdominal body fat, glucose intolerance, blood fat disorders, and elevated blood pressure, the prevalence of metabolic syndrome has increased within industrial societies and has been linked to evolutionary changes in modern lifestyles and human development (Matheson, 2007).

Various malignancies, including breast, endometrial, and ovarian cancers, have been linked with the changes in fertility patterns noted in the foregoing section. It is argued that Stone Age women ovulated and menstruated much less regularly than modern women, so today's women have much greater exposure to estrogen and other reproductive hormones than their ancient sisters. In addition, exposure to environmental toxins that mimic estrogen contributes to the estrogen load of women in industrial countries. This long-term exposure to estrogen is suggested as contributing to the increase in reproductive cancers in modern populations (Worthman, 1999).

Childbirth and infant feeding patterns are also drastically changed today compared with earlier times, with, some argue, significant health consequences. For example, current technological birth practices and loss of childbirth social support are cited as contributing to certain labor complications and increased caesarian section rates. Finally, researchers have implicated the replacement of breast-feeding with artificial feeding in the rise of childhood allergies and other disorders (Trevathan & McKenna, 1994). In a large epidemiologic study of more than 8,900 infants in the United States followed from birth to 1 year, researchers examined the relationship between infant feeding practices and postnatal deaths. Infants who were only breast-fed had a 20% lower risk of death at 1 year compared with infants who were never breast-fed (Chen & Rogan, 2004).

In addition to changes in infant-feeding practices, environmental modifications have been linked to the increased prevalence of allergic disease, including asthma, in developed country settings. In particular, modern domestic architecture creates tightly closed spaces that accumulate substances (dust mites, animal dander, insect pests, mold) that trigger allergic reactions in some people. The allergic response to inhaled substances may include bronchial constriction (wheezing), coughing, sneezing, and mucous secretion, while food allergies may cause vomiting or diarrhea. Such reactions are mediated by the immunoglobulin IgE, which triggers the bodily reactions when it comes into contact with allergens to which the host is sensitive. Evolutionary researchers suggest that the allergic response serves (or served in the past) to protect people from various toxins they encounter in the environment. Some theorists propose that the IgE system evolved as a backup mechanism to quickly rid the body of harmful substances when other defenses fail (Profet, 1991). Others propose that the IgE-mediated allergic response may be linked to a protective mechanism from our evolutionary past, that is, as a defense against the highly prevalent helminthic (parasitic worm) infections in prehistoric populations (Barnes, Armelagos, & Morreale, 1999; Hurtado, Arenas de Hurtado, Sapien, & Hill, 1999). The role of IgE antibodies in controlling damage from parasitic disease has been demonstrated. Furthermore, contemporary populations that carry a heavy parasitic load have very low rates of allergy, while those with low helminthic infestation have experienced a marked increase in allergic disease in recent decades. Proponents of the second theory argue that as changes in living conditions and disease patterns reduce the risk of parasites, the IgE system has been redirected to respond to other environmental toxins.

Child care practices related to infant sleeping arrangements have been linked to sudden infant death syndrome (SIDS). Infant mortality from SIDS has declined significantly since health authorities began recommending that infants be positioned on their backs or sides, but not prone, during sleep. Research on infant sleeping patterns suggests that there may be a link between the risk of SIDS and solitary sleep, and conversely, infants sleeping with their mothers or parents (cosleeping) may be protective. In laboratory experiments, infants cosleeping with their mothers exhibited breathing patterns that have been associated with lower rates of SIDS (McKenna, Mosko, & Richard, 1999; Mosko, Richard, McKenna, & Drummond, 1996). The Western practice of solitary infant sleep, often in a separate room, contrasts sharply with the historical and cross-cultural norm for infants to sleep next to their parents.

The evolutionary perspective offers new ways to analyze public health problems and design interventions to improve population health. Eaton and colleagues (2002) have proposed such an approach, which they call "evolutionary health promotion," one based on a conceptual framework that addresses issues of health and disease through the lens of long-term culture change. Building on this notion, Lieberman (2008) argues for expanding evolutionary health promotion beyond the conventional realms of diet and physical activity to include early-life prevention, pharmacologic therapies, psychosocial stress reduction, and focused interventions such as increasing sleep duration.

2. Settled Village (15,000 BP)

Roughly 10,000 to 15,000 years ago, a very different form of cultural adaptation evolved within the human species. In response to population pressure, people began to settle down in small villages to grow staple crops and raise livestock for consumption and production of raw materials. The shift to a sedentary population concentrated in a permanent community created a whole new set of ecological interactions, with significant health consequences. With increased population density came problems of waste accumulation and the breeding of disease pathogens. Domestic animals living in close proximity to humans became a new reservoir for zoonotic diseases. Modifications to the natural environment for agricultural and settlement purposes altered the ecological relationships among local plant and animal species, sometimes creating health hazards. Most important, the increased population density allowed the continuous transmission of communicable diseases in the population, marking the beginning of a long-term public health problem, which is with us even today.

The first, and least complex, system of agriculture is called *horticulture*. Horticulture is a nonmechanized system that relies solely on human labor to cultivate plants in small gardens. It is characterized by reliance on human energy and a limited inventory of simple tools. Digging sticks and hoes are used rather than plows; neither irrigation nor terracing is employed. In traditional horticultural groups, food production is intended for home consumption rather than commercial sale. Each farmer controls his or her own production, and there is little interdependence between groups. Horticulture is still practiced by a large number of people throughout the world.

Today, many people relying on horticulture to produce crops for sale as well as home consumption are no longer independent. These farmers, sometimes called peasants, participate in a national and international marketplace. Peasants use the cash they obtain from these sales to pay tax or rent and buy necessities and luxury items produced outside their communities. Typically, the elite or wealthy members of the society rely on trade with peasants to enhance their own standard of living. This link between peasants and the elite is a key factor distinguishing peasants from more autonomous agriculturists. Most farmers in developing countries fit the above pattern of the peasant economy.

As peasant societies shift from subsistence food crops to cash crops, their diets change radically, usually with deleterious effects. Typically, the most fertile land is used for cash crops (coffee, peanuts, cotton, cocoa), thus lowering the production capacity of the land under food cultivation. The shift to a cash economy also means that a large part, if not the majority, of food is purchased instead of produced. The high cost of purchased protein-rich foods often makes them prohibitive, thereby forcing people into an affordable high-carbohydrate diet deficient in many vitamins and minerals as well as protein.

In contrast to the varied food consumption of foraging society, fewer types of foods make up the agrarian diet, and high-carbohydrate grains and root crops are their main staples. Because horticulturalists rely primarily on one or two crops, typically high in carbohydrates and low in protein, they are more vulnerable to episodic famines and nutritional deficiencies than hunters and gatherers. A high-carbohydrate diet also affects the health of infants, children, and adults.

Easy access to cereal grains enabled the production of soft baby foods that made earlier weaning of infants possible. Young children fed on high-carbohydrate diets without adequate protein and specific nutrients are vulnerable to nutritional disorders such as kwashiorkor and micronutrient deficiencies. Dental caries become a problem.

Increased sedentary lifestyle in villages, coupled with the above noted dietary changes, led to fertility increases and population growth. Menarche in young girls occurred earlier because of increased fat stores in youth. Shorter breast-feeding duration and early introduction of supplementary infant foods reduced the natural child-spacing anovulatory intervals among postpartum women. Children were born closer together in families, and larger numbers of children were desired to provide household agricultural labor. The net effect of these demographic changes was larger family size and increase in population.

⊠ **Focus:** Culture Change, Malaria, and Sickle-Cell Disease ⊠

The most significant public health consequence of the Neolithic Revolution was the creation of more densely settled populations, which could sustain the presence of infectious diseases. In addition, agricultural land clearing often led to environmental changes that affected the concentration of disease vectors such as insects. One such case, which is often cited as a classic example of such linkages, is the introduction of agriculture in sub-Saharan Africa 2,000 years ago, including its impact on the emergence of more lethal forms of malaria and the evolution of sickle-cell disease.

Prior to the domestication of food crops, foraging groups subsisted through traditional hunting and gathering of edibles within the thick rainforests of the region. Then, Bantu-speaking horticultural tribes began moving into the forest zones, gradually clearing the land for planting and, in the process, removing the trees and shady canopy that had heretofore blocked out the tropical sun. The reduction of tree cover left many wet areas exposed to the warm rays of the sun, just the right conditions for breeding *Anopheles gambiae* mosquitoes, the vectors for a severe form of malaria. Although malaria was present in the preagricultural populations, it was the introduction of the particular strain of malaria caused by *Plasmodium falciparum* that led to markedly increased mortality from this parasitic disease. The proliferation of the mosquito vector, coupled with the closer proximity of more numerous human hosts, quickly led to a serious problem. Caused by a protozoan that reproduces in red blood cells, malaria not only causes extreme debilitation from fever and chills, it also greatly increases the incidence of low-birth-weight infants and miscarriage and stillbirths in pregnant women, and it is particularly lethal among young children. Mortality from the disease was high, often killing 25% of the infected individuals.

The malaria situation might have had even more devastating consequences had it not been for the opportune presence of a genetic mutation in the population, which protected heterozygous human hosts from the most devastating effects of the disease.

The anomaly in question is the abnormal hemoglobin condition we know today as the sickle-cell trait. Unlike normal hemoglobin (A), sickle-cell hemoglobin (S) molecules cannot carry oxygen well and tend to clump together and distort the red blood cells into their characteristic "sickle" shape. Individuals with the sickle-cell gene produce fewer red blood cells, thus preventing the Plasmodium organisms from completing their full life cycle, so these people are spared the more severe effects of malaria.

Since human beings are born with a pair of chromosomes for each gene (one from each parent), it makes it possible to have three different hemoglobin combinations in the population (AA, AS, and SS). In the normal form (AA), individuals do not have impaired red blood cells, but they remain vulnerable to malaria. In the heterozygous form (AS), the sickle-cell trait remains recessive, yet still confers significant immunity to malaria, while the homozygous form (SS) leads to sickle-cell anemia and a short life expectancy. Thus, the heterozygote has selective advantage over both homozygous forms of the gene. In heavy malaria zones, a "balanced polymorphism" between the two genes has evolved within the population, so that the proportion of each hemoglobin type is maximally advantageous for survival of the group.

Thus, what began as a large-scale culture change in Africa had profound biological repercussions involving complex disease-genetic adaptations. The social ecology of malaria in Africa dramatically illustrates the interaction of physical environment and culture in the production of disease patterns. Yet this story has a more recent chapter that highlights the consequences of other social changes for the sickle-cell trait. The forced migration of African slaves to the New World has led to a situation where, in North America today, the sickle-cell gene persists in the African American population, in a setting where malaria is now eradicated, and the genetic anomaly confers no health advantages, only serious risks. Homozygous sickle-cell individuals, like their African counterparts, suffer anemia and a high risk of early death. Heterozygous "carriers," on the other hand, face discrimination in employment opportunities within occupations requiring high-altitude or physically demanding work. They also face difficult fertility decisions when the risk of conceiving a sickle-cell child is present (Reese & Smith, 1997).

3. Preindustrial Cities (1200–1700 CE)

The public health problems that first emerged in settled village life became intensified in preindustrial cities as a result of even denser populations in urban areas. The Middle Ages are marked by the demands of food, water, shelter, and waste management, as even larger numbers of people had to live together in confined spaces. For the first time, pollution became a serious public problem. Food security, water supply, and sanitation became a challenge for local municipalities as the state increasingly assumed responsibility for social welfare. This was also the age of exploration, and expanded trade contacts with the outside world introduced new diseases into the European populations. Many infectious diseases reached the endemic state in medieval societies, with constant transmission among new hosts. Devastating epidemics also coursed through the population regularly during this age of the great pandemics. The Great Plague alone wiped out a third of the world's population in the 14th century.

⧽⧽ **Focus:** Early Public Health Practices ⧽⧽

Organized public health actions have roots in the ancient cities of Greece and Rome. There, under the authority of government regulation, complex systems of water supply and waste disposal were built and operated to meet the municipal needs of urban populations. An awareness of the concept of community health was evident in the early medical texts, most prominently in the Hippocratic book *Airs, Waters and Places.* This classic work outlines the environmental conditions believed to affect human health at that time, most notably the noxious vapors emitted from fetid swamps and marshes, a view sometimes described as the miasma theory of disease. The book also introduced the notions of *endemic* and *epidemic* disease and laid out guidelines for public health practice that remained largely unchanged until the end of the 19th century.

During the Middle Ages (500–1500), understanding of health and disease was closely intertwined with religious dogma. When a person became ill, the misfortune was attributed to moral or spiritual transgression, a form of punishment from God. Likewise, epidemics were assumed to manifest divine wrath hurled down on people for their depraved and evil ways. However, it was believed that the human body, vessel of the soul, could be fortified against the work of the Devil by hygienic practices. Efforts to promote community health, too, were common in medieval cities, particularly the enforcement of codes designed to keep the waterways clean and prevent the accumulation of waste. A huge amount of refuse was produced in the preindustrial cities, which often housed livestock within their borders, where all food and material goods were prepared from raw materials. Dirt streets thick with mud, trash, animal dung, household sewage, rotting food waste, and foul-smelling water were commonplace. Marketplaces were particularly important centers for enforcement of sanitation measures such as disposal of rotten food and contaminated goods.

Among the diseases that menaced the population were bubonic plague, tuberculosis, typhus, diphtheria, leprosy, smallpox, measles, influenza, anthrax, and scabies (Rosen, 1993). Organized responses to two of these diseases, leprosy and plague, helped shape the medieval emergence of a basic public health strategy—that is, the use of isolation and quarantine. The Christian church took the lead in isolation of lepers based on scriptural prescriptions to avoid the contagious impurity of spiritually unclean, diseased persons. Lepers were cast out of their communities to protect the healthy members and forced to live in segregated areas outside the cities. They were required to wear special identifying clothing and to announce their approach to other persons.

Efforts to protect cities from plague, on the other hand, led to the institution of quarantine. First noted in mid-14th-century Venice, the practice consisted of a time-limited sequestering of people and goods suspected of being infected. Ships coming into the harbor from the Orient, believed to be the source of plague, were kept at bay for an interim to allow the sick to die. Persons who came in contact with a plague victim were quarantined for 2 weeks in their homes or special facilities. Later, the period of sequester was extended to 30 days, then 40 days, the latter being the Italian derivative of the term *quarantine.* Organized efforts involving observation stations, isolation hospitals, and disinfection procedures laid the groundwork for this public health practice, which remains important today.

4. Industrial Cities (1750–1950 CE)

The Industrial Revolution transformed human society in dramatic ways, with profound repercussions both life saving and hazardous to health. Many forces underlie the complex changes involved in the transformation process, including the mechanization of work, the emergence of the factory, mass production of goods and services, increasing urbanization, rapid transportation, and the enlarged role of government in public welfare. European colonization of the New World, Africa, and other areas laid the groundwork for present-day geopolitical issues. The Modern Era brought the demise of feudalism, the promise of human progress through technological innovation, the advent of Western medicine, and improvements in the standard of living and life expectancy of the population.

Urban life was still fraught with the ongoing problems of food, water, shelter, and sanitation, which only intensified with the growth of large cities and metropolitan areas. Epidemics remained common, and endemic diseases held on tenaciously. Added to this were new sources of pollution from industrial wastes unregulated by government legislation, now contaminating air and land as well as water. Beginning in the 19th century, however, the sanitary reform movement in Europe sparked the beginning of organized public health efforts to improve health. Improvements in living conditions, not the emergence of scientific medicine as sometimes assumed, accounted for most of the decline in mortality that began during this period. Most important, infant and child mortality from infectious diseases declined, improving overall life expectancy. As people began to live longer as well, chronic diseases emerged as the major public health problems.

⬛ **Focus:** Cholera Epidemics of the 19th Century ⬛

By the 19th century, the major cities of Europe and North America had been transformed by industrialization into teeming centers of commerce and manufacturing, home to large populations of factory workers, merchants, and tradesmen. Sanitary and living conditions in the cities had improved dramatically from medieval times, with organized waste disposal services and access to drinking water from municipal pumps. Such improvements made a significant impact on the morbidity and mortality of the urban residents. It was an era of enlightened thinking and optimism about addressing social problems through progress and reason. Officials believed that the health of the populace could be protected through environmental controls and healthful living conditions. The prevailing explanations of disease continued to be miasma theory and contagionism, with the corollary that people living under oppressive conditions (poverty, crowded housing, overwork, inadequate diet, and intemperance and immorality) were especially vulnerable to the deleterious effects of miasma and contagion. Outbreaks of infectious disease were controlled through public health measures such as isolation of the sick, quarantine, and hygienic procedures.

Against this backdrop, the cholera epidemics of the 19th century in Europe and the United States caused great consternation because the disease did not conform to prevailing views of contagion. A swift-acting bacterial infection spread by water contaminated with human feces, cholera causes severe diarrhea, dehydration, and death in a large percentage of its victims. Most perplexing was the fact that the epidemics affected diverse and geographically dispersed populations, including middle-class neighborhoods and communities far removed from miasmatic conditions. Moreover, traditional efforts to control the epidemic, such as quarantine of vessels and seaports, seemed to have little impact on its spread.

The cholera riddle challenged medical thinking and led to the physician John Snow's famous epidemiologic studies of the London public water supply. He was able to show that cases of cholera were highest among people whose drinking water derived from the most polluted sections of the Thames River. In particular, his investigation of the Broad Street pump provided confirmation of this theory that cholera was transmitted through water infested with the excreta of cholera victims. He published his thesis in a pamphlet dated 1849, *On the Mode of Communication of Cholera* (Rosen, 1993). He also showed that cholera could be transmitted from person to person through soiled hands, food, and clothing. His ideas were accepted by some people and repudiated by others. However, in 1883, Koch successfully isolated and cultivated the cholera pathogen, *Vibrio cholera,* proving the correctness of Snow's ideas. The discovery of waterborne diseases led to important improvements in sewerage and control of water pollution in the late 19th century.

5. Postindustrial Society (1950 to the present)

Following the end of World War II, tremendous changes took place in the industrial regions of the world. Improvements in sanitation, disease prevention, medical care, and overall quality of life have reduced mortality at all ages. Most of the infectious diseases that contributed to mortality in the past have been controlled by large-scale immunization programs and an array of antibiotic drugs (although some are reemerging). People are living longer and healthier lives, and the health needs of the elderly have emerged as a new public health concern (see Chapter 12). Chronic, degenerative diseases have replaced infectious diseases as the main health problems, although the AIDS epidemic of the late 20th century dispelled the notion that global pandemics were a thing of the past.

Pollution from industrial manufacturing and massive reliance on automobile transportation continue to pose threats, but government regulation of waste and emissions is much tighter than before. Maintaining an adequate and safe water supply is an increasingly troublesome challenge for local and regional jurisdictions. We are running out of space for disposal of solid waste, and toxic chemicals threaten our land and waterways. In addition, we now live in the Atomic Age, in which radioactive contamination is a serious risk, not to mention the possibility of mass destruction from nuclear weapons.

Our extremely sedentary lifestyle, coupled with a diet that is high in fat and low in fiber, has contributed substantially to the chronic disease burden of our times, including obesity, cardiovascular disease, and diabetes. Tobacco use constitutes a major threat to health, either directly or indirectly contributing to the leading causes of death, such as lung, breast, and other cancers; heart disease; stroke; and chronic obstructive pulmonary disease. Mental illness and substance abuse are highly prevalent. Unintentional injury and violent behavior are rampant, accounting for major proportions of deaths in certain age groups. Chronic stress and an unrelenting accelerated pace of life take its toll on the emotional and physical well-being of the population.

Industrialization turned agriculture into a large-scale business enterprise requiring large amounts of capital and energy. It relies heavily on fossil fuels rather than human labor, making it energy intensive and technologically complex. For example, in the United States, more than 500 million gallons of gasoline are used annually to move fresh vegetables and produce to market, and 1,300 million gallons are needed to move manufactured food products from processors to warehouses and supermarkets. Many scientists question the ability of intensive agriculture to feed the world's population without damaging the earth's ability to produce food for future generations. Industrialized agriculture also relies heavily on mechanical equipment, chemicals, and a complex system of food distribution. Global energy demands have increased oil and gas prices, which in turn have elevated world food prices, straining the ability of people everywhere to afford healthy diets. One response to the energy crisis is the shift to production of biofuels, which diverts agricultural production into energy sources instead of food staples, further exacerbating food prices and availability of food.

Increasing concern has arisen over the impact of global warming, natural and man-made disasters, warfare, terrorism, food shortages, and a host of other large-scale public health threats. Many of these threats fall within the scope of what are called complex humanitarian emergencies (CHEs), and disaster management has emerged as an important area of specialization within the field of environmental health. Experts predict that CHEs will occur with increasing frequency in the coming years and will pose major challenges to public health systems worldwide. The following section highlights some of the social and behavioral aspects of CHEs.

⊠ Focus: Complex Humanitarian Emergencies ⊠

Complex humanitarian emergencies have been defined by the Centers for Disease Control and Prevention (CDC) as "a humanitarian crisis in a country, region or society where there is a *breakdown of authority* due to internal or external conflict and *requires an international response* that goes beyond the capacity of any single agency and/or the UN country program" (CDC, 2008; emphasis in original). Common characteristics include war or civil strife, food shortages, population displacement, political impediments to delivery of assistance, and inability to pursue normal social and economic activities, all resulting in significant health problems and mortality (Burkholder & Toole, 1995). The causes of CHEs are rooted in the political sphere and since World War II have been associated with human rights violations and genocide in many parts of the globe (Toole, Waldman, & Zwi, 2001). Some well-publicized examples include the killing fields of Cambodia; genocide in Rwanda; repression of Mayan communities in Guatemala; and, most recently, starvation in Darfur, Sudan. In many instances, the violence involves calculated attacks against particular ethnic or tribal groups, sometimes referred to as "ethnic cleansing." International response in such emergencies varies markedly, ranging from full-scale relief efforts to total neglect and apathy.

The public health challenges associated with CHEs are similar to those accompanying natural disasters, including the provision of food, water, sanitation, shelter, and medical assistance; resettlement of displaced individuals; rebuilding of infrastructure; and intersectoral collaboration in long-term recovery. Women and children often bear the greatest burden of adverse consequences in emergency situations (Al Gasseer, Dresden, Keeney, & Warren, 2004). Women and girls are exposed to sexual violence, and infants and children are particularly vulnerable to infectious diseases and malnutrition. Psychosocial impacts have acute and long-term effects on child well-being, particularly when children are forced into perpetrator roles (Williams, 2007). Special attention to the needs of racial and ethnic groups has been noted, such as in the case of the Hurricane Katrina disaster in New Orleans (Andrulis, Siddiqui, & Gantner, 2007).

CONCLUSION

Taking a historical perspective on population and disease enlarges our understanding of the complex interaction of human culture and social organization with the technological and physical environment in shaping disease patterns and societal responses to health threats. Population dynamics underpin demographic features that affect disease epidemiology, nutrition, and reproduction. Classic public health concerns, such as waste disposal, water supply, food security, and control of infectious diseases, emerged with the first demographic transition, the shift from foraging society to settled village life and food growing. These issues remain important today, as well as new problems created by the processes of industrialization and urbanization. Although technological developments have enabled profound advances in medicine and areas such as food production, technology has also created new health risks. Contemporary industrial nations face challenges posed by high rates of injury, violence, and chronic disease, along with new threats related to global warming and CHEs.

There are many lessons to be learned from human history, both in the general sense of understanding issues within a larger time frame and, more specifically, through specialized areas of study such as evolutionary medicine. Knowing where we have come from can help us envision the constellation of old and new problems that will encompass the public health agenda of the 21st century.

REFERENCES

Al Gasseer, N., Dresden, E., Keeney, G. B., & Warren, N. (2004). Status of women and infants in complex humanitarian emergencies. *Journal of Midwifery & Women's Health, 49*(4), 7–13.

Andrulis, D. P., Siddiqui, N. J., & Gantner, J. L. (2007). Preparing racially and ethnically diverse communities for public health emergencies. *Health Affairs, 26*(5), 1269–1279.

Armelagos, G., & Dewey, J. R. (1978). Evolutionary response to human infectious diseases. In M. H. Logan & E. E. Hunt (Eds.), *Health and human condition: Perspectives on medical anthropology* (pp. 101–106). North Scituate, MA: Duxbury Press.

Barnes, K. C., Armelagos, G. J., & Morreale, S. C. (1999). Darwinian medicine and the emergence of allergy. In W. R. Trevathan, E. O. Smith, & J. J. McKenna (Eds.), *Evolutionary Medicine* (pp. 209–244). New York: Oxford University Press.

Burkholder, B. T., & Toole, M. J. (1995). Evolution of complex emergencies. *Lancet, 346,* 1012–1015.

Caldwell, J. C. (1993). Health transition: The cultural, social and behavioural determinants of health in the Third World. *Social Science and Medicine, 36,* 125–135.

Centers for Disease Control and Prevention. (2008). *Frequently asked questions.* Retrieved April 22, 2008, from www.cdc.gov/nceh/ierh/FAQ.htm

Chen, A., & Rogan, W. J. (2004). Breastfeeding and the risk of postneonatal death in the United States. *Pediatrics, 113*(5), E435–E439.

Cohen, J. E. (1995). *How many people can the earth support?* New York: Norton.

Cohen, M. N. (1989). *Health and the rise of civilization.* New Haven, CT: Yale University Press.

Cohen, M. N., Malpass, R. S., & Klein, H. G. (Eds.). (1980). *Biosocial mechanisms of population regulation.* New Haven, CT: Yale University Press.

Crocker, D. A., & Linden, T. (1998). *Ethics of consumption: The good life, justice and global stewardship.* Lanham, MD: Rowman & Littlefield.

Eaton, S. B., Strassman, B. I., Neese, R. M., Neele, J. V., Ewald, P. W., Williams, G. C., et al. (2002). Evolutionary health promotion. *Preventive Medicine, 34,* 109–118.

Fabrega, H., Jr. (1997). *Evolution of sickness and healing.* Berkeley: University of California Press.

Handwerker, W. P. (1983). The first demographic transition: An analysis of subsistence choices and reproductive consequences. *American Anthropologist, 85*(1), 5–27.

Hill, J. O., & Peters, J. C. (1998). Environmental contributions to the obesity epidemic. *Science, 280,* 1371–1374.

Hurtado, A. M., Arenas de Hurtado, I., Sapien, R., & Hill, K. (1999). The evolutionary ecology of childhood asthma. In W. Travathan, E. Smith, & J. McKenna (Eds.), *Evolutionary medicine* (pp. 101–134). New York: Oxford University Press.

Imhoff, M. L., Bounoua, L., Ricketts, T., Loucks, C., Harriss, C., & Lawrence, W. T. (2004). Global patterns in human consumption of net primary production. *Nature, 429,* 870–873.

INFO Project. (2003). Desired family size. *Information and Knowledge for Optimal Health Project, 31*(2), (Series M, No. 17, Special Topics). Baltimore: John Hopkins University, Bloomberg School of Public Health. Retrieved April 22, 2008, from www.infoforhealth.org

Lee, R. B. (1968). What hunters do for a living, or how to make out on scarce resources. In R. B. Lee & I. Devore (Eds.), *Man, the hunter* (pp. 30–48). Chicago: Aldine.

Lee, R. B. (1980). Lactation, ovulation, infanticide, and women's work: A study of hunter-gatherer population regulation. In M. N. Cohen, R. S. Malpass, & H. G. Klein (Eds.), *Biosocial mechanisms of population regulation* (pp. 321–348). New Haven, CT: Yale University Press.

Lieberman, L. S. (2008). Diabesity and Darwinian medicine: The evolution of an epidemic. In W. R. Trevathan, E. O. Smith, & J. J. McKenna (Eds.), *Evolutionary medicine and health: New perspectives* (pp. 72–95). New York: Oxford University Press.

Maren, M. (1997). *The road to hell: The ravaging effects of foreign aid and international charity.* New York: Free Press.

Matheson, A. (2007). From syndrome to spectrum: What evolution suggests about the status of the metabolic syndrome. *Clinical Chemistry, 53,* 2218–2219.

McKenna, J. J., Mosko, S., & Richard, C. (1999). Breastfeeding and mother-infant cosleeping in relation to SIDS prevention. In W. R. Trevathan, E. O. Smith, & J. J. McKenna (Eds.), *Evolutionary medicine* (pp. 53–74). New York: Oxford University Press.

Mosko, S., Richard, C., McKenna, J., & Drummond, S. (1996). Infant sleep architecture during bedsharing and possible implications for SIDS. *Sleep, 19,* 677–684.

Mosley, W. H., Jamison, D. T., & Henderson, D. A. (1990). The health sector in developing countries: Problems for the 1990s and beyond. *Annual Review of Public Health, 11,* 335–358.

Neese, R. M., & Williams, G. (1996). *Why we get sick: The new science of Darwinian medicine.* New York: Vintage Books.

Notestein, F. (1983). On population growth and economic development. *Population and Development Review, 9*(2), 345–360.

Omran, A. R. (1983). The epidemiologic transition theory: A preliminary update. *Journal of Tropical Pediatrics, 29*(6), 305–316.

Polgar, S. (1964). Evolution and the ills of mankind. In S. Tax (Ed.), *Horizons of anthropology* (pp. 200–211). Chicago: Aldine.

Profet, M. (1991). The function of allergy: Immunological defense against toxins. *Quarterly Review of Biology, 66,* 23–62.

Reese, F. L., & Smith, W. R. (1997). Psychosocial determinants of health care utilization in sickle cell disease patients. *Annals of Behavioral Medicine, 19*(2), 171–178.

Rosen, G. (1993). *A history of public health.* Baltimore: Johns Hopkins University Press.

Stuart-Macadam, P., & Dettwyler, K. A. (Eds.). (1995). *Breastfeeding: Biocultural perspectives.* New York: Aldine.

Toole, M. J., Waldman, R. J., & Zwi, A. B. (2001). Complex humanitarian emergencies. In M. H. Merson, R. E. Black, & A. J. Mills (Eds.). *International public health: Diseases, programs, systems, and policies* (pp. 439–514). Gaithersburg, MD: Aspen.

Trevathan, W. R., & McKenna, J. J. (1994). Evolutionary environments of human birth and infancy: Insights to apply to contemporary life. *Children's Environments, 11*(2), 88–104.

Trevathan, W. R., Smith, E. O., & McKenna, J. J. (Eds.). (1999). *Evolutionary medicine.* New York: Oxford University Press.

Trevathan, W. R., Smith, E. O., & McKenna, J. J. (Eds.). (2008). *Evolutionary medicine and health: New perspectives.* New York: Oxford University Press.

Ungar, P. S., & Teaford, M. F. (Eds.). (2002). *Human diet: Its origin and evolution.* Westport, CT: Bergin & Garvey.

United Nations Population Fund. (2007). *State of the world population, 2007.* Retrieved April 24, 2008, from www.unfpa.org/swp/2007/english/introduction.html

Williams, R. (2007). The psychosocial consequences for children of mass violence, terrorism and disasters. *International Review of Psychiatry, 19*(3), 263–277.

Worthman, C. M. (1999). Epidemiology of human development. In C. Panter-Brick & C. M. Worthman (Eds.), *Hormones, health, and behaviour: A socio-ecological and lifespan perspective* (pp. 47–104). Cambridge, UK: Cambridge University Press.

3

Social Epidemiology

Jeannine Coreil

The core discipline of public health is epidemiology, the study of disease patterns in defined populations. Epidemiologists investigate the distribution of health conditions across time, space, and social groups, analyzing the factors associated with the incidence and prevalence of disease. *Incidence* is defined as the number of new cases of illness occurring within a certain time period, usually per 100,000 persons over a year's time, while *prevalence* refers to the total number of cases in a population at a particular time. Epidemiologic research seeks to identify the factors associated with the causes, or etiology, of disease, which are often referred to as "risk factors." For example, currently recognized risk factors for heart disease include genetic predisposition, diet, use of alcohol and tobacco, exercise habits, and distribution of body fat.

The aims of epidemiologic research are usually very pragmatic. By identifying the correlates of disease, studies can be designed to test hypotheses about causal mechanisms, which then can guide the design of interventions to prevent illness or reduce the burden of disease. Knowledge of epidemiologic patterns is also useful in planning health services and formulating public health policies to meet the needs of various populations (Friis & Sellers, 1999). Health agencies at national, state, and local levels use diverse sources of epidemiologic data to carry out the basic public health functions of assessment, policy development, and assurance of health care. Examples of such data sources include vital statistics (i.e., births and deaths), disease registries and surveillance systems, and periodic health surveys, such as the Health and Nutrition Examination Survey (HANES) and the Behavioral Risk Factor Surveillance System (BRFSS). It is usually necessary to draw from multiple sources to obtain comprehensive epidemiologic information about a problem. In addition, an in-depth understanding of a health problem draws on multiple indicators that describe different dimensions of the problem. For example, *mortality rates* indicate the number of deaths within a defined population and within a certain time period, as noted in the previous chapter. *Morbidity rates,* on the other hand, report the magnitude of a problem affecting a population at a point in time.

Social epidemiology is a more recently developed subfield, concerned with the social characteristics or psychosocial risk factors associated with patterns of disease within and across populations (Berkman & Kawachi, 2000). Even newer is the field of *behavioral epidemiology,* which focuses on the specific behaviors that contribute to the etiology of disease (Sallis, Owen, & Fotheringham, 2000). While social epidemiologic research often poses questions about differences in morbidity and mortality by gender, age, socioeconomic status (SES), and race/ethnicity, behavioral epidemiology usually targets lifestyle factors such as sleep habits, stress management, risk taking, and other health-related behaviors. *Cultural epidemiology,* on the other hand, investigates the relationship between disease patterns and cultural factors such as religion, cultural models of illness (see Chapter 8), and ritual practices (e.g., circumcision) (Trostle, 2005). Both behavioral epidemiology and cultural epidemiology include studies of the determinants and distribution of the risk factors themselves. For example, studies of smoking patterns and the determinants of who smokes in a population are included within the rubric of behavioral epidemiology. Likewise, cultural epidemiology includes research on the distribution of cultural beliefs within a population, such as looking at gender differences in explanatory models of illness (Weiss, 2001).

Some of the most common factors investigated as independent (etiologic) variables in social epidemiology include sociodemographic characteristics (e.g., age, education, income, occupation), cultural traits (ethnicity, religion), behavior patterns (diet, exercise), and social environmental factors (family structure, neighborhood, racism). Dependent or health outcome variables studied, on the other hand, often include measures of morbidity, mortality, incidence, and prevalence, usually expressed as a rate or a ratio. While the foregoing variables typically are disease specific, more generalized health indicators, such as overall mortality and life expectancy, are also used. Health status measures sometimes include quality-of-life variables, such as ability to function in everyday life, and include indicators such as loss of workdays due to illness. Finally, as noted above, risk behaviors can also be studied as dependent variables, such as looking at the predictors of seat belt use. While it is not possible to present a comprehensive overview of social epidemiologic research in this chapter, selected examples are provided to illustrate the scope of investigations in this field.

THE CAUSAL CONTINUUM

In Chapter 1, we presented the social ecology of health model for understanding multilevel determinants of disease. Here, we introduce a related framework, the Causal Continuum, which is particularly relevant for social epidemiologic research. Borrowing the terminology of social science research methods, the social ecology of health model can be seen as a kind of "cross-sectional" or synchronic view of interacting factors. In contrast, the Causal Continuum (see Figure 3.1) is based on differing degrees of directness of effect for various etiologic factors affecting health. Variables that have a close, direct influence on health and illness are considered "proximate" in their effect, while "distal" variables are more removed and affect problems more

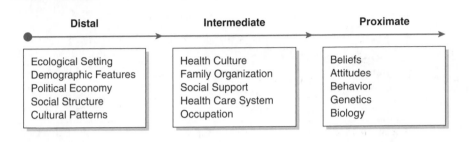

FIGURE 3.1 Causal Continuum Model

Distal	Intermediate	Proximate
Ecological Setting Demographic Features Political Economy Social Structure Cultural Patterns	Health Culture Family Organization Social Support Health Care System Occupation	Beliefs Attitudes Behavior Genetics Biology

indirectly, that is, through the linkages and pathways of "intermediate" and ultimately proximate variables. *Proximate variables* have the most direct effects on biological processes or situational events that precipitate ill health or other undesirable outcomes. *Distal variables,* on the other hand, derive from the macrolevel sociocultural and environmental context and are often described as background factors that predispose people to greater or lesser health risks. *Intermediate variables* can serve as buffers for distal factors, thereby mitigating their potential impact, or they can operate as intervening variables that channel the negative influence of distal factors through specific mechanisms. The relationship between the distal, intermediate, and proximate factors of the Causal Continuum and the levels of the social ecology of health model are shown in Figure 1.1 of Chapter 1.

Various categories of risk factors can be positioned at different points along the continuum, depending on the relative directness or indirectness of their impact on the health outcome under investigation. Of course, etiology never involves such a simplified linear chain of causality, and current epidemiologic models use more complex multilevel schema, such as the "web of causation" (Duncan, Gold, Basch, & Markellis, 1988) and the "scaffolding and bush" configuration (Krieger, 1994). Here, we intentionally use a simple model to highlight the relative directness of effects of different categories of factors. As noted previously, distal determinants such as urban residence, poverty, or educational level are sometimes discussed as "structural" or "fundamental" causes, because they operate through large-scale social structural processes that affect large groups of people in complex ways (Link & Phelan, 1995). Intermediate determinants of illness correspond to what we would categorize as local or community-level risk factors, such as occupation, social support, and health care resources. Proximate determinants, on the other hand, tend to fall mainly in the realm of behavioral epidemiology and involve specific activities linked to biological mechanisms (e.g., eating, sleeping, use of drugs). Figure 3.2 presents a diagram of pathways of influence on health between social structural conditions, social networks, psychosocial mechanisms, and proximate variables.

When we consider the use of models such as the Causal Continuum for planning prevention programs, it is worth noting that the further one moves away from the proximate factors and the closer one moves toward the distal determinants, the more difficult it is to intervene in the chain of causality. The reason for this is that structural determinants tend

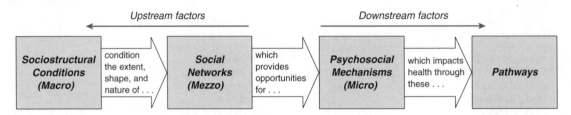

Upstream factors | **Downstream factors**

Sociostructural Conditions (Macro) → condition the extent, shape, and nature of . . . → *Social Networks (Mezzo)* → which provides opportunities for . . . → *Psychosocial Mechanisms (Micro)* → which impacts health through these . . . → *Pathways*

Culture:
- Norms and values
- Social cohesion
- Racism
- Sexism
- Competition/cooperation

Socioeconomic Factors:
- Relations of production
- Inequality
- Discrimination
- Conflict
- Labor market structure
- Poverty

Politics:
- Laws
- Public policy
- Differential political enfranchisement/participation
- Political culture

Social Change:
- Urbanization
- War/civil unrest
- Economic "depression"

Social Network Structure:
- Size
- Range
- Density
- Boundedness
- Proximity
- Homogeneity
- Reachability

Characteristics of Network Ties:
- Frequency of face-to-face contact
- Frequency of nonvisual contact
- Frequency of organizational participation (attendance)
- Reciprocity of ties
- Multiplexity
- Duration
- Intimacy

Social Support:
- Instrumental and financial
- Informational
- Appraisal
- Emotional

Social Influence:
- Constraining/enabling influences on health behaviors
- Norms toward help-seeking/adherence
- Peer pressure
- Social comparison processes

Social Engagement:
- Physical/cognitive exercise
- Reinforcement of meaningful social roles
- Bonding/interpersonal attachment
- "Handling" effects (children)
- "Grooming" effects (adults)

Person-to-Person Contact:
- Close personal contact
- Intimate contact (sexual, IDU, etc.)

Access to Resources and Material Goods:
- Jobs/economic opportunity
- Access to health care
- Housing
- Human capital
- Referrals/institutional contacts

Health Behavioral Pathways:
- Smoking
- Alcohol consumption
- Diet
- Exercise
- Adherence to medical treatments
- Help-seeking behavior

Psychological Pathways:
- Self-efficacy
- Self-esteem
- Coping effectiveness
- Depression/distress
- Sense of well-being

Physiological Pathways:
- HPA axis response
- Allostatic load
- Immune system function
- Cardiovascular reactivity
- Cardiopulmonary fitness
- Transmission of infectious disease

SOURCE: Berkman, L. F., Glass, T., Brissette, I., & Seeman, T. E. (2000). From Social Integration to Health: Durkheim in the New Millennium. *Social Science & Medicine, 51,* 847. Used by permission from Elsevier.

to be less amenable to change than individual risk factors. For example, factors such as urban residence, SES, and gender at the population level are, practically speaking, not amenable to change. Intermediate factors tend to have greater modifiability, but the easiest risk factors to change are behavioral patterns involving individual choice. This is one reason why many public health interventions focus on individual behavior change. It also helps explain why so few programs focus on changing the social conditions that are the fundamental cause of illness.

To illustrate how the Causal Continuum model can be applied to a specific health problem, we turn to the case of breast cancer. In the United States, incidence rates for breast cancer have been increasing at a rate of nearly 2% per year since 1973. Better detection through improved screening accounts for some of this increase, but the specific causes of the rise in breast cancer remain unclear. On the distal end of the causality continuum, we note that high SES is associated with an increased incidence of breast cancer (in contrast to most other diseases). Possible mediating factors for SES include delayed marriage—and therefore late age at first full-term pregnancy, breast-feeding experience, and fat consumption affecting age at menarche and hormone levels. The larger physical and social environment, also distal in level, includes technological aspects that affect type of and age at exposure to exogenous carcinogens through the workplace, community, and home (intermediate). A variety of socially mediated factors may ultimately affect dietary patterns, which can have a more proximate effect on disease risk.

In the following sections, some of the major social determinants of health are reviewed, including possible pathways of effect through intermediate and proximate factors influencing health. The examples presented illustrate current social epidemiologic research and the implications for understanding the impact of social structure on health.

GLOBAL DISEASE PATTERNS

In recent years, increasing attention has been given to global inequalities in health conditions and the interrelationships between disease patterns and complex world systems linking all the regions of the globe. The distinction between developed and developing countries has become increasingly blurred as many less developed countries make important strides in social conditions as well as economic development. It long has been recognized that the nations of the world do not fall neatly into two categories of "more" and "less" developed but instead extend across a wide continuum of socioeconomic diversity; in addition, health and quality-of-life indicators can be quite variable within countries traditionally considered underdeveloped (Pillai & Shannon, 1995). Some very poor countries have made remarkable improvements in the health of their populations, while comparatively wealthier nations have not fared so well (Caldwell, 1990).

The criteria used to define development have included economic, demographic, social, and political indicators. According to World Bank (2007) definitions, national economies are divided according to *gross national income* (GNI) per capita. GNI includes the total value of products and services produced within a country (gross domestic product, or GDP) plus income received from other countries and minus payments made to other countries. Low-income countries are those with GNI of $905 or less; lower-middle-income countries have GNI between $906 and

$3,595; upper-middle-income countries have GNI between $3,596 and $11,115; and high-income countries have GNI of $11,116 or more. The term *developing economies* refers to those falling within the low to middle range of GNI per capita. Low- and middle-income countries are also defined as demographically developing, in the sense that their age distributions are young compared with industrialized nations owing to their high fertility rate. Composite social/health indicators have been devised to measure quality-of-life conditions, such as the Physical Quality of Life Index (PQLI) and the Index of Suffering (Pillai & Shannon, 1995). In some contexts, the term *Third World* is used synonymously with developing countries in the economic sense; however, the original use of the term was primarily political in meaning, growing out of the Cold War era, when the three worlds of development corresponded to democratic, communist, and nonaligned nations (Horowitz, 1966).

In discussions related to health, it is helpful to consider the social and health-related indicators that often are cited in discussions of the health conditions in developing countries. These include urban/rural population distribution, literacy rate, access to clean water, infant and under-5 mortality, maternal mortality, fertility rate, and life expectancy. While developed countries are highly urbanized and industrialized, developing countries have predominantly agricultural economies supported by rural-dwelling populations with little education. Access to clean water and modern medical services is comparatively low, with infant mortality, child malnutrition, and maternal mortality being very high in the less developed areas. Life expectancy is considerably lower and fertility much higher. (See Table 3.1.)

Societal Factors

Socioeconomic Status

One of the most widely used indicators of social position within a society is SES. Typically, SES is measured in terms of income, education, and/or occupational status, but most often simply by income. People who lack the money and material resources to meet the basic needs of living are said to live in poverty. Obviously, poverty can be defined only in relation to the normative standards of living in a particular society. For example, in the United States, a family of four that had a total income less than $21,200 in 2008 was considered "below the poverty line" (Department of Health and Human Services, 2008). In Haiti, however, where 78% of the adult population earn less than $2.00 per day (World Bank, 2007), such a family income could provide a middle-class standard of living. While acknowledging that deprivation is relative, nevertheless, it is worth noting that poverty is one of the most pervasive risk factors for ill health in all countries.

Despite the documented far-reaching health effects of poverty, the U.S. government does not routinely report health statistics by income level. For example, the National Center for Health Statistics provides periodic reports on mortality rates from all causes for the nation. These data are routinely broken down by age, race, and sex, but rarely by income or educational level. Although SES data are more difficult to obtain than the basic demographics reported on death certificates, specialized surveys could be used to complement the vital statistics data by analyzing the impact of poverty, but such analyses are seldom performed.

TABLE 3.1 Ten Leading Causes of Mortality in Low- and Middle-Income and High-Income Countries

Low- and Middle-Income Countries			High-Income Countries		
Cause	Deaths (millions)	% of Total Deaths	Cause	Deaths (millions)	% of Total Deaths
Ischaemic heart disease	5.70	11.8%	Ischaemic heart disease	1.36	17.3%
Cerebrovascular disease	4.61	9.5%	Cerebrovascular disease	0.78	9.9%
Lower respiratory infections	3.41	7.0%	Trachea, bronchus, lung cancers	0.46	5.8%
HIV/AIDS	2.55	5.3%	Lower respiratory infections	0.34	4.4%
Perinatal conditions	2.49	5.1%	Chronic obstructive pulmonary disease	0.30	3.8%
Chronic obstructive pulmonary disease	2.38	4.9%	Colon and rectum cancers	0.26	3.3%
Diarrhoeal diseases	1.78	3.7%	Alzheimer's disease and other dementias	0.21	2.6%
Tuberculosis	1.59	3.3%	Diabetes mellitus	0.20	2.6%
Malaria	1.21	2.5%	Breast cancer	0.16	2.0%
Road traffic accidents	1.07	2.2%	Stomach cancer	0.15	1.9%

SOURCE: Reprinted by permission from Lopez, A. D., Mathers, C. D., Ezzati, M., Jamison, D. T., and Murray, C. L. (2006). Global and Regional Burden of Disease Risk Factors, 2001: Systematic Analysis of Population Health Data. *Lancet, 367,* 1747–1757.

Consequently, racial disparities tend to be overemphasized, and economic influences downplayed, in official reports. In the absence of economic breakdowns, race becomes a proxy for SES, thereby reinforcing stereotypes about racial minorities.

One reason for our society's reluctance to address the relationship between poverty and health is our discomfort with social class differences (Dutton, 1987). We do not like to openly acknowledge the extreme differences in wealth that underlie many social problems. Instead, we substitute proxy measures of social disadvantage, such as race and ethnicity, which redefine economic inequality in terms of biological and cultural differences (see Chapter 9).

The lack of good data on SES and health makes it difficult to formulate health policies that adequately address the effects of poverty (Farmer, 1999). For example, epidemiologic data document excess rates of HIV and AIDS among African Americans and Hispanics. A closer analysis of intervening variables reveals that most of this excess is related to intravenous drug use in these populations. Drug use, in turn, has been linked to lack of opportunity for occupational and economic success in disadvantaged populations, as well as perceptions of deprivation relative to the majority.

Research from industrial countries on the relationship between life expectancy and income has revealed some interesting findings regarding the distribution of income within societies. Several cross-national comparative studies have demonstrated a robust, statistically significant relationship between *income inequality* within a single society and its overall life expectancy rate, which is linked to mortality. Countries with a more egalitarian income distribution have a higher life expectancy than countries in which there is a wide gap between the upper- and lower-income range (Wilkinson, 1996). Surprisingly, overall per capita income does not appear to affect life expectancy, so that in the developed world, there is no linear relationship between the wealth of a nation and mortality. Rather, health is adversely affected when the gap between the "rich" and the "poor" is large. The negative health effects of income inequality are also seen in rates of infant mortality. Among wealthy, industrial countries, relative poverty within countries has a stronger impact on infant mortality than variation in the level of economic development between countries. Moreover, public policies related to family welfare, such as medical care and family leave benefits, also affect infant mortality (Wennemo, 1993).

The intervening variables that may account for the impact of relative wealth on health are not entirely clear; however, some interesting hypotheses have been suggested. First, because of market forces, there is a tendency for the material infrastructure and organization of a society to be geared to people close to the average income. For this reason, people with lower incomes are often unable to afford the goods and services that would allow them to manage day-to-day tasks without a lot of additional effort, which could affect health. Second, one's income must be adequate to maintain self-respect and to participate in the social life of a society where most people are much better off. Consequently, poor people often skimp on food, heating, and even use of health services to maintain the visible symbols of acceptability, such as clothing and participation in social activities. A related issue here is the notion of "financial stress" among both low- and middle-income people, who constantly strive to support a costly "normative" lifestyle that is skewed toward the wealthier end of the income spectrum. Third, relative wealth deprivation has been shown to be socially isolating (Townsend, 1979), so that the health benefits of social support may be enjoyed less by lower-income groups. Fourth, relative poverty is widely understood to be a demeaning and devaluing experience that can affect one's sense of self-worth and, indirectly, health status. Taken together, these hypotheses suggest a relationship between perceived relative deprivation and psychosocial stress, which contributes to ill health and mortality. Alternative hypotheses suggest the possible role of social ordering or "dominance status" within groups. Hierarchical position may have direct effects on physiological processes and neuroanatomic structures that may increase biologic vulnerability to disease (Adler et al., 1994).

Public health professionals have long recognized the relationship between SES and health. SES is one of the strongest and most consistent predictors of morbidity and premature mortality. Everywhere, poor people suffer disproportionately from most diseases and die younger than their wealthier counterparts. SES has been associated with infant mortality, cardiovascular disease, many types of cancer, arthritis, diabetes, and numerous infectious diseases. Particularly puzzling is the fact that this relationship runs across the entire population, so that people who enjoy the greatest wealth live longer and experience lower rates of many diseases than those in the middle class.

As early as the 1840s, Edwin Chadwick reported significant differences in the life expectancy of the gentry (36 years), tradesmen (22 years), and laborers and servants (16 years) (Morley, 2007). More recently, four large population studies found similar health disparities between people in the lower and upper socioeconomic brackets. The first Whitehall Study was conducted among British civil servants employed in white-collar jobs between 1930 and 1982. A follow-up study of the same employees, Whitehall Study II, examined these employees between 1985 and 1988. The Wisconsin Longitudinal Study (WLS) studied men and women who graduated from Wisconsin high schools in 1957 and were followed until the early 1990s. The National Survey of Families and Households (NSFH) was conducted among a national sample of adults living in the United States, including people who were extremely poor. Despite differences in samples and methodologies, all four studies found a strong association between social position and mortality rates. In the first Whitehall Study, for example, mortality rates were three times higher among men working in the lowest civil service grades than those in the highest classifications. More important, social differentials in mortality were discovered in most of the major causes of death. The follow-up study of these men revealed that socioeconomic differences in health persisted even into retirement (Marmot, Bobak, & Smith, 1995).

These four studies also documented significant differences based on SES and a variety of other health indicators, including self-reported health status, depression, and psychological well-being. For example, SES was strongly correlated with research subjects' answers to a three-question self-esteem measure used in the NSFH, a question about finding "little meaning in life" in Whitehall II, and a seven-question purpose-of-life scale used in the WLS (Marmot, Ryff, Bumpass, Shipley, & Marks, 1997)

Although the association between SES and health status is well established, the factors at work in the relationship are poorly understood. Why do people who live at the top of the socioeconomic ladder enjoy a longer and healthier life than those below them? How do income, occupation, and education—the major components of SES—affect health? A variety of answers to these questions have been vigorously debated. These explanations include limited resources, psychosocial stress, health selection, early-life experiences, access to health care, and health behavior, and each will be discussed briefly in turn.

Limited Resources. As a family's income drops, they have an increasingly difficult time obtaining the clean, safe housing needed to maintain good health. Crowding, rat and insect infestation, leaky roofs, and lead paint are among the many health hazards associated with low-income housing. Poor people also have difficulty purchasing an adequate diet. In fact, notions of a "poverty line" date back to the turn of the century, when nutrition surveys revealed that no matter how wisely very poor families managed their budgets, they did not have enough purchasing power to consume an adequate diet. Since that time, many countries, including the United States, have calculated an income level, known as the poverty threshold, below which malnutrition will eventually result. This amount is adjusted for household size and then used to determine eligibility for federal assistance programs and to estimate poverty rates.

No one argues against the proposition that absolute deprivation leads to poor health. However, lack of resources only explains the relationship between health and the social standing of people living on the lowest rungs of the SES ladder. If lack of material resources were the key factor, an income threshold would exist below which people would have poor health but above which there would be no detectable effect. However, this threshold does not exist. As mentioned above, a gradient runs across the entire population, with people at each position better off than those immediately below them and worse off than those immediately above them. It is easy to understand why someone in the middle of the SES scale has better health than someone at the bottom, but it is less clear why a corporate executive who makes $250,000 per year enjoys better health than managers in the same organization who make $100,000.

Psychosocial Stress. This theory is related to the previous explanation in that people with limited economic resources experience higher levels of stress in daily life. Many have to work long hours in order to make ends meet, sometimes holding down two jobs, and the kinds of employment associated with low income are often physically demanding and offer little autonomy. Job insecurity, underemployment, and periodic unemployment are also characteristic of the low-paid workforce. Related challenges include access to quality education, finding affordable child care, maintaining a reliable vehicle, and a host of similar strains inherent in living on a tight budget. Low-income persons also report higher levels of depression and anxiety and, overall, have lower levels of mental health and subjective well-being. In a society with strong materialist values and high expectations for everyone achieving the "good life," difficulties in attaining a comfortable lifestyle can be an unremitting source of stress.

Health Selection. The health selection theory postulates that poor health status determines social position rather than the reverse. This explanation posits that people who are unhealthy are less productive and drift down the socioeconomic ladder, while those who are healthier are more productive and migrate upward. As people drift downward socially and economically, a disproportionate number of unhealthy people end up at the bottom. The theory has received some support from studies of people with specific diseases, such as schizophrenia, and studies of children who are ill before their education has been completed who subsequently enter the labor market (Marmot et al., 1995; Wadsworth, 1986). Both groups are more likely to experience downward social mobility than their healthier counterparts. However, the effect of these cases is limited and does not account for the more general relationship that exists in adulthood (Marmot et al., 1995; Wadsworth, 1986; West, 1991). As a result, this theory has been largely rejected as the major cause of social inequities in health (Sudano & Baker, 2006).

Early-Life Exposures. Another explanation posits that the factors operating early in life, such as genetic and other biological factors, education and cultural advantages, and psychosocial factors, affect both social standing and health status in later life. Known as the "indirect selection" theory, this explanation claims that the relationship between SES and health status is actually an artifact of the other forces that affect them both. It is difficult to test this hypothesis because it is so hard to separate early-childhood factors from those operating in adulthood. Not surprisingly, little evidence has been accumulated to support this proposition. None of the four major studies described above followed people from early childhood into adulthood and, therefore, could not test this theory directly; however, each study was able to control for measures of early-childhood disadvantage to determine if it influenced the SES-health gradient. The Whitehall II study, for instance, found that the gradient did not change when the social background of parents was taken into account. The WLS found that the strength of the relationship between health and SES was reduced, but only slightly, when parents' education, whether the person grew up in an intact family, and IQ measured in high school were controlled. And the NSFH showed that the association between SES and mortality remained the same after parents' education and nonintact family composition during childhood were accounted for (Marmot et al., 1997).

Access to Health Care. A third explanation for the SES-health gradient is differential access to health care between people in different socioeconomic strata. In the United States, people who cannot afford health care are at a greater risk for a wide variety of health problems that could be treated, if not prevented altogether. Early detection of cancer and other diseases, for example, greatly improves the odds of cure and extends survival time. Poor people are less likely than more affluent people to have health insurance and the means to pay for drugs and medical procedures not covered by their insurance policies.

Although this argument explains the difference between insured and uninsured people's health status, it, too, provides an insufficient explanation for the socioeconomic gradient that runs across the broader SES scale. How do we account for differences between insured people in the middle- and upper-income brackets? Can the rich really buy medical care that is so much better that it gives them lower morbidity and mortality than those with slightly less income and social standing? Most scholars do not think so. Evidence suggesting that more is at work than differential access to health comes from nations that offer their citizens universal access to health care yet still show the same SES-health gradient as found in the United States (Adler, Boyce, Chesney, Folkman, & Syme, 1997). The United Kingdom offers one of the best illustrations: During the 30 years after universal health care access was granted to British citizens, inequalities in health status actually widened. Finally, this theory fails to account for socioeconomic differences that exist in rates of diseases not amenable to medical care, again suggesting that other factors are at work (Marmot et al., 1995).

Health Behavior. Another common argument is that poor people behave in ways that make them more likely to get sick and die than affluent people. Advocates of this view point to well-known socioeconomic differences in rates of smoking, alcohol consumption, physical activity, seat belt usage, fat intake, and other health behaviors, which place the poor at greater risk than affluent people (Frankish, Milligan, & Reid, 1998). While no one would argue that health behaviors are not an important pathway between SES and health outcomes, again, this explanation alone cannot account for the linear relationship between SES and health status (Adler et al., 1997). In the Whitehall II study, for example, the strength of the relationship between SES and health was reduced only slightly when smoking and other health behaviors were held constant. When looking just at nonsmokers or just at smokers, a gradient still existed between SES and health (Marmot et al., 1997).

The Social Ecology of Inequality

To explain the relationship between SES and health, many scholars have turned to an ecological explanatory model, one in which health status and social standing are linked to a combination of interrelated social, cultural, and psychological factors. Although each of the factors already mentioned plays a role in explaining this conundrum, other social, psychological, and environmental factors must also be taken into consideration.

An important additional factor is *relative deprivation*. When income disparities are pronounced and highly visible, citizens feel deprived relative to those who have more than they do. Even people who have abundant resources to meet their subsistence needs and maintain good health may feel resentful and frustrated when they cannot share the riches they see others enjoying. In societies such as the United States, which view competitive achievement and economic affluence as the result of personal qualities, relative deprivation may also lead to feelings of failure and hopelessness. Relative deprivation may also trigger hostility, depression, and other psychological reactions that adversely affect health. The impact of prolonged depression, stress, and hostility on vulnerability to disease is now widely recognized.

Support for the psychological effects of relative deprivation comes from studies of the relationship between hypertension and ability to achieve a socially normative material style of life. Using cultural consensus analysis, a technique for measuring the degree to which individuals achieve in their own behavior a culturally shared model of lifestyle indicative of "success," Dressler and colleagues (Dressler, Balieiro, & Santos, 1999; Dressler & Bindon, 2000) found a strong association between the latter measure and arterial blood pressure among African Americans living in the U.S. South and among Brazilians living in urban areas. The researchers describe the observed level of lifestyle concordance as "cultural consonance." Interestingly, cultural consonance was a stronger predictor of hypertension than conventional indicators of SES including income, education, and occupation. The investigators interpret these findings as evidence that feelings of deprivation relative to cultural norms play a role in the link between poverty and health (see Chapter 9).

In addition to psychological responses associated with relative deprivation, the social environment responds in ways that affect health. In societies with wide gaps in income levels, people's comparison of themselves with others and their sense that they have failed to achieve enough can lead to discontent, distrust, and strained social relations. Society becomes less cohesive, and people have access to less social support—changes known to have an adverse impact on health (Patrick & Wickizer, 1995). Relative deprivation has also been linked to another health hazard—violent crime (Kawachi, Kennedy, & Wilkinson, 1999). Meta-analyses of 34 studies of crime found that places with large income gaps experienced significantly higher crime rates than more egalitarian communities (Wilkinson, 1998).

A large part of current research on social structural factors, such as SES, and health focuses on variables believed to mediate the relationship between income inequality and health. Some of the mediating factors that have been addressed include social integration, social support, and social capital. These concepts are discussed from a theoretical perspective in Chapter 6. Here, we will briefly review research findings for the relationship between social capital and health. *Social capital* is a characteristic of collectivities such as communities, neighborhoods, and populations and can be viewed as an aspect of social cohesion or integration. It is typically measured by variables such as civic engagement and participation in associations, interpersonal trust, and norms of reciprocity that enable collective action (Putnam, 2000). Studies have found a positive association between social capital and a variety of health outcomes, including overall mortality (Kawachi, Kennedy, Lochner, & Prothrow-Smith, 1997), cardiovascular disease (Franzini & Spears, 2003), violent crime (Kennedy, Kawachi, Prothrow-Smith, Lochner, & Gupta, 1998), adolescent childbearing (Gold, Kennedy, Connell, & Kawachi, 2002), sexually transmitted infections, including HIV (Holtgrave & Crosby, 2003), self-rated health (Greiner, Li, Kawachi, Hunt, & Ahluwalia, 2004), and mental distress (Phongsavan, Chey, Bauman, Brooks, & Silove, 2006). The mechanisms through which social capital is thought to affect health include more proximate determinants, such as social support, as well as access to resources through social networks of enduring, trusting relationships (Coleman, 1990).

Further evidence that relative deprivation affects health status comes from studies comparing life expectancy and income distributions between and within nations and other geographical units. As one would expect, life expectancy is lower in poorer nations than in wealthier ones. However, once countries have attained a certain level of wealth, the relationship between the absolute income level as measured by income or gross national product (GNP) per capita and life expectancy disappears. In more affluent countries, the size of the income gap replaces GNP as the predictor of life expectancy. Countries with large income disparities have shorter life expectancies than more egalitarian countries (Wilkinson, 1996). Also, when changes in six nations' income disparity was examined (Wilkinson, 1992), Japan experienced both the greatest increase in equality of income dispersion and the greatest increase in life expectancy. In contrast, the United Kingdom experienced declining equity in income distribution and the smallest gains in life expectancy. Looking at the 50 states in the United States, Kawachi and Kennedy (1997) documented a strong association between mortality rates and income inequity. Americans living in relatively egalitarian states outlive citizens living in states with large income gaps.

CASE STUDY   Infant Mortality, Preterm Birth, and Low Birth Weight

The case of infant mortality provides a good illustration of the complexity of the social and behavioral factors along the Causal Continuum that cause adverse health outcomes. Infant mortality is generally considered one of the most sensitive indicators of the general health status of a population, and it is reflective of the standard of living at the societal level. In this example, we are concerned with cross-ethnic differences in infant mortality rates and what such comparisons reveal about social and behavioral risk factors for this outcome. The *infant mortality rate* is defined as the number of deaths among infants during the first year of life per 1,000 live births. It is closely associated with low birth weight (LBW) and preterm delivery. *Low birth weight,* defined as a weight of less than 2,500 grams or 5.5 pounds at birth, is the single greatest cause of infant mortality in the United States. In recent years, attention has focused on *preterm delivery* as the primary risk factor for LBW. Figure 3.3 presents data on rates of infant mortality and preterm-related mortality for various ethnic groups in the United States during 2004. Both infant mortality, and LBW and preterm delivery are consistently highest for African Americans and are notably high compared with other ethnic groups. However, while infant mortality is high among Native Americans (American Indians and Alaska Natives), their rates of preterm births are comparable with the rates for whites, Hispanics, and Asian Americans. In addition, despite socioeconomic disadvantages, Mexican American populations have lower rates of infant mortality, LBW, and preterm delivery than non-Hispanic whites and all other ethnic groups except Asian/Pacific Islanders (see Hispanic Paradox, below).

Both preterm delivery and LBW can be reduced by improved interconceptual health, that is, maternal health status between pregnancies, as well as early, appropriate prenatal care, good maternal nutrition, and adequate weight gain during pregnancy. On the other hand, living in stressful neighborhoods, single-parent families, lack of social support, and high prevalence of drug use and HIV/AIDS increase the risk of preterm birth and LBW (Behrman & Butler, 2007).

FIGURE 3.3 Total and Preterm-Related Infant Mortality Rates by Race and Ethnicity of Mother: United States, 2004

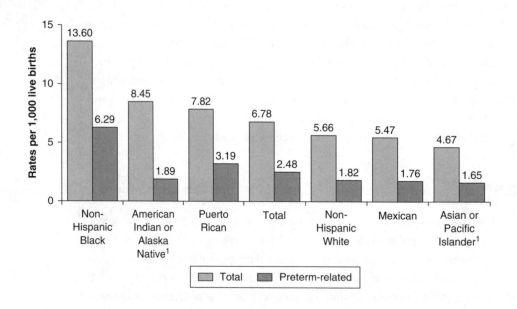

SOURCE: MacDorman, Callaghan, Mathews, Hoyert, and Kochanek (2007).

NOTE: Preterm-related deaths are those where the infant was born preterm (before 37 completed weeks of gestation), with underlying cause of death assigned to one of the following International Classification of Diseases Tenth Revision categories: K550, P000, P010, P011, P015, P020, P021, P027, P070-P073, P102, P220-P229, P250–279, P280, P281, P360-P369, P520-P523, P77.

1. Includes persons of Hispanic and non-Hispanic origin.

Looking first at the distal end of the continuum, social contextual factors associated with preterm births and LBW include low socioeconomic position, racism and discrimination, and residential segregation in unfavorable neighborhoods. These structural factors in turn influence intermediate factors such as low social support and social capital, higher prevalence of childbearing among unmarried/unpartnered and younger women, and exposure to the secondary effects of living in unhealthy neighborhoods. Unhealthy neighborhoods are concentrated in urban areas and are characterized by high crime and violence and poor access to goods and services such as health care, grocery stores, recreational facilities, and police and fire protection. These neighborhoods also expose pregnant women to environmental toxins, pollutants, substandard housing, and poorer-quality public space. At the proximal end of the continuum, individual-level factors associated with preterm birth and LBW include chronic stress, maternal anxiety, nutritional status/weight gain, infection, physical activity, and health-related behaviors (use of alcohol, tobacco, and illicit drugs; diet; and physical activity).

Determining the pathways of influence across the various distal, intermediate, and proximate factors found to be associated with birth outcomes has proven extremely challenging. The pathways are complex and multifactorial, making it difficult to disentangle the most important elements and locate points of intervention to improve outcomes. Current models emphasize the role of chronic, long-term stress related to the social conditions discussed above (Lu & Halfon, 2003). These stress-inducing conditions affect African American populations disproportionately and at least partly explain the racial differences observed. Although much of the research has focused on factors during pregnancy, the chronic stress model takes a life-course perspective that considers cumulative wear and tear on the body from coping with long-term stressors. The physiological processes underlying unremitting stress are sometimes referred to as *allostatic load,* or the body's inability to maintain homeostasis across nervous, hormonal, metabolic, and immune systems. Strain on the adaptive responses of the body in turn can affect a variety of health outcomes, including pregnancy.

⊠ **Focus:** Hispanic Health Paradox ⊠

The apparent health advantage of Mexican origin populations in the area of birth outcomes is part of a broader phenomenon that has been called the Hispanic Health Paradox, or the "epidemiologic paradox" (Markides & Coreil, 1986). The paradox is based on the observation that unlike other socioeconomically disadvantaged minority groups, Mexican Americans fare better than would be expected on a number of health indicators. The evidence is found most strongly in Southwestern Hispanics, who are predominantly of Mexican origin, though it has also has been shown in other, but not all, Hispanic groups (Finch, Hummer, Reindl, & Vega, 2002; Franzini, Ribble, & Keddie, 2001; Hummer, Powers, Pullum, Gossman, & Frisbie, 2007; Sudano & Baker, 2006). However, studies reporting contrary evidence and methodologic issues have called into question the true extent of the apparent health advantages (Hunt et al., 2003; Palloni & Morenoff, 2001; Smith & Bradshaw, 2006).

First noted half a century ago in relation to mental health (Jaco, 1960), Hispanic health advantages have been documented in the areas of infant mortality, LBW and preterm births, life expectancy, and mortality from cardiovascular diseases and several major types of cancer. Mortality and longevity advantages are particularly evident in elderly Hispanic populations. On the other hand, self-reported health status has been shown to be consistently low for Mexican Americans, and rates of diabetes and infectious diseases are higher, further compounding the issue. The paradox remains a puzzle, although numerous explanations have been proposed. For example, it has been suggested that the high value placed on children and the strong tradition of care for pregnant and parturient women contribute to favorable birth outcomes in this ethnic group. For other health advantages, hypotheses include the influence of cultural practices, family support systems, selective migration, diet, and genetic heritage. Potential migration effects are twofold: (1) immigrants must be healthy enough to relocate and adapt to a new country, and they must pass health screenings to obtain legal status, and (2) return migration (the "salmon effect") of less healthy older persons to their country of origin may result in distorted mortality rates for the population remaining in the United States. Further research is needed to untangle the causal factors in such anomalous epidemiologic patterns. A better understanding of this paradox will expand our understanding of the complex links between social factors and health. Investigation of situations characterized by more positive outcomes than would be expected is sometimes referred to as positive deviance analysis. It contrasts with the more usual approach to deviance as a negatively sanctioned social problem (see Chapter 7).

Race, Ethnicity, and Discrimination

Many minority and socially disadvantaged groups experience a higher mortality rate than is found in the general population (Feldman & Fulwood, 1999; Nazroo, 2003). Explanations for health disparities in racial and ethnic groups have focused on "upstream" social structural factors, including social stratification, residential segregation, and racism or racial discrimination (Anderson, Bulatao, & Cohen, 2004; Schulz, Williams, Israel, & Lempert, 2002; Sudano & Baker, 2006). These theories invoke the kind of pathways of effects discussed in the previous section on SES. Structural (distal) factors are viewed as limiting financial resources, educational opportunities, access to health care, and occupational status (intermediate determinants), which in turn affects individual- and interpersonal-level influences such as stress, social support, and personal health behaviors (proximate determinants).

The mechanisms through which racial and ethnic groups experience the negative effects described above, especially the structural impacts, are complex and difficult to assess. In recent years, increasing attention has been given to the role of discrimination and racism, both institutional and interpersonal, in mediating health disadvantages for minority groups. Institutional racism and discrimination occur through social policies that treat social groups unfairly or limit access to opportunities and resources. For example, the Tuskegee Study is often cited as an example of health-related institutional racism (Pence, 2008). In this famous case, a group of African American men diagnosed with syphilis were deceived and denied treatment for their condition over a period of several decades, ostensibly for purposes of documenting the natural history of the disease, until the study was halted in 1972. The study is now viewed as most instructive for what it taught us about racism, not syphilis. Another well-documented example of institutional discrimination was the exclusion of women and minorities from most medical research until such practices were outlawed by the National Institutes of Health Revitalization Act of 1993 (Department of Health and Human Services, 1994). Such blatant racism and discrimination would be quickly challenged today, but other groups continue to experience discrimination in policies such as the denial of medical insurance coverage for domestic partners.

Interpersonal racism and discrimination are less overt but may still affect health in important ways. Social interactions in everyday life can be imbued with racist and bigoted attitudes, employee-hiring practices may be subtly discriminatory, and people may be excluded from social networks on the basis of skin color, to give just a few examples. To study these personal experiences, researchers have relied heavily on self-reported racism and discrimination. A recent review by Paradies (2006) of 138 studies addressing self-reported racism and health identifies several key patterns. In addition to interpersonal racism, some studies addressed racism-related stress (i.e., the experience of racism as a form of stress), systemic racism (i.e., racism encountered through interaction with organizations), and internalized racism (i.e., the incorporation of racist attitudes, beliefs, or ideologies into an individual's worldview), while others focused on general discrimination nonspecific to a particular race or ethnicity. The most consistent health-related outcomes associated with racism were poor mental health status and health-related behaviors. Some studies found an interaction effect between self-reported racism and gender, age, ethnicity, stress, or coping response (e.g., passive vs. active response to racism). Little is known about the mechanisms through which racism affects health; however, the strength of evidence for mental health effects suggests that physiological processes may be involved.

CONCLUSION

Like the central position that epidemiology holds in public health, social epidemiology constitutes a core component of the subject matter of this book. Understanding the ways in which health problems are differentially distributed among social groups helps clarify the etiology of such conditions and can inform policy development and intervention design. In this chapter, we present the Causal Continuum model as a way to depict the relative effects of distal, intermediate, and proximate determinants of health status. We illustrate the applicability of the model to problems such as breast cancer etiology, infant mortality and preterm births, and the relationship between racism and health. Special attention is devoted to the economic factors that have prominence in public health, poverty, and SES, exploring the links that mediate the effects of these more distal determinants on proximate causes of illness. Despite common trends in the social epidemiology of disease, some anomalous patterns are noted, such as the overall positive health status of Mexican American populations.

We present the Causal Continuum as a simplified representation of the concepts of distance and directness of effect in etiologic processes, recognizing that current epidemiologic approaches incorporate more complex models of causality. In the real world, the impact of multiple factors at different levels of the ecosystem is not linear, as the continuum might suggest, but multilevel with complex causal pathways. Nevertheless, it is helpful to view social and behavioral determinants of health in terms of their relative proximity to the outcome of interest, particularly since this relative position is so significant in evaluating the modifiability of the factor.

REFERENCES

Adler, N. E., Boyce, T., Chesney, M. A., Cohen, S., Folkman, S., Kahn, R. L., et al. (1994). Socioeconomic status and health: The challenge of the gradient. *American Psychologist, 49*(1), 15–24.

Adler, N. E., Boyce, W. T., Chesney, M. A., Folkman, S., & Syme, S. L. (1997). Socioeconomic inequalities in health: No easy solution. In P. R. Lee & C. L. Estes (Eds.), *The nation's health* (pp. 15–24). Sudbury, MA: Jones & Bartlett.

Anderson, N. B., Bulatao, R. A., & Cohen, B. (Eds.). (2004). *Critical perspectives on racial and ethnic differences in health in late life.* Washington, DC: National Academies Press.

Behrman, R. E., & Butler, A. S. (Eds.). (2007). *Preterm birth: Causes, consequences and prevention* (Committee on Understanding Premature Birth and Assuring Healthy Outcomes). Washington, DC: National Academies Press.

Berkman, L. F., Glass, T., Brissette, I., & Seeman, T. E. (2000). From social integration to health: Durkheim in the new millennium. *Social Science & Medicine, 51,* 847.

Berkman, L. F., & Kawachi, I. (2000). *Social epidemiology.* New York: Oxford University Press.

Caldwell, J. C. (1990). Cultural and social factors influencing mortality levels in developing countries. *Annals of the American Academy of Political and Social Sciences, 510,* 44–59.

Coleman, J. S. (1990). *Foundations of social theory.* Cambridge, MA: Harvard University Press.

Department of Health and Human Services. (1994). NIH guidelines for the inclusion of women and minorities in clinical research. *Federal Register, 59,* 14508–14513.

Department of Health and Human Services. (2008). Annual update of the HHS poverty guidelines. *Federal Register, 73*(15), 3971–3972.

Dressler, W. W., Balieiro, M. C., & Santos, J. E. D. (1999). Culture, skin color, and arterial blood pressure in Brazil. *American Journal of Human Biology, 11,* 9–59.

Dressler, W. W., & Bindon, J. R. (2000). The health consequences of cultural consonance: Cultural dimensions of lifestyle, social support and arterial blood pressure in an African American community. *American Anthropologist, 102,* 244–260.

Duncan, D. F., Gold, R. J., Basch, C. E., & Markellis, V. C. (1988). *Epidemiology: Basis for disease prevention and health promotion.* New York: Macmillan.

Dutton, D. B. (1987). Social class, health, and illness. In L. H. Aiken & D. Mechanic (Eds.), *Applications of social science to clinical medicine and health policy* (pp. 31–62). New Brunswick, NJ: Rutgers University Press.

Farmer, P. (1999). *Infections and inequality.* San Francisco: University of California Press.

Feldman, R. H., & Fulwood, R. (1999). The three leading causes of death in African Americans: Barriers to reducing excess disparity and to improving health behaviors. *Journal of Health Care for the Poor and Underserved, 10,* 45–71.

Finch, B. K., Hummer, R. A., Reindl, M., & Vega, W. A. (2002). Validity of self-rated health among Latino(a)s. *American Journal of Epidemiology, 155,* 755–759.

Frankish, C. J., Milligan, C. D., & Reid, C. (1998). A review of relationships between active living and determinants of health. *Social Science & Medicine, 47*(3), 287–301.

Franzini, L., Ribble, J. C., & Keddie, A. M. (2001). Understanding the Hispanic Paradox. *Ethnicity & Disease, 11,* 496–518.

Franzini, L., & Spears, W. (2003). Contribution of social context to inequalities in years of life lost to cardiovascular disease in Texas. *Social Science & Medicine, 57,* 1847–1861.

Friis, R. H., & Sellers, T. A. (1999). *Epidemiology for public health practice* (2nd ed.). Gaithersburg, MD: Aspen.

Gold, R., Kennedy, B., Connell, F., & Kawachi, I. (2002). Teen births, income inequality, and social capital: Developing an understanding of the causal pathway. *Health & Place, 8*(2), 77–83.

Greiner, K. A., Li, C., Kawachi, I., Hunt, D. C., & Ahluwalia, J. S. (2004). The relationships of social participation and community ratings to health and health behaviors in areas with high and low population density. *Social Science & Medicine, 59*(11), 2303–2312.

Holtgrave, D. R., & Crosby, R. A. (2003). Social capital, poverty, and income inequality as predictors of gonorrhoea, syphilis, chlamydia and AIDS case rates in the United States. *Sexually Transmitted Infections, 79*(1), 62–64.

Horowitz, I. L. (1966). *Three worlds of development.* New York: Oxford University Press.

Hummer, R. A., Powers, D. A., Pullum, S. G., Gossman, G. L., & Frisbie, W. P. (2007). Paradox found (again): Infant mortality among the Mexican-origin population in the United States. *Demography, 44*(3), 441–457.

Hunt, K. J., Resendez, R. G., Williams, K., Haffner, S. M., Stern, M. P., & Hazuda, H. P. (2003). All-cause and cardiovascular mortality among Mexican-Americans and non-Hispanic white older participants in the San Antonio Heart Study: Evidence against the "Hispanic Paradox." *American Journal of Epidemiology, 158,* 1048–1057.

Jaco, E. G. (1960). *The social epidemiology of mental disorders.* New York: Russell Sage.

Kawachi, I., & Kennedy, B. P. (1997). The relationship of income inequality to mortality: Does the choice of indicator matter? *Social Science & Medicine, 45*(7), 1121–1127.

Kawachi, I., Kennedy, B. P., Lochner, K., & Prothrow-Smith, D. (1997). Social capital, income inequality, and mortality. *American Journal of Public Health, 87,* 1491–1498.

Kawachi, I., Kennedy, B. P., & Wilkinson, R. G. (1999). Crime: Social disorganization and relative deprivation. *Social Science & Medicine, 48,* 719–731.

Kennedy, B. P., Kawachi, I., Prothrow-Smith, D., Lochner, K., & Gupta, V. (1998). Social capital, income inequality, and firearm violent crime. *Social Science & Medicine, 47*(1), 7–17.

Krieger, N. (1994). Epidemiology and the web of causation: Has anyone seen the spider? *Social Science & Medicine, 39*(7), 887–903.

Link, B. G., & Phelan, J. (1995). Social conditions as fundamental causes of diseases. *Journal of Health and Social Behavior, 35*(Extra issue), 80–94.

Lopez, A. D., Mathers, C. D., Ezzati, M., Jamison, D. T., & Murray, C. L. (2006). Global and regional burden of disease risk factors, 2001: Systematic analysis of population health data. *Lancet, 367,* 1747–1757.

Lu, M. C., & Halfon, N. (2003). Racial and ethnic disparities in birth outcomes: A life-course perspective. *Maternal and Child Health Journal, 7*(1), 13–30.

MacDorman, M. F., Callaghan, W. M., Mathews, T. J., Hoyert, D. L., & Kochanek, K. D. (2007). *Trends in preterm-related infant mortality by race and ethnicity: United States, 1999–2004.* Retrieved August 4, 2008, from www.cdc.gov/nchs/products/pubs/pubd/hestats/infantmort99–04/infantmort99–04.htm

Markides, K. S., & Coreil, J. (1986). The health of Southwestern Hispanics: An "epidemiologic paradox"? *Public Health Reports, 101*(3), 253–265.

Marmot, M., Bobak, M., & Smith, G. D. (1995). Explanations for social inequalities in health. In B. C. Amick, S. Levine, A. R. Tarlov, & D. Chapman Walsh (Eds.), *Society and health* (pp. 172–210). New York: Oxford University Press.

Marmot, M., Ryff, C. D., Bumpass, L. L., Shipley, M., & Marks, N. F. (1997). Social inequalities in health: Next questions and converging evidence. *Social Science & Medicine, 44*(6), 901–910.

Morley, I. (2007). City chaos, contagion, Chadwick and social justice. *Yale Journal of Biology and Medicine, 80*(2), 61–72.

Nazroo, J. Y. (2003). The structuring of ethnic inequalities in health: Economic position, racial discrimination, and racism. *American Journal of Public Health, 93,* 277–284.

Palloni, A., & Morenoff, J. D. (2001). Interpreting the paradoxical in the Hispanic Paradox: Demographic and epidemiologic approaches. *Annals of the New York Academy of Science, 954,* 140–174.

Paradies, Y. (2006). A systematic review of self-reported racism and health. *International Journal of Epidemiology, 35,* 888–901.

Patrick, D. L., & Wickizer, T. M. (1995). Community and health. In B. Amick, S. Levine, A. R. Tarlov, & D. Chapman Walsh (Eds.), *Society and health* (pp. 64–92). New York: Oxford University Press.

Pence, G. E. (2008). *Medical ethics: Accounts of the cases that shaped and define medical ethics.* Boston: McGraw-Hill.

Phongsavan, P., Chey, T., Bauman, A., Brooks, R., & Silove, D. (2006). Social capital, socio-economic status and psychological distress among Australian adults. *Social Science & Medicine, 63*(10), 2546–2561.

Pillai, V. K., & Shannon, L. W. (1995). Introduction: Definition and distribution of developing areas. In V. K. Pillai & L. W. Shannon (Eds.), *Developing areas: A book of readings and research* (pp. 1–13). Oxford, UK: Berg.

Putnam, R. D. (2000). *Bowling alone: The collapse and revival of American community.* New York: Simon & Schuster.

Sallis, J. F., Owen, N., & Fotheringham, M. J. (2000). Behavioral epidemiology: A systematic framework to classify phases of research on health promotion and disease prevention. *Annals of Behavioral Medicine, 22*(4), 294–298.

Schulz, A. J., Williams, D. R., Israel, B. A., & Lempert, L. B. (2002). Racial and spatial relations as fundamental determinants of health in Detroit. *Milbank Quarterly, 80,* 677–707.

Smith, D. P., & Bradshaw, B. S. (2006). Rethinking the Hispanic Paradox: Death rates and life expectancy for U.S. non-Hispanic white and Hispanic populations. *American Journal of Public Health, 96*(9), 1686–1692.

Sudano, J. J., & Baker, G. W. (2006). Explaining racial/ethnic disparities in health declines and mortality in late middle age: The roles of socioeconomic status, health behaviors and health insurance. *Social Science & Medicine, 62*(4), 909–922.

Townsend, P. (1979). *Poverty in the United Kingdom.* Harmondsworth, UK: Penguin Books.

Trostle, J. A. (2005). *Epidemiology and culture.* New York: Cambridge University Press.

Wadsworth, M. E. J. (1986). *Serious illness in childhood and its association with later-life achievement.* London: Tavistock.

Weiss, M. G. (2001). Cultural epidemiology: An introduction and overview. *Anthropology & Medicine, 8*(1), 5–29.

Wennemo, I. (1993). Infant mortality, public policy and inequality: A comparison of 18 industrialized countries 1950–85. *Sociology of Health and Illness, 15*(4), 429–446.

West, P. (1991). Rethinking the health selection explanation for health inequalities. *Social Science & Medicine, 32*(4), 373–384.

Wilkinson, R. G. (1992). Income distribution and life expectancy. *British Medical Journal, 304,* 165–168.

Wilkinson, R. G. (1996). *Unhealthy societies. The afflictions of inequality.* London: Routledge.

Wilkinson, R. G. (1998). Letter to the editor. *Social Science & Medicine, 47*(3), 411–412.

World Bank. (2007). *World development indicators 2007.* Washington, DC: Author.

PART II

Theoretical Foundations

This section overviews the theoretical foundations of social and behavioral science contributions to public health by describing the guiding frameworks, approaches to health-related behavior, and components of the social environment.

Chapter 4 reviews the core concepts, theories, and models in the field by first presenting the four broad theoretical traditions of social ecology, health promotion, interpretive studies, and critical perspectives and then identifying the core concepts that have received most attention in research and practice. The remainder of the chapter discusses important theories and models that can be applied at different levels of the social ecology of health model.

Chapter 5 organizes the discussion of health-related behavior into three categories: health behavior, illness behavior, and disease management behavior. These categories can be conceptually linked to primary, secondary, and tertiary prevention. Examples are presented to illustrate the illness recognition and help-seeking process and adherence to therapeutic regimens.

Although in some respects the entire book focuses on the social environment and health, Chapter 6 presents the theoretical underpinnings of the field in greater depth. The content is organized by social environmental levels, including interpersonal (family systems, social support), community (social capital, support groups), and societal (social roles, social structure, social construction). A particular focus on gender relations and men's health illustrates the use of theory to explain health differences in men and women.

CHAPTER

4

Behavioral and Social Science Theory

Jeannine Coreil

A *theory* is a set of interrelated concepts, constructs, and propositions that present a systematic view of a domain of study for the purpose of explaining and predicting phenomena. A *model*, on the other hand, is a heuristic device for organizing components of a domain of phenomena to show relationships between the parts and the outcome of interest. Scholars from different disciplines distinguish between theories and conceptual models in contrasting ways; however, common distinctions emphasize the degree of generality, formalization, coherence, and causality involved. Theories tend to encompass broad classes of phenomena, while models are applied to more narrowly defined domains, have less formalization, and make more tentative claims about causality. For example, the social ecology of health model draws on general systems and social science theories, but it is a model and not a theory. It organizes component factors according to levels of influence on health and uses the heuristic device of the iceberg-type figure to depict the relationship between deep structural factors, intermediate factors, and individual factors. Different theories can be used to explain phenomena at different ecological levels, a topic to which we will return later in this chapter.

Public health professionals who work in areas unrelated to the social and behavioral sciences often become overwhelmed by the multiplicity of theoretical and conceptual "models" that are found in the behavioral science literature. Many of the frameworks and the constructs they contain appear very similar but go by different names, and the component concepts seem

Author's Note: Parts of this chapter are reprinted by permission from Coreil, J. (2008). Social Science Contributions to Public Health: Overview. In K. Heggenhougen & S. Quah (Eds.), *International Encyclopedia of Public Health* (Vol. 6., pp. 101–114). Oxford, UK: Oxford University Press.

vague, abstract, and difficult to grasp. Some are called "theories" but seem more like models, while others are called "models" but seem more like simply a list of concepts or variables shown to influence health.

Habituated to a work environment that emphasizes "hard evidence" and "facts," public health professionals in technical fields often muddle their way through this abstract conceptual territory, searching for clear anchors on which to hang the many theoretical constructs. In this chapter, we aim to provide a roadmap to behavioral and social science theory that may help simplify and clarify the complexity and help those who come from a non–social science background to understand the role of social and behavioral theory in public health research and practice.

THEORETICAL TRADITIONS IN PUBLIC HEALTH

In Chapter 1, we discussed the history of behavioral and social science contributions to public health, including the emergence of social perspectives in the 19th century and the accelerated growth of a sociobehavioral paradigm in the second half of the 20th century. We noted the importance of theoretical and conceptual advances during the latter period, which shifted the focus of research and practice to sociocultural context and behavioral underpinnings of public health problems. In this chapter, we describe some of the most important theoretical contributions to this shift in greater depth and discuss how they offer tools for understanding the complex etiology of health problems in today's world and translate into different approaches to problem amelioration. These can be grouped into four broad categories: (1) *social ecology,* (2) *health promotion,* (3) *interpretive studies,* and (4) *critical perspectives.* Next, we examine selected key concepts that have gained prominence in the field, giving examples of their application and usefulness in public health work. The third section presents an overview of selected theories and models according to the different levels of social ecological systems.

Social Ecology

The social ecology of health model serves as the organizing framework of this book. The model is rooted in the traditional public health model of host-agent-environment, which was developed to study the relationship between human populations (host), disease pathogens (agent), and the physical setting (environment) in which people live and work. For instance, the transmission of waterborne illnesses can be studied in terms of the relationship between a human (host) exposed to a disease-causing pathogen (agent) through the use of a contaminated water source (environment). The traditional public health model can be contrasted with the traditional biomedical model, which assumes that illness can be explained by the presence of pathogens in the body (germ theory of disease) and abnormal physiological processes or biochemical imbalances. The biomedical model accords only a minor role to psychological and social processes, and it views mental and social phenomena as largely independent of biological processes (mind-body dualism). The social ecology of health model expands the traditional public health model to incorporate aspects of the *social environment* as fundamental contributors to health problems.

Health Promotion

Theoretical approaches to health promotion have tended to rely on social psychological models of behavior change. These models seek to identify determinants and pathways of influence for health-related behaviors, such as diet and exercise, smoking, safe-sex practices, contraceptive use, and screening behavior. Some of the most widely used approaches among these are the theory of reasoned action, later modified as the theory of planned behavior (Ajzen, 2002); social learning theory, later renamed social cognitive theory (Bandura, 2001); and the transtheoretical model, based on the stages of change construct (Prochaska, DiClemente, & Norcross, 1992). What the various models have in common is the focus on individual behavior change to improve health through the adoption of health-enhancing practices, such as smoking cessation, contraceptive use, and mammography screening. A key construct that emerged through various applications and elaborations of these models is the notion of *self-efficacy,* the degree to which an individual feels competent to perform a health practice. Originally proposed as part of social cognitive theory (Bandura, 1977), the construct proved to be a strong predictor of behavior that required sustained lifestyle change. Thus, this notion was incorporated into the expanded health belief model, the theory of planned behavior (recast as "perceived behavioral control"), and the transtheoretical model (see below).

Interpretive Studies

Several strands of theoretical development across disciplines can be subsumed under the interpretive studies rubric. In anthropology, it includes cognitive approaches to illness, such as the study of explanatory models of illness (Kleinman, 1978), and cultural consensus analysis (Romney, Weller, & Batchelder, 1986). Related sociological perspectives include social constructionism (Berger & Luckmann, 1967) and symbolic interactionism (Blumer, 1969). In psychology, relevant examples include self-regulatory models of illness and the notion of illness representations (Leventhal, Brissette, & Leventhal, 2003) as well as attribution theory for explaining beliefs about illness causation. The common denominator of these approaches is a focus on subjective, perceptual, and cognitive dimensions of illness. It is assumed that meanings are neither "correct" nor fixed but are constructed or negotiated through cognitive, social, and cultural filtering. Anthropological distinctions between the concepts of emic and etic, and illness and disease are relevant here. *Emic* refers to the insider's view (e.g., the patient's subjective experience of illness) and *etic* to the objective view of outsiders (e.g., the health care provider's and biomedical understanding). In recent years and across disciplines, increased attention has been given to illness "narratives," that is, the ways in which people weave their illness experiences into stories incorporating events and themes from related aspects of their lives (Hurwitz, Greenhalgh, & Skultans, 2004). Qualitative studies of illness narratives reveal the nuanced meanings that people assign to the process of becoming sick, including understanding its ramifications, coping with the adaptations required, and negotiating the health care system as they seek help in its management. For example, narratives of breast cancer survivors often invoke themes of empowerment, personal growth, and the significance of a new life journey.

Critical Perspectives

Critical perspectives are those that challenge the dominant paradigms of public health practice and argue for alternative approaches to improving the health of populations. They can be grouped into at least two general categories: those that fault the political-economic organization of health systems and those influenced by postmodern perspectives on the role of the state and regulatory practices in producing healthy citizens. The first school of critical theory has historical roots in Marxist theory, critiques of capitalism, and the emergence of the medical-industrial complex (Navarro, 1986). This tradition traces the causes of health inequalities to broad social structural arrangements, such as global systems of trade and neocolonial domination of less developed countries by economic power elites. Likewise, health disparities are attributed to the deleterious effects of the market economy on health issues. Examples include critiques of the disproportionate distribution of the global burden of disease across different regions of the world. Ethical critiques about unequal availability of life-saving drugs would also fit into this category. An example within the United States would be the explanation of health inequalities across racial and ethnic groups in terms of economic structures, racism, and discrimination. Feminist perspectives on the health status of women would also fall within this genre.

The second category of critical perspectives emerged more recently within the post-structuralist paradigm, which analyzes social problems from a constructivist perspective, giving primacy to how we frame health-related issues and how this leads to various control strategies. For example, in modern industrial societies, the state has assumed an increasingly larger role in health surveillance and monitoring, constantly urging the populace to adopt healthy lifestyles and conform to the regimes of a healthy citizenship (Petersen & Lupton, 1996) in the pursuit of "perfect health" (Hours, 2001). Threats to public health are constructed as emanating from the unhealthy "other," such as immigrant groups, and "risks" are seen as ubiquitous and constant; therefore, citizens must remain continually vigilant. The latter tradition includes critiques of the "riskfactorology" approach to public health thinking as a misguided oversimplification of problems that produces a false sense of security and control (McKinlay & Marceau, 2000).

Critical theorists have challenged ecological models for accepting the status quo of the social context and for failing to challenge the unequal distribution of resources across groups. In an attempt to integrate critical and ecological perspectives, some theorists have developed synthetic models that incorporate aspects of both traditions. For example, the ecosocial model (Krieger, 1994, 2001) attempts to link a social production of disease perspective with the multilevel framework of social ecology. It focuses on patterns of inequalities in health across the ecological levels of biological processes, the individual, family systems, community, populations, society, and global systems. It also incorporates the notion of embodiment, that is, how social inequalities are expressed through biological processes. Others have advocated for the development of similar synthetic models along the lines of a "critical ecological perspective" (Leatherman, 2005).

KEY CONCEPTS

Knowledge and Attitudes

In terms of sheer volume, the bulk of social science research and practice has centered on cognitive factors related to health and illness. There are a number of reasons for this. First, the most accessible, simple, and least costly variables to measure are cognitive; perceptions, attributions, attitudes, and knowledge can be studied through survey and interview techniques as opposed to more time-consuming and labor-intensive methods such as behavioral observation. Second, until recently, the prevailing paradigm for social research assumed that the most important obstacles to program success resided in the minds and dispositions of the target audience. Hence, the goal was to uncover faulty understandings so that correct information could be provided, thereby leading to more enlightened behavior. Third, psychological theories have strongly influenced research in this field, and anthropological approaches have also emphasized cultural beliefs as central. The combination of these influences has created a huge body of literature on cognitive factors in health. Some of the key concepts have been previously touched on, such as basic health beliefs and attitudes, explanatory models of illness, and illness representations. Related concepts that have received particular attention include locus of control (e.g., internal vs. external to the individual), self-efficacy (perceived ability to successfully execute), expectancies (anticipated outcomes), and intentions (anticipated action). However, along with the volume of research on cognitive factors has come the recognition that beliefs often do not lead to behavior and it is necessary to study behavior itself as well as its varied influences.

Health Behavior

The attention accorded to behavior change models in the field of health promotion has stimulated the development of quite a few concepts and methods for the toolkit of the behavioral scientist. To begin with, considerable attention has been accorded to the development of reliable and valid measures of specific health behaviors, such as the use of alcohol, tobacco and drugs, injury prevention practices, food consumption, physical activity, and sexual behavior. Likewise, precision has been introduced for measuring frequency, intensity, salience, and other dimensions. Health behavior has also been conceptualized according to different stages, such as initiation, maintenance, and relapse, as well as positive versus negative behavior, such as adoption or acceptance versus cessation or refusal. The field of health behavior research has incorporated principles and techniques of testing and measurement to a notable degree, and it is common for researchers to use standardized instruments, structured scales, quantitative indices, and similar tools. In addition, many analyses use secondary data sources, such as the periodic surveys sponsored by the National Center for Health Statistics. The reliance on specific indicators has come to be described as the "risk factor approach" to health behavior. Even when study designs include higher-level influences, such as social structural and cultural variables, the focus is on "predicting" specific health behaviors by showing a statistical association with structural risk factors. This orientation is favored among researchers from a social psychological and health education background. In contrast, anthropological and sociological research accords greater attention to understanding the sociocultural context in and of itself.

Culture

The concept of culture refers to shared patterns of thought and behavior that characterize a social group, which are learned through socialization processes and endure through time. As will be discussed in Chapter 8, cultural concepts can be applied to different kinds of social groups including families, communities, ethnic groups, organizations and societies. Culture can also be studied in terms of cultural domains such as diet, child rearing, or health. In public health research and practice, culture is often treated as a contextual variable influencing health-related behavior and outcomes. The concepts of ethnicity, and to a lesser extent race, are often used as proxy variables for cultural background (see Chapter 9). In addition, acculturation, or the degree to which a minority group has adopted the culture of the majority group, is often taken into account in research studies. Processes of culture change have received attention in analyzing the impact of interventions such as applications of the diffusion of innovation theory, discussed in a later section of this chapter. Finally, the notion of cultural competence, or the ability of health care providers to deliver culturally appropriate services to members of different ethnic and linguistic groups, has figured importantly in public health programs (see Chapter 9).

In research on health, cultural concepts have focused on analytic and linguistic categories for understanding the illness process and health behavior. Anthropologists make the distinction between *disease* and *illness*, with disease referring to the physiological pathology associated with a biomedically defined diagnosis and illness describing the complex biopsychosocial experience of feeling sick or unwell. Research has shown that while medical practitioners focus primarily on treating disease, patients often respond to their conditions in terms of different perceptions of the illness process. Related concepts include the distinction between *emic* and *etic* beliefs about health conditions, where emic beliefs are specific to a particular cultural group (the "insider" perspective) and etic beliefs derive from some external standard (e.g., the International Classification of Diseases). Patient explanatory models of illness focus on emic perceptions of the causes, consequences, and appropriate treatment for specific illness episodes. Cultural models of illness, on the other hand, refer to shared understandings, or shared explanatory models, for locally recognized illness categories. In Chapter 8, we discuss the concept of cultural model in greater depth and provide examples of its application to health-related problems.

Social Environment

A large body of literature has accumulated relating to social environmental factors and health, including the effects of social stress, social support, social networks, and social capital. Beginning in the 1970s, researchers took a serious interest in the health effects of stress, and over the decades, the weight of evidence has shown conclusively that stress affects not only chronic disease but also almost every health condition imaginable. Early studies of stress investigated the impact of major life events such as bereavement, divorce, and loss of job on morbidity and mortality (Lazarus & Folkman, 1984). Subsequent studies expanded this line of inquiry to include "daily hassles," job-related stress (see also Chapter 21), and other, more day-to-day kinds of stress, developing various instruments to measure the varieties of stress. Concomitantly, researchers also began to investigate the health protective benefits of social support and social networks (Berkman, Glass, & Brisette, 2000). Often studies of social support investigated its mitigating effects on the impact of stress, developing alternative hypotheses about whether social support operated directly on a health outcome or whether its protective effects occurred primarily because it buffered the negative impact of stress. The literature on social support identifies at least four major types of support: (1) emotional, (2) instrumental, (3) informational, and (4) appraisal. Other related concepts include direct and indirect support and formal and informal support. Studies attempted to identify the variable impact of different kinds of support on particular health outcomes.

A related line of research focuses on the concept of social networks, that is, the connections people have through relationships with others. Researchers have furthered the development of various measures of social integration and isolation, including network structure (size, density, and dispersion of linkages), and the relational content of support such as sources, types of demands, conflicts, role expectations, and social regulation of behavior. An important milestone study in this genre came out of the previously mentioned Alameda County Study, which documented prospectively the significant positive impact of social connectedness (Berkman & Syme, 1979; House, Robbins, & Metzner, 1982). Similar findings have been documented in other studies in the United States and Europe. More complex research designs have further documented the differential impact that social integration and social support have on subgroups in the population, such as comparing men and women and rural and urban dwellers. As the health effects of social support became well established, researchers shifted their attention to better understanding the biopsychosocial processes that mediate the association with health (see Chapter 6).

In recent years, social epidemiologic studies have focused on the concepts of social capital and collective efficacy as explanatory variables in population-level health. Growing out of a renewed interest in the influence of neighborhoods on health conditions, researchers have investigated how shared norms, mutual trust, and reciprocal obligations (social capital) influence diverse health outcomes, including crime and mortality rates (Kawachi & Berkman, 2003). Whereas individuals may not be conscious of the beneficial effects of social capital, collective efficacy refers to a group's perceived ability to successfully take action for the benefit of the common good (e.g., crime prevention). Studies have associated collective efficacy with lower rates of violence, for example (Sampson, 2003). However, the ability to achieve common goals also depends on the wider political environment or institutional capacity through linkages among organizations within and outside the focal community.

A TYPOLOGY OF THEORIES AND MODELS

At the beginning of this chapter, some distinctions were presented between theories and models. However, to simplify the following review, both theories and models are discussed under the rubric of "models." In the following sections, different conceptual frameworks are grouped according to the level of the social ecology of health model in which it fits most closely. A number of the models reviewed might be grouped under more than one level; the decision to place them in a particular level was based on the dominant emphasis of the approach and how they have been used in practice. The first category describes Level I models, or *intrapersonal models* that emphasize mental constructs about how people think about a health-related domain. The second category describes aspects of an individual's social environment within Level II models, or *interpersonal models* of health-related behavior. The third category includes Level III models, or *organizational models* for research and interventions to improve the health status of groups. The fourth category addresses Level IV models, or *community models* for health intervention. The fifth category, *societal-level models,* includes approaches that stress the social structural and national policy influences on health problems. Finally, the sixth category encompasses *multilevel models,* or frameworks that transcend any single level of influence within the social ecology of health model and, therefore, are treated separately. It brings together multilevel models of health behavior change, which address all levels of the social ecology of health model, including societal and global-level influences. Although many of the models to be reviewed within the categories of intrapersonal, organizational, and community, in fact, include components that overlap more than one level, multilevel models encompass the full model or several levels and place explanatory emphasis on more than two levels.

Intrapersonal-Level Models

A large number of health behavior models fall within the intrapersonal level of influence because they emphasize cognitive and behavioral factors and are often referred to as cognitive models. The term *cognitive models* comes from the root word *cognition,* which denotes the process of knowing or perceiving. Thus, cognitive models focus on people's knowledge, attitudes, and perceptions about a topic. As noted previously, much of the early work on health behavior emphasized individuals' understanding of the factors involved in producing a healthy or unhealthy outcome. Over the years, more specific constructs have been identified to denote more narrowly defined cognitions, such as expectancies and intentions.

The Health Belief Model

The earliest framework in this tradition is the health belief model (Janz, Champion, & Stretcher, 2002), depicted in Figure 4.1. The model posits that the decision to take action to

FIGURE 4.1   Health Belief Model

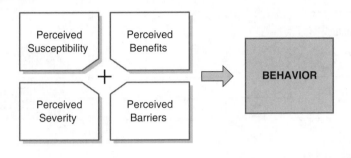

protect one's health is determined by four factors: (1) whether people consider themselves susceptible to the condition (perceived susceptibility), (2) whether the condition is perceived as having serious personal consequences (perceived severity), (3) whether a specific action is expected to reduce the risk of getting the condition or the consequences of it (perceived benefits), and (4) whether the perceived benefits of the action outweigh the subjective costs or barriers to taking action (perceived barriers).

For example, a middle-aged woman in good health may think that she has a very low chance of getting the flu because she hasn't had a bout in many years (susceptibility), and her recollection of the last episode is that it was not that debilitating (severity). She has doubts that the generic flu shot actually protects someone from acquiring the infection (benefit), and she would have to take time off work and drive across town to get one (barrier). In this scenario, the woman's "decisional balance" would probably lead her to decide not to get the immunization. In contrast, another middle-aged woman with a family history of breast cancer might consider herself at risk for the disease (susceptibility), which she fears as a "death sentence" because several of her relatives have died from it (severity). She has faith that a mammography exam can detect cancerous growths at an early stage (benefit), her health care plan provides full coverage of the costs, and the mammography service is located in the same building as her primary provider (no barriers). In addition, her doctor provides what the health belief model calls a "cue to action"; that is, he reminds her to get a mammogram when she goes in for an annual checkup. Not surprisingly, this woman receives mammography screening on a regular basis.

Theory of Planned Behavior

The theory of planned behavior, which grew out of the theory of reasoned action, gives primary attention to cognitive factors that influence an individual's "intention" to perform a behavior (Ajzen, 1991). Intention is singled out as the most proximate determinant of behavior because health-related actions are usually adopted in a conscious or "planned" manner. This model posits that intentional behavior is determined by three factors: (1) attitude toward the behavior, (2) subjective social norms, and (3) perceived behavioral control. The relationship among the model's components is depicted in Figure 4.2.

FIGURE 4.2   Theory of Planned Behavior

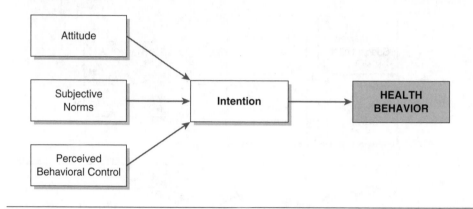

An attitude differs from a belief in that it reflects some form of disposition toward the object of attention. Thus, an individual's attitude toward making a dietary change may range from negative to positive on a continuum. Subjective norms refer to people's perceptions of how their reference groups (people they think about when assessing what is normal or socially approved) feel about the behavior. Someone living in a community where others rarely get an annual checkup but instead go to the doctor only when they are obviously sick might feel that getting a specific screening test is unnecessary, too much trouble, and a luxury he or she cannot afford. Perceived behavioral control refers to individuals' assessment of how easy or difficult it will be for them to successfully perform a behavior, a construct that is similar to what other models call "self-efficacy." Early trials at using a condom, for example, may have been problematic for an adolescent, leading to low perceived behavioral control when contemplating future use of condoms. Putting the parts together, the model predicts that people will plan and carry out a health behavior when their attitude toward the behavior is positive, the people important to them endorse the behavior, and they expect to be able to perform the behavior successfully.

Transtheoretical Model

The transtheoretical model is an example of a "stage model" of behavior change. Stage models of health behavior are built around the principle that people rarely make significant changes in their health-related behavior all at once. Instead, they tend to go through predictable sequences of thinking about, trying out, and then adopting a behavior. For example, smokers rarely abandon cigarettes overnight; most quitters go through periods of thinking about cessation, making plans for how to do it, and multiple attempts to stop before becoming permanent nonsmokers. One of the most important practical applications of stage models is the idea that interventions should be tailored to address the unique constellation of influences on different stages of behavior change. According to this model, people move from no motivation to change through incremental phases of thinking about adopting a behavior, preparing to do it, initiating the behavior, and finally reaching a stage of regular performance (Prochaska & DiClemente, 1984). These phases are labeled precontemplation, contemplation, preparation, action, and maintenance (see Figure 4.3).

The process of moving through the stages is not always linear; that is, people may not progress directly from one stage to the next in the sequence. They may remain stationary in one stage or even revert back to a prior phase if their attempts to advance to the next stage are unsuccessful. For example, a substance abuser who has managed to remain drug-free for a long period may still "relapse" and begin using drugs again. Moreover, the factors that propel successful movement through the sequence, called "processes" in the model, vary across the different stages of change. For example, perceived risk is an important determinant of movement from precontemplation to contemplation, perceived self-efficacy is important in movement to action, and social support is important to reaching maintenance. This model has proved very useful in explaining cessation of addictive behaviors and has been applied successfully to other health-promoting behaviors as well.

Self-Regulatory Models

The term *self-regulation* comes from the field of psychology and is concerned with the ways in which individuals monitor their behavior and its consequences and continually make adjustments to "regulate" their actions to achieve life goals (Cameron & Levanthal, 2003). If

FIGURE 4.3   Transtheoretical Model

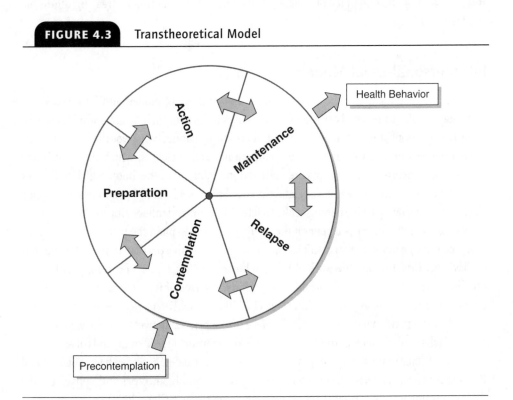

someone's goal is to maintain a certain weight range, for example, he or she may engage in a variety of behaviors and pay attention to certain things in day-to-day living, such as getting on the scale the first thing in the morning, observing how his or her clothes fit, and watching what he or she eats. If one notices that his or her clothes seem tighter than usual, this may trigger more heightened self-monitoring about food consumption. Self-regulatory models attempt to explain the factors that come into play during this regulation process. One approach is to focus on the specific "scripts" people follow to accomplish goals (Schank & Abelson, 1977). Take the general goal of "staying healthy," for example; most people have in their heads a certain script for maintaining overall health that might include eating a balanced diet, exercising regularly, consuming alcohol in moderation, managing stress levels, getting regular checkups, and following physicians' recommendations when they get sick. More specific scripts might be identified for maintaining sexual health, coping with a serious illness, or learning to perform a specific behavior, such as strength training.

One particular self-regulatory model that has been used in health behavior research is the common sense model developed by Leventhal and colleagues (2003). The model is based on two general propositions. First, people react to health threats in commonsense ways, by constructing representations about the threat that include, for example, ideas about its causes, consequences, and control. Second, these representations generate goals for managing the problem and suggest actions for achieving the goals as well as criteria for assessing the effectiveness of one's response to the threat. Over time, representations are shaped and modified by the outcomes of specific procedures for preventing or treating illness, as in a feedback loop.

Interpersonal-Level Models

Interpersonal theories of health encompass a wide range of models and frameworks for understanding how the social context of people's lives influences their health. Individuals have important relationships with others through their family connections, work settings, friendships, organizations, as well as the wider community and society in which they live. Many interpersonal theories and concepts are reviewed in Chapter 6 of this book, which addresses the social environment of health. For example, social roles, social support, and family systems all play an important part in shaping health-related behavior and influencing health outcomes.

Social support theory is a general theory that seeks to explain the process of assistance provided through human relationships. It is not associated with a particular individual but has evolved over time through the work of many scholars. The concept of social support has figured importantly in research on health, particularly in terms of its protective effects against stress and adverse life events (Berkman et al., 2000; Cassel, 1976; Heaney & Israel, 2002). Supportive interpersonal transactions take place through social networks, or the web of interpersonal relationships surrounding an individual, and may include different kinds of assistance, such as emotional or instrumental (practical) support. A great deal of research has documented the positive effects of social support on a broad range of health outcomes and, conversely, the deleterious impact of low social support on health (Berkman & Glass, 2000).

One widely used theory of social influence is social cognitive theory (Bandura, 2001). As suggested by its name, social cognitive theory describes how social relationships influence cognitions and behavior in a reciprocal process of dynamic interaction. The theory includes quite a few constructs and processes and has grown more complex over the years. Although we have chosen to present the model within the category of interpersonal models, because of its emphasis on social influence, it could also be considered a multilevel model because it addresses dynamic interactions with higher ecological levels. A simplified version is presented here that highlights the components that have received more attention in public health applications. Key constructs within the theory include modeling, outcome expectations, self-efficacy, and behavioral capability (see Figure 4.4). Modeling refers to the process of vicarious learning from observing significant others in our social environment. For example, a teenage boy may have observed his elder brother carrying condoms in his wallet and heard his brother's stories about using a condom. This modeling may lead him to carry condoms when he begins to think about initiating sex. Outcome expectations refer to beliefs about the consequences of taking a certain action. For example, the adolescent may believe that using a condom will protect him from a sexually transmitted disease. Self-efficacy refers to one's perceived ability to carry out a behavior. The adolescent in this example may believe that he can use a condom because it was demonstrated for him on a banana at school. Behavioral capability, on the other hand, refers to someone's actual ability to perform the behavior in real-life situations. For example, a teenager may believe that he can use a condom properly when the situation requires it (self-efficacy), but when the time comes to act, he lacks the knowledge and skills (behavioral capability) to use the condom effectively.

Organizational-Level Models

Much of the work of public health takes place through organizations, whether these are local or state health departments, community coalitions, civic associations, schools, health care

FIGURE 4.4 Social Cognitive Theory

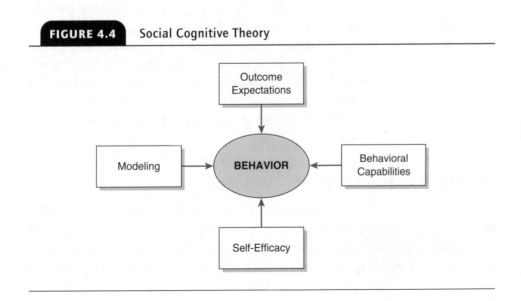

organizations, nonprofit corporations, professional associations, government agencies, or international organizations. Thus, organizational theory can be useful in understanding the workings of these complex entities, and it can help plan programs that involve the collaboration of different organizations and sectors of society. For example, in Chapter 8, organizational culture theory is applied to the professions of medicine and public health, showing how basic values and principles differ in the practices of these institutions. In this section, we describe the diffusion of innovation theory, which can be applied to both organizations and individual behavior change.

Diffusion of Innovation Theory

When introducing a new behavior into a population or a new program into an organization, it is helpful to understand how the adoption of the innovation will proceed over time. Like individual behavior change, new health practices and programs are not adopted overnight by the target group. They tend to be adopted in predictable stages, and the determinants of adoption at different stages also tend to be patterned. One theory that attempts to model the change process within populations and organizations is the diffusion of innovation theory (Rogers, 1995). The theory was originally developed to explain individual adoption of technological innovations, such as the use of contraception, but in recent years has shifted to organizational change. Early formulations identified distinct groups of adopters in the innovation process (early adopters, early majority, late majority, and laggards), as well as characteristics of the innovation itself that affected patterns of acceptance. For example, early adopters tend to be open to risk taking, and innovations that are highly compatible with existing practices are more readily adopted. When applied to organizations, the change process tends to be more complex because of embedded bureaucratic and decision-making structures; however, stages of change analogous to individual innovation have been identified. One formulation defines the stages as following a pattern of dissemination, adoption, implementation, maintenance, and institutionalization (Oldenberg & Parcel, 2002). For example, a school district may consider adopting a coordinated program for improving healthy food choices in its schools. It may disseminate information about the program to its member schools and invite interested schools to participate in a pilot project. Evaluation of the first year of implementation in the demonstration schools may show impressive results, which leads more schools to adopt the program in succeeding years. Sustained success with the program and support from parent and teacher groups eventually may lead to districtwide institutionalization of the program.

Community-Level Models

Because so much of public health work is community based and conducted within defined local populations, community-level models offer useful approaches to research and program design. In Chapter 14, Bryant discusses the application of community organization theory to planning community-based health interventions, which emphasize the principle of local participation in the planning and implementation of programs. In recent years, increasing attention has been accorded to cultural diversity within target communities and the importance of incorporating cultural competence in program design through an in-depth understanding of the cultural factors that influence responses to planned interventions (see Chapter 9). The study of cultural models of illness, and how these shape behavior, offers one approach to gaining a deeper understanding of the cultural context of behavior.

Cultural Models

Cultural models of health and illness focus on identifying the components of health-related beliefs and behavior that are shared by members of a social group. The group may be very small, such as when we look at family culture; medium sized, such as when we look at organizational culture; or large scale, such as when we refer to "American" culture. Cultural models outline common ways of thinking about and acting on a defined area of concern. Like other aspects of culture, they are learned through processes of socialization within the group, and they guide human action in responding to life events. For example, most Americans subscribe to a common model of what is involved in "going to the doctor" when sick. One makes an appointment in advance, signs in on arrival, sits in the "waiting room" until called, gets weighed and has one's blood pressure taken, and is then taken to an exam room to wait for the doctor. The doctor comes in to take a history of the problem, a medical assistant takes samples for diagnostic tests, and then the doctor returns to give a diagnosis and prescribe treatment. Cultural models are similar to the notion of action scripts discussed in the previous section, but while scripts may be idiosyncratic to particular individuals, cultural models are shared across members of a group. However, similar to the way psychologists apply the idea of scripts, anthropologists use the concept of "explanatory models" of illness to describe an individual's understanding of a particular illness episode in terms of its etiology, symptoms, and treatment.

Societal-Level Models

Approaches to understanding health that emphasize societal-level influences include those that encompass social structural, political, and economic influences on health. Research and practice of this type focus on distal determinants of health, such as social class, economic inequality, and national health policy. The approach taken may be descriptive, such as the perspectives on social epidemiology presented in Chapter 3, or it may take a more critical stance on health policy and the organization of services. For example, in discussing different approaches to policy and advocacy in Chapter 16, Whiteford applies political-economic perspectives in analyzing the Cuban health care system.

Societal-level models draw on various sociopolitical theories, such as world systems theory and political economy of health theory, to help explain variation in health conditions and risk behavior through analysis of upstream, macrolevel forces. All these theories have roots in the work of Karl Marx and his critique of capitalism as an economic system. World systems theory (Wallerstein, 1974) expands the critique of capitalism to a global scale, arguing that relations of production create economic inequalities not only within countries but also among nations, through expropriation of resources away from "peripheral" economies and toward the dominant "core" economies of capitalism. Applied to health, the theory posits that the unequal flow of resources to the global North explains a great deal about worldwide health disparities. This theory and other similar formulations grew out of attempts to describe the nature of social change in postindustrial society, including processes of modernization and globalization. In recent years, a body of ideas has developed around the study of globalization, the process of movement toward worldwide integration of not only economic systems but also sociocultural systems, communications media, sports, education, entertainment, and many other social institutions. Within such a broad context, public health problems can be analyzed in terms of the forces of globalization, such as understanding drug use in one part of the world as intricately connected to world economic systems and global politics as well as youth and celebrity culture communicated through television and the Internet.

Political-economic theory can also be applied to health within single societies to understand how the relations of economic production shape public health problems. For example, some argue that the medical-industrial complex in the United States fuels ever higher production and spending on health care, leading to an out of control situation in which many citizens fall through the cracks (Waitzman, 1983). A related perspective is sometimes referred to as the social production of health (Turshen, 1989), a model of disease causation that views health outcomes as socially generated and nonspecific. In other words, the same set of disadvantageous social conditions (poverty, homelessness, incarceration, and discrimination) can be linked to a variety of health outcomes, including malnutrition, infectious diseases, drug use, violence, infant mortality—the list is quite long. The social production of health model further posits that intervening on a single health outcome without addressing deeper fundamental causes will invariably lead to failure in the long term.

More recently, critical medical anthropologists have proposed a "syndemic model" of disease causation that stresses both the co-occurring nature of multiple health problems in disadvantaged populations and the co-occurrence of predictable social conditions associated with these problems (Singer & Clair, 2003). The traditional biomedical view of disease, and to some extent the view of public health as well, is to study and intervene with individual diseases as if they were distinct entities that exist separately from other diseases and independent of the social contexts in which they occur. The syndemic model emphasizes the biosocial interconnections between multiple health problems and their antecedent social conditions. For example, it is no surprise that in Haiti, which is the poorest and least developed country in the western hemisphere, one finds very high rates of malnutrition and infectious diseases and that the HIV/AIDS epidemic hit very hard there (Baer & Singer, 2006). In general, the poor and disenfranchised bear a disproportionate share of disease burden throughout the world.

Societal-level influences are also emphasized in multilevel models of health problems, to which we now turn.

Multilevel Models

Multilevel frameworks that address distal, intermediate, and proximate factors have become increasingly important for understanding all kinds of health conditions, and they are essential for analyzing public health problems. As noted in the Preface to this volume, one of the core competencies for training public health students is the ability to analyze determinants of health and disease using an ecological, or multilevel, framework. One of the earliest multilevel models developed in the health field was the biopsychosocial model (Suls & Rothman, 2004). Developed primarily to explain the complex interplay of biological and social factors in disease etiology, the model depicts multiple levels above and below the individual, arranged hierarchically from the most macrolevel at the top (global systems) down to the most microlevel at the bottom (genetic systems). Figure 4.5 shows the different levels in this model.

There are obvious similarities between the biopsychosocial model and the social ecology of health model presented in Chapter 1. However, the biopsychosocial model gives greater attention to different levels of biological systems within the human body, while the social ecology of health model elaborates macrolevel differentiation within higher-order social systems.

Another multilevel model based on systems theory is Bronfenbrenner's (1979) ecological model of child development. In this formulation, child development is viewed within the

FIGURE 4.5   Biopsychosocial Model

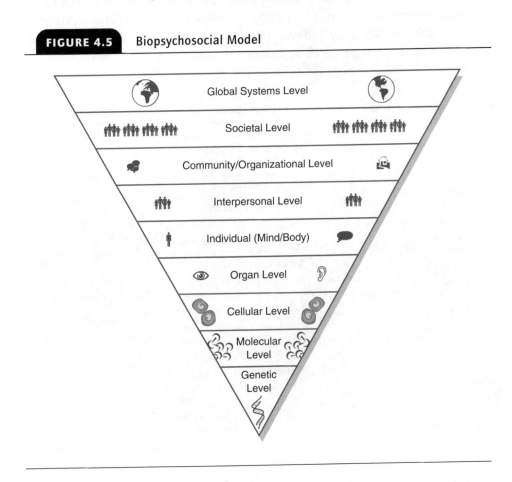

context of relationships that form the child's environment. These relationships are organized into three-tiered systems: the microsystem, mesosystem, and exosystem. Similar to other ecological models, the microsystem encompasses individual biology and behavior as well as cognitive and emotional dimensions; the mesosystem encompasses child-relevant institutions such as family, school, and religion; and the exosystem incorporates broader community, societal, and cultural systems affecting the child's development. These complex layers of the child's environment interact with the child's biological endowment to shape development in predictable ways.

MAPPING THEORIES TO THE SOCIAL ECOLOGY OF HEALTH MODEL

In this final section, the theories reviewed in this chapter and elsewhere in the book are matched with the ecological level to which they correspond most closely[1] (see Figure 4.6). Some theories might be placed at more than one level. For example, diffusion of innovation theory can be applied to individual behavior as well as to organizational change. Likewise, multilevel models, such as the biopsychosocial model, cut across multiple levels of the ecosystem. While an ecological framework is useful as an analytic tool for understanding complex influences on a problem, it is rather unwieldy to apply in a comprehensive fashion within a single research study or intervention. The complexity and costliness of a project that might address all levels of the model within the scope of a single program or study would be unmanageable. In practice, research

---

FIGURE 4.6   Theories and Levels in the Social Ecology Framework

Level	Theories and Models
INDIVIDUAL	Health Belief Model Theory of Planned Behavior Transtheoretical Model Self-Regulatory Models
INTERPERSONAL	Social Support Theory Social Cognitive Theory
ORGANIZATIONAL	Organizational Culture Theory Diffusion of Innovation Theory
COMMUNITY	Community Organization Cultural Models
SOCIETY	Social Determinants of Health Political Economy of Health

and interventions typically address a single level or at best a partial subset of the entire framework, although the importance of other levels may be taken into consideration in the design of the project. In addition, most studies and programs focus on a narrowly defined problem and seek to understand or affect a circumscribed set of influences. Therefore, to analyze public health problems in their complexity, it is necessary to review a range of different kinds of research and programs conducted at different levels and think through how the different results might fit together. Likewise, knowledge generated through different theories can provide a multifaceted understanding of problems and their solutions.

The choice of theories to use in designing a study, planning a program, or formulating a policy will be informed by the aims of the study, the resources available to achieve one's goals, and the preferences and background of the researcher/planner. Although many professionals develop allegiances to a particular theory because the kind of explanation it offers makes the most sense to them, it is the target problem itself that counts the most in determining which theory or model fits best. For example, if the aim of the study is to better understand why some community coalitions are more successful than others, the health belief model is not likely to offer much useful theoretical guidance. On the other hand, if the goal is to understand the process that persons with diabetes go through to learn how to regulate their blood sugar levels, a behavior change or self-regulation model might prove highly useful in planning the study. In the same way that research methods should fit the problem under study, theories, models, and frameworks must "fit" the problem.

In recent years, refinements of behavior change models have taken two directions, one focused on developing problem-specific conceptual models and the other in the direction of synthesizing multiple models to produce more generic frameworks applicable across a wide range of problems. For example, the information-motivation-behavioral skills (IMB) model was developed to study HIV-/AIDS-related behavior and to design preventive interventions related to sexually transmitted diseases (Fisher, Fisher, Bryan, & Misovich, 2002). It posits that for health protective action to take place, relevant information and motivation must first be present. Under these conditions, five types of skills necessary for reduction of sexual risk behavior can be identified. This model has been applied to a range of sexual health issues and has applicability to an even broader range of health behaviors. An example of the synthetic approach is the development of the integrated model of health behavior (Fishbein et al., 2001). This model grew out of a workshop sponsored by the National Institute of Mental Health, which brought together leading theorists in the field of health behavior to review the state of knowledge and try to reach consensus on what were the most important factors to consider in understanding and predicting health-related behavior. The outcome of the workshop was a formulation given the name of the integrated model, which incorporates external variables, beliefs, norms, efficacy expectations, motivation, skills, and intentions.

Development of new conceptual models and refinement of existing frameworks for understanding health behavior will continue undoubtedly in the coming years. The professional reward system fosters the production of conceptual reformulations that can be published as "new" models claiming to offer advantages over existing ones, and there is a tendency for researchers to assume that what is new is better than the old. However, investigators rarely compare the utility of more than one model in a single study, so there is limited evidence to support the relative advantages that one model has over another. This issue is discussed further in the Afterword, which looks to future directions of scholarly work in the social and behavioral sciences applied to public health.

NOTE

1. A similar mapping of theories to ecological levels can be found in Bartholomew, Parcel, Kok, and Gottlieb (2001, p. 80).

REFERENCES

Ajzen, I. (1991). The theory of planned behavior. *Organizational Behavior and Human Decision Processes, 50,* 179–211.

Ajzen, I. (2002). Perceived behavioral control, self-efficacy, locus of control, and the theory of planned behavior. *Journal of Applied Social Psychology, 32,* 665–683.

Baer, H., & Singer, M. (2006). *Introducing medical anthropology.* Lanham, MD: AltaMira Press.

Bandura, A. (1977). *Social learning theory.* New York: General Learning Press.

Bandura, A. (2001). Social cognitive theory: An agentive perspective. *Annual Review of Psychology, 52,* 1–26.

Bartholomew, L. K., Parcel, G. S., Kok, G., & Gottlieb, N. H. (2001). *Intervention mapping: Designing theory- and evidence-based health promotion programs.* Mountain View, CA: Mayfield.

Berger, P. L., & Luckmann, T. (1967). *The social construction of reality.* New York: Anchor.

Berkman, L. F., & Glass, T. (2000). Social integration, social networks, social support, and health. In L. F. Berkman & I. Kawachi (Eds.), *Social epidemiology* (pp. 137–173). Oxford, UK: Oxford University Press.

Berkman, L. F., Glass, T., & Brisette, I. (2000). From social integration to health: Durkheim in the new millennium. *Social Science & Medicine, 51,* 843–857.

Berkman, L. F., & Syme, S. L. (1979) Social networks, host resistance, and mortality: A year follow-up study of Alameda County residents. *American Journal of Epidemiology, 109,* 186–204.

Blumer, H. (1969). *Symbolic interactionism: Perspective and method.* Berkeley: University of California Press.

Bronfenbrenner, U. (1979). *The ecology of human development: Experiments by nature and design.* Cambridge, MA: Harvard University Press.

Cameron, L. D., & Leventhal, H. (Eds.). (2003). *The self-regulation of health and illness.* London: Routledge.

Cassel, J. (1976). The contribution of the social environment to host resistance. *American Journal of Epidemiology, 104,* 107–123.

Fishbein, M., Triandis, H. C., Kanfer, F. H., Becker, M., Middlestadt, S. E., & Eichler, A. (2001). Factors influencing behavior and behavior change. In A. Baum, T. A. Revenson, & J. E. Singer (Eds.), *Handbook of health psychology* (pp. 3–17). Mahwah, NJ: Lawrence Erlbaum.

Fisher, J. D., Fisher, W. A., Bryan, A. D., & Misovich, S. J. (2002). Information-motivation-behavioral skills model-based HIV risk behavior change intervention for inner-city high school youth. *Health Psychology, 21*(2), 177–186.

Heaney, C. A., & Israel, B. A. (2002). Social networks and social support. In K. Glanz, B. K. Rimer, & F. M. Lewis (Eds.), *Health behavior and health education: Theory, research, and practice* (3rd ed., pp. 185–209). San Francisco: Jossey-Bass.

Hours, B. (2001). Pour une anthropologie de la santé et sociétés. In B. Hours (Ed.), *Systèmes et politiques de santé: De la santé publique à l'anthropologie* (pp. 5–21). Paris: Karthala.

House, J. S., Robbins, C., & Metzner, H. M. (1982). The association of social relationships and activities with mortality: Prospective evidence from the Tecumseh Community Health Study. *American Journal of Epidemiology, 116,* 123–140.

Hurwitz, B., Greenhalgh, T., & Skultans, V. (2004). *Narrative research in health and illness.* Malden, MA: Blackwell.

Janz, N. K., Champion, V. L., & Strecher, V. J. (2002). The health belief model. In K. Glanz, B. K. Rimer, & F. M. Lewis (Eds.). *Health behavior and health education: Theory, research and practice* (3rd ed., pp. 45–66). San Francisco: Jossey-Bass.

Kawachi, I., & Berkman, L. F. (Eds.). (2003). *Neighborhoods and health.* New York: Oxford University Press.

Kleinman, A. (1978). *Patients and healers in the context of culture: An exploration of the borderland between anthropology, medicine and psychiatry.* Berkeley: University of California Press.

Krieger, N. (1994). Epidemiology and the web of causation: Has anyone seen the spider? *Social Science & Medicine, 39,* 887–903.

Krieger, N. (2001). Theories for social epidemiology in the 21st century: An ecosocial perspective. *International Journal of Epidemiology, 30,* 668–677.

Lazarus, R. S., & Folkman, S. (1984). *Stress, appraisal, and coping.* New York: Springer.

Leatherman, T. (2005). A space of vulnerability in poverty and health: Political-ecology and biocultural analysis. *Ethos, 33,* 46–70.

Leventhal, H., Brissette, I., & Leventhal, E. A. (2003). The common-sense model of self-regulation of health and illness. In L. D. Cameron & H. Levanthal (Eds.), *The self-regulation of health and illness* (pp. 42–65). London: Routledge.

McKinlay, J. B., & Marceau, L. D. (2000). To boldly go. *American Journal of Public Health, 90*(1), 25–33.

Navarro, V. (1986). *Crisis, health, and medicine: A social critique.* New York: Tavistock.

Oldenberg, B., & Parcel, G. S. (2002). Diffusion of innovations. In K. Glanz, B. K. Rimer, & F. M. Lewis (Eds.), *Health behavior and health education: Theory, research and practice* (3rd ed., pp. 312–334). San Francisco: Jossey-Bass.

Petersen, A., & Lupton, D. (1996). *The new public health: Health and self in the age of risk.* Thousand Oaks, CA: Sage.

Prochaska, J. O., & DiClemente, C. C. (1984). The *transtheoretical approach: Crossing traditional boundaries of therapy.* Homewood, IL: Dow Jones-Irwin.

Prochaska, J. O., DiClemente, C. C., & Norcross, J. C. (1992). In search of how people change: Applications to addictive behaviors. *American Psychologist, 47,* 1102–1114.

Rogers, E. M. (1995). *Diffusion of innovations* (4th ed.). New York: Free Press.

Romney, A. K., Weller, S. C., & Batchelder, W. H. (1986). Culture as consensus: A theory of cultural and informant accuracy. *American Anthropologist, 88,* 313–339.

Sampson, R. J. (2003). Neighborhood-level context and health: Lessons from sociology. In I. Kawachi & L. F. Berkman (Eds.), *Neighborhoods and health* (pp. 132–146). New York: Oxford University Press.

Schank, R. C., & Abelson, R. P. (1977). *Scripts, plans, goals and understanding: An inquiry into human knowledge structures.* Hillsdale, NJ: Lawrence Erlbaum.

Singer, M., & Clair, S. (2003). Syndemics and public health: Reconceptualizing disease in bio-social context. *Medical Anthropology Quarterly, 17*(4), 423–441.

Suls, J., & Rothman, A. (2004). Evolution of the biopsychosocial model: Prospects and challenges for health psychology. *Health Psychology, 23*(2), 119–125.

Turshen, M. (1989). *The politics of public health.* New Brunswick, NJ: Rutgers.

Waitzman, H. (1983). *The second sickness: Contradictions of capitalist health care.* New York: Free Press.

Wallerstein, I. (1974). *The modern world system.* New York: Academic Press.

5

Health and Illness Behavior

Jeannine Coreil

In public health research and practice, problems are often analyzed by the point of intervention in the illness process—that is, in terms of *primary, secondary,* and *tertiary prevention* (see Chapter 1). Social and behavioral scientists take a similar approach to examining the factors that influence different kinds of *health-related behaviors,* differentiated by where they occur in the illness process. Three types of health-related behavior have been identified (Gochman, 1997). *Health behavior* refers to actions taken in the absence of observable illness and includes primary prevention, such as diet and exercise, as well as some secondary prevention, such as screening for specific diseases. The term *illness behavior* is used to designate help-seeking behavior and diagnostic testing for obvious or suspected illness and includes consulting health care providers and engaging in self-care activities. The third type of health-related behavior traditionally addressed is *sick-role behavior;* this category encompasses all the things people do in response to a diagnosed illness. It includes adherence to prescribed treatment regimens as well as management of long-term chronic disease.

In the past 20 years, use of the term *sick role* has declined because of its limited applicability to chronic disease (see Chapter 7). Instead, attention has increasingly been focused on long-term coping, self-regulation, and disease management (Clark, 2003). This category corresponds to tertiary prevention in public health, or control of disease progression and prevention of disability and complications resulting from a condition. This chapter presents an overview of significant research findings in the area of sociobehavioral factors affecting health, illness, and disease management behavior. It differs from the approach taken in Chapter 3, "Social Epidemiology," in that it focuses on the determinants of health-related behavior as opposed to the determinants of health status, morbidity, and mortality. To give a specific example of this distinction, it is analogous to the distinction between "determinants of successful smoking cessation" and "smoking as a risk factor for disease."

HEALTH BEHAVIOR

As we saw in the preceding chapter, the most widely used theories and models focus heavily on intrapersonal or individual factors that influence health-related behavior. For example, cognitive factors such as knowledge about disease risks and protective behavior, beliefs related to personal susceptibility, attitudes and intentions regarding health-related behavior, and confidence in one's ability to perform preventive actions have been associated with health behavior across many studies (Rimer, 2002). Another individual-level focus of investigation has been the identification of personality types and/or traits and dispositional coping styles associated with health behavior. Although most research of this genre has focused on disease outcomes rather than health behavior per se, many health behaviors have been associated with psychological constructs such as negative affect, anger/hostility, pessimism/optimism, and conscientiousness (Booth-Kewley & Vickers, 1994). However, as research has accumulated, it has become clear that individual factors alone have limited explanatory power in understanding health behavior. The influence of contextual factors on individual behavior and the dynamic interplay between social, environmental, and intrapersonal factors increasingly have emerged as critical components in the health-illness process.

Interpersonal-level determinants of health behavior include factors such as parental role models, communication with peers and health care providers, social support, and other types of social influence. One particular behavior and population that has received much attention is the adoption of smoking among adolescents. Most smokers pick up the habit while still in their teens; thus, an important focus of primary prevention is to reduce initiation of tobacco use among youth. Parental behavior in general has been identified as an important social influence on adolescent smoking, not only in terms of directly modeling the behavior themselves but also, more indirectly, through parenting style. For example, an authoritative parenting style has been associated with a lower use of tobacco and alcohol in teenagers (Jackson, Henriksen, & Foshee, 1998). In Chapter 11, Mimi Nichter examines a variety of interpersonal influences on adolescent smoking, including the role of family members and peers in monitoring smoking patterns and providing feedback about observed escalation or inappropriate use.

The influence of more distal factors on health behavior, such as community and organizational context, and societal and policy influences, is less directly linked to health behavior and often operates through mediating variables such as social support and access to information, opportunities, and services. For example, as discussed more thoroughly in Chapter 17, children's food choices are often influenced by policies affecting school lunch menus as well as commercial marketing of dietary products to youth. Across all age groups, physical activity is influenced by societal norms for sedentary leisure pursuits, such as time spent watching television and access to safe places for outdoor recreation in different community settings.

Perhaps the most striking example of contextual influences on health behavior can be found in the realm of early detection of health problems through the use of screening services. Early detection is particularly relevant in the area of cancer control. Cancer-screening rates in the United States are comparable or higher than those found in other industrialized countries. A review of cancer-screening trends in the United States found that the most important determinants of cancer screening were having insurance coverage and a regular source of care, the organization of services, including the use of reminder systems, and policies affecting provider practices, such as routine recommendations for screening from physicians (Breen & Meissner, 2005). Insurance coverage for cancer screening is heavily influenced by what tests are covered by Medicare. Only relatively recently has Medicare coverage been extended to the major cancer-screening tests, including cervical cancer (1990), breast cancer (1991), colorectal cancer (1998), and prostate cancer (2000) (National Cancer Institute, 2008).

The newest trend in screening for disease has arrived in the form of genetic testing to identify persons who carry genes associated with specific conditions. Although genetic testing for certain conditions (e.g., sickle cell, see Chapter 2) has been around for decades, recent advances in biotechnology have greatly expanded the number of conditions for which tests are becoming available, generating a host of ethical, policy, and practice issues (Williams, Skirton, & Masny, 2006). This rapidly growing field promises to produce a new class of "at-risk" individuals who do not as yet have clinical signs of the disease, and may never develop it, but nevertheless may benefit from the knowledge of their risk status. Research on determinants of who chooses to have genetic testing is at an early stage (Anderson, 2007; Diefenbach & Hamrick, 2003) but, undoubtedly, will grow in the coming years.

CASE STUDY Physical Activity

Physical activity is one type of health behavior that is often studied using a multilevel ecological approach because of the importance of the built environment in which people live (Sallis & Owen, 1999). For example, physical "walkability" and perceived safety of neighborhoods have been correlated with level of physical activity. In addition to physical environments, research has documented the importance of individual perceptions such as exercise self-efficacy and psychosocial factors including social support for engaging in physical activity (Trost, Owen, Bauman, Sallis, & Brown, 2002).

One study investigated the relationships among neighborhood built environment characteristics, psychosocial factors, perceived and objective proximity to public trails, and use of the trails for exercise in a West Virginia community (Abildso, Zizzi, Abildso, Steele, & Gordon, 2007). The researchers found that perceptions of neighborhood walkability (e.g., presence or absence of sidewalks, heavy traffic, streetlights, enjoyable scenery, and high crime) influenced perceptions of trail proximity and use independent of objective distance from the trail. Use of the trail was also related to reported psychosocial barriers, such as lacking the time or energy to exercise. Another study focused on the social and cognitive correlates of leisure-time physical activity in a Latino population of central Illinois (Marquez & McAuley, 2006). Study participants with high levels of physical activity reported greater self-efficacy for exercising and overcoming the barriers to physical activity, received more social support from friends to exercise, and placed greater importance on the beneficial outcomes of activity compared with participants having low levels of physical activity. The above two studies are examples of empirical research demonstrating the importance of different levels of influence on health behavior.

Type A Behavior and Coronary Heart Disease

The behavioral epidemiology of coronary heart disease (CHD) is distinctive in that more than any other major public health problem, research has emphasized psychological risk factors in addition to sociocultural variables (Jenkins, 1988). CHD, the leading cause of death in the United States since about the mid-20th century, has been a primary national concern. Research has documented a number of behavioral factors that predispose individuals to hypertension, cardiac arrest, stroke, and other circulatory problems. Most of these behaviors cover the usual broad-spectrum health risks, such as age, socioeconomic status (SES), race, cigarette smoking, alcohol consumption, dietary fat consumption, sedentary lifestyle, blood lipids, and obesity. However, in addition, research has focused on psychological factors such as the Type A behavior pattern, hostility, and anger expression.

First described in the 1950s, the classic features of the Type A pattern included competitiveness, intense striving for achievement, easily provoked hostility, a sense of urgency, quick actions, punctuality, impatience, abrupt and rapid speech, emphatic gestures, and concentration on self-selected goals to the exclusion of other aspects of the environment (Prokop, Bradley, Burish, Anderson, & Fox, 1991). Numerous studies from 1960 to 1980 showed strong associations between Type A symptoms and CHD in diverse populations. After 1980, however, empirical results became more inconsistent, and researchers began investigating the effects of specific components of the behavior pattern, including chronic anger and hostility (King, 1997). In recent years, research has tended to focus particularly on hostility, expression of hostility, and cardiovascular reactivity (Taylor, 2006). People who tend to express hostile emotions, such as anger and cynicism, may be more at risk, and they may have stronger physiological responses to provoking situations. Researchers now suspect that the Type A behavior pattern itself may not cause CHD but it may increase exposure to acute stress because of the way individuals react to stressful situations (Gallacher, Sweetnam, Yarnell, Elwood, & Stansfield, 2003).

Depression and anxiety have also been suggested as important risk factors, although it is not clear whether Type A behavior and anger lead to depression and anxiety or whether the latter are independent risk factors for disease. A person who is anxious about meeting deadlines and feels in competition with others may begin to view the world in a hostile and cynical fashion and may eventually become emotionally exhausted by the struggle. Some have suggested that chronic arousal associated with confronting the world as an enemy is the common thread among the psychological risk factors for CHD.

Given the complexity of factors that interact in the process of chronic disease development, it is not surprising that studies attempting to isolate individual-level risks have found inconsistent results. For example, the characteristics of Type A behavior are reinforced by the environmental demands of many work settings of modern industrial societies, where there is unrelenting pressure to produce more, faster, and with fewer resources. In contrast to predictions that people would spend less time working as technology changed the workplace, the opposite has occurred, with people spending more and more time on the job and less time in leisure activities. Not surprisingly, work overload has been linked to increased risk of CHD. This association holds good for white-collar jobs as well as assembly-line work and seems to be particularly strong for occupational stress related to conflicting demands and low flex-ibility and control over the organization of work. The Japanese term *Karoshi* has been applied to describe this phenomenon of death from overwork. It has been implicated in 30,000 deaths per year in that country, and it has served as the basis for some wrongful-death suits filed against employers (Bowman, 2008).

Some critics have argued that if there is a "coronary-prone behavior pattern," it is not a personality defect but a conditioned way of acting that is embedded in social relationships (Radley, 1994). For this reason, it has been suggested that the Type A behavior pattern is a "culture-bound syndrome," that is, a disorder that occurs primarily and can be understood only within the context of a particular culture—in this case, Western culture, with its inexorable time urgency and capitalist competitiveness.

ILLNESS BEHAVIOR

When people experience bodily sensations, they often go through a process of appraising the symptoms as a possible sign of sickness. Then they react to what they perceive in a variety of ways. Some consult their doctor at the first sign that something might be wrong, while others put off seeking help until it is absolutely necessary or until others pressure them into taking action. Between the initial event of symptom recognition at the start of the illness process and being prescribed a treatment by a health care professional, many steps and sequences may take place. Social scientists have devoted considerable attention to the complex pathways through which sick persons evaluate and manage their health problems, for better or for worse. They have found that these pathways tend to follow predictable courses, and they have devel-oped conceptual models to explain the influence of factors at different points along the way. Central to all models is the assumption that illness behavior is a culturally and socially learned response pattern.

Researchers have approached the study of illness behavior from two general perspectives. One approach focuses on the process that unfolds over the course of the illness, including the appraisal stage, self-care activities, and patterns of help seeking. The unit of study is the entire illness episode. Studies of this type tend to be more subjective, descriptive, and qualitative in nature. Another approach focuses on identifying objective factors that predict utilization or choice of health services. The unit of study is a specific outcome or event, such as consulta-tion of a physician, the amount of health services used, or therapeutic choice among alterna-tives. The goal of such studies is to specify which variables predict the behavior in question. More often than not, quantitative analysis is used, guided by conceptual models of health service utilization.

The Illness Episode

When someone experiences troubling bodily sensations, the illness appraisal process usually begins with some kind of evaluation of the symptoms based on personal experience and culturally shared knowledge. Different disciplines use various terminologies to describe this interpretive process of attributing meaning to the sensations. For example, psychologists refer to illness representations (Leventhal, Brissette, & Levanthal, 2003) to describe the interpretation and elaboration of meaning assigned to somatic sensations. This occurs at an early stage in the appraisal process and may involve consultation with others in one's network or watching to observe changes in the sensation over time. The person may decide that the sensation is not a real symptom of illness and end the appraisal process without taking action. However, once a symptom is identified, or "recognized," and a tentative diagnostic label applied, a patterned response typically ensues, involving further assessment of the cause, duration, consequences, and appropriate remedial action. Some theorists, mostly from psychological backgrounds, use the term *attributions* (Lewis & Daltroy, 1990) to describe this evaluative process, while anthropologists have favored the term *explanatory model* of illness (see Chapter 8). Psychologists tend to emphasize the subjective and emotional dimensions of attribution, such as self-assessed level of health and the effects of mood states (e.g., depression, stress, and anxiety) on symptom interpretation. A good illustration of this approach is the study of older U.S. adults by Haug, Musil, Warner, and Morris (1998) to identify the effects of external stresses, psychological factors, health attitudes, and contextual variables on three types of illness representations (applying an illness label, consulting a physician, and engaging in self-care). Taking a different approach, anthropologists more often frame the appraisal process in terms of how people apply cultural models to recognized symptom constellations. For example, a study of Mexican American causal models of diabetes (Hunt, Valenzuela, & Pugh, 1998) identified the importance of *provoking factors,* such as self-indulgent behaviors and life crisis events, in the shared cultural models of the disease.

Earlier studies of illness behavior used various models of the help-seeking process based on stages, strategies, or categories of determinants. Stage models identify predictable sequences of therapeutic action, evaluation of outcomes, and subsequent decision making (Chrisman, 1977; Romanucci-Ross, 1969; Suchman, 1965). These models often incorporate the notion of *referral systems,* involving advice and recommendations from both professionals and nonprofessionals in one's social network. For example, Pescosolido (1992) applied a social network model to identify eight distinct strategies of health care use involving different combinations of consultation and behavior involving family, friends, coworkers, classmates, physicians, nonprescription drugs, home remedies, and no action. An example of a model using categories of determinants is Mechanic's general theory of help seeking (1978), which identifies four sources of influence: (1) salience and evaluation of symptoms; (2) degree of disruption in one's usual activities; (3) competing needs of those affected, including family and significant others; and (4) available coping resources, including treatment options.

More recently, research on the illness process has shifted toward a *narrative approach* that describes the experience in terms comparable to "telling a story." The account might be told or written by the person(s) directly involved, or it may be constructed through interaction with the primary parties. The focus is on understanding the meaning of the illness for those affected (Good & Good, 2000; Kleinman, 1988). For example, illness narratives often ascribe spiritual meaning to sickness (Koss-Chioino & Hefner, 2006). When interviewing is used to elicit the illness narrative, an attempt is made to allow the story to develop with minimal direction from the researcher in a "collaborative" fashion, where the interviewee is actively involved in the process. Autobiographical accounts of illness also fall under the narrative umbrella. For example, Kolker (1996) gives a first-person account of her experience with health care rationing, when her insurance company refused to pay for a bone marrow transplant recommended by her oncologist for treating breast cancer.

HEALTH CARE UTILIZATION

A large body of research has accumulated on the determinants of health care utilization. Utilization research is useful in assessing population needs for health care and in planning and evaluating health programs. In general, utilization studies have focused on three categories of factors: (1) patient characteristics and behavior, (2) provider characteristics and behavior (including interaction between provider and patient), (3) and health system factors.

By far, the greatest attention in research on illness behavior has been focused on utilization of formal medical services. There are probably many reasons for this, including the interests of funding agencies, concern for the economic aspects of health services, and a bias toward giving priority to "official" or "orthodox" therapy as opposed to self-help or alternative care. Nevertheless, interest in "complementary and alternative medicine" has steadily grown over the past two decades, among both consumers and researchers (Goldstein, 2000).

Patient-focused research has found that the main reasons people seek treatment for illness are when the troubling symptom is unusual or perceived to be serious and when the problem causes disability or disruption in important areas of life (Cameron, Levanthal, & Levanthal, 1995). The very young and the elderly use medical services more than other age groups, and as discussed in Chapter 6, women use more health services than men. Underutilization of services by persons of low SES and among minority groups is also discussed in other chapters of the book. People also sometimes overuse medical services, such as when they seek care to meet emotional needs unrelated to physical illness (De Jonge, Latour, & Huyse, 2003). In addition, because of the emphasis placed on attaining "high-level wellness" in Western culture along with constant media attention to health problems and marketing of new treatments, consumers are seeking care more often than is necessary (Petrie & Wessely, 2002).

The most influential and widely used model of health care utilization is Andersen's behavioral model of health services use (Aday & Andersen, 1974; Andersen, 1968, 1995). Originally devised to explain individual utilization of health services, the model identified three categories of influence: predisposing, enabling, and need characteristics. Over time, the model was expanded to encompass health care system variables as well as external environmental characteristics in explaining service utilization, and it has been applied as an intervention framework to promote equitable access to care. In using the model for improving access, the concept of mutability becomes important—that is, the degree to which a factor can be intentionally modified. For example, demographic and social structural variables are very difficult to change, while health beliefs and resources are much easier to modify, as noted in Chapter 3. The most recent formulation of the model also incorporates feedback from the perceived outcome of service use, such as evaluated health status and consumer satisfaction. In this version, the focus is on evaluating the performance of the medical care system (Aday & Awe, 1997).

Anthropological models of health care utilization have emphasized choice among pluralistic health options, including home-based and folk sector care, as well as bureaucratic medicine. This is not surprising given the continued reliance on nonprofessional therapy in developing-country settings, where many anthropologists continue to work. Early anthropological work on treatment choice applied a hierarchical model to explain the sequence of help seeking from home therapy to traditional healing and then modern medicine. As Western medicine became increasingly available and accepted, treatment choice patterns were better explained by applying decision modeling to individual episodes of illness. A good example of such decision models is Young's (1981) ethnomedical choice-making approach, which applied the four criteria of (1) illness gravity, (2) knowledge of a home remedy, (3) faith in the efficacy of a treatment, and (4) accessibility of a service. The utility of the model was assessed by comparing actual treatment choices with those predicted by the four criteria for a sample of illness episodes.

CASE STUDY   Illness Behavior

In a health systems model, such as Andersen's (1995) model, the focus of the study is the aggregate population, and it typically involves multivariate regression modeling of factors that "predict" aggregate patterns of health service use. The statistical model can be used to develop a conceptual model identifying which set of factors predicts the use of services. With a decision-theoretic model, on the other hand, the focus of study is the individual illness episode, in which the goal is to determine whether a particular case of help seeking correctly fits a predetermined set of decision criteria. In a sample of cases examined this way, the researcher can calculate the proportion of episodes "correctly" classified by the decision model.

Typically, researchers select a utilization model based on the goals of the study; however, in some instances, they are interested in comparing the relative utility of different models. Such was the case in Weller, Ruebush, and Klein's (1997) investigation of treatment-seeking behavior in Guatemala. Illness case histories ($N = 736$) were collected from a random sample of 270 households in six villages. Using the same data set, two predictive models, Andersen's health systems model (1968, 1995) and Young's (1981) decision-theoretic approach, were compared to determine which model better predicted health care choices among four main categories: (1) home- or store-bought remedies, (2) pharmacy medicines, (3) health post services, or (4) physician/hospital care. In this study, the health systems model better predicted illness behavior than the decision-theoretic approach. The systems model correctly classified 60% of cases, which was 23% better than chance, while the decision model correctly classified 48% of cases, only 9% better than chance. The authors noted that both models identified similar predictor variables (e.g., illness severity and loss of work) and that the two approaches have different strengths and weaknesses.

DISEASE MANAGEMENT BEHAVIOR

Once a person has been diagnosed with a specific illness and prescribed an appropriate treatment regimen, he or she is expected to follow the medical advice given. Failure to comply with treatment is socially disapproved and may even lead to negative sanctions, such as loss of the privileges associated with the sick role (see Chapter 7). Given such consequences, you might expect that patient compliance is usually very high, but in fact it often is not. It is estimated that 30% to 60% of patients fail to comply fully with treatments, and only about 50% of patients adhere to long-term-care regimens. About half of all patients also do not take medications properly, and for asymptomatic conditions, noncompliance rates rise to 75% (Becker & Maiman, 1975, 1980).

Concern for improving patient compliance was an important impetus for the early involvement of social scientists in medical settings. Seeking answers to questions such as "How can we get more patients to follow regimen X appropriately?" or "Why don't more people in the target population use our services?" a huge body of literature has been generated on patient compliance, or adherence to treatment. Between 1960 and 1995, close to 12,000 articles were published on this topic (Trostle, 1997). Studies have identified consistent determinants related to illness characteristics, patient variables, aspects of the medical encounter, and regimen factors. However, the concept of "compliance" and the literature focused on it have been the target of critical deconstruction in recent years. Central to this critique is the need to expose an implicit ideology of hierarchical power relations in compliance-oriented conceptualizations of patient behavior (Kotarba & Seidel, 1984; Trostle, 1997). In response to such criticisms, some researchers have adopted a less authoritarian terminology, such as "acceptance" of medical therapy, which accords greater latitude for patient agency in responding to recommended advice. As populations worldwide are living longer and health systems are challenged with the burden of chronic disease, attention in public health has increasingly focused on the control of chronic diseases, or tertiary prevention. Chronic conditions such as diabetes, asthma, hypertension, and obesity require long-term management strategies on the part of patients and their health care providers. The concept of self-regulation (See Chapter 4 for an overview of self-regulation theory) can be applied within a multilevel ecological framework of factors influencing patient management of chronic disease (Clark, 2003). This approach assumes the following:

> That intrapersonal and external factors give rise to and are modified by the observations, judgments, and reactions of the individual, leading him or her to undertake disease management strategies (including modification of the physical and social environments) to achieve a desired endpoint or goal. (Clark, 2003, p. 293)

The management of asthma, for example, may involve individual knowledge and beliefs about the condition; family support for appropriate administration of medication; and modifications in the home, work, or school environment. Living conditions and the ability to purchase special products, such as air-filtering systems, may constrain or enable desired actions.

Research on chronic disease has also focused on psychological adjustment and quality of life for patients living with long-term health problems. While most research has emphasized the negative consequences of chronic disease for mental health and well-being, some studies also highlight the positive aspects of adjustment, such a personal growth and development. Indeed, reviews of existing research note the heterogeneity of individual response to chronic disease across multiple life domains (Stanton, Revenson, & Tennen, 2007). Common concerns of patients include fear, pain, disruption of usual activities, physical limitations, and impact on social relationships. Persons living with chronic conditions are at an elevated risk for depression. Studies of adjustment have tended to focus on proximal factors—for example, personality attributes such as dispositional optimism, which has been found to positively influence coping strategies (Schou, Ekeberg, & Ruland, 2005). However, increasing attention also has been accorded to more distal contextual factors, including SES, culture, and ethnicity. For example, among African American and Latino cancer patients, faith and spirituality are notably more important aspects of adjustment compared with European cancer patients (Lee, Lin, Wrensch, Adler, & Eisenberg, 2000).

Research on patient adherence has identified several types of problems. To begin with, there are those individuals who fail to get their prescriptions filled or to begin treatment. More commonly, it is the interruption of the medication or regimen before completion that is problematic. Then there are those who take an incorrect dosage, do not follow the right schedule, or do not ingest medicines improperly. Finally, there is the problem of "supercompliance" with prescriptions received from multiple caregivers (Griffith, 1990).

Compounding the nonadherence problem is the fact that clinicians overestimate the extent to which their patients follow the recommended treatment. When clinicians do recognize noncompliance, they tend to see it as a problem residing with the patient and having little to do with their own interaction, or communication, with the patient. This view is reinforced by the fact that adherence research has emphasized patient variables and has neglected aspects of the medical encounter (Svarstad, 1987). Also, there are persistent methodological difficulties involved in monitoring patient compliance both in clinical practice and in research (Turk & Meichenbaum, 1991). Most studies have relied on patient self-report or physician estimation to measure compliance, but both of these approaches are subject to bias. Likewise, indirect assessments, such as measuring the remaining contents of medication supply, can also be unreliable because they can be manipulated. The most objective approach is the measurement of a medication or its metabolites in body fluids, but this technique can only be used with certain kinds of drugs and has limited applicability for behavioral regimens.

With regard to illness characteristics, adherence has been found to be lower for chronic illnesses, asymptomatic or minimally disruptive disorders, less severe disorders, socially unacceptable conditions, and incorrectly diagnosed problems. Less compliant patients tend to be at the older or younger extremes in age, have low health motivation, and perceive as slight both their own susceptibility to the illness and the seriousness of the illness. Some of the regimen factors that lower compliance are prolonged treatment, use of multiple medications or therapies, frequent administration of a drug or performance of an activity, costly treatment, side effects, and interference with one's usual lifestyle (DiMatteo, Giordani, Lepper, & Croghan, 2002).

Attention has been given to the dynamics of the medical encounter as sources of influence on patient adherence. For example, effective communication between practitioner and patient, as well as the degree of concern and supportiveness demonstrated by the clinician, improves patient adherence (Svarstad, 1987). Other findings point to the importance of providing patients the opportunity and encouragement to ask questions and express their feelings. The extent to which patient expectations are met also affects compliance, as does the level of congruence between the patient and the clinician's explanatory models of the illness.

Efforts to use research findings to devise strategies for improving patient adherence have generated several successful approaches (Becker & Maiman, 1980). One strategy is tailoring the regimen to the patient's daily activities so that following the treatment is less disruptive. Another technique is to introduce graduated regimen plans, which start out at a minimal level and then slowly build to full strength. With some patients, written or oral contracts have been found to be effective incentives, while with others the use of environmental cues works well. Attention to the social environment has also proved beneficial, such as enlisting family support and involvement in the patient's regimen (DiMatteo, 2004). With the specific problem of multiple medications, the use of fixed-ratio-combination drugs can reduce the number and simplify the schedule of pills prescribed.

In keeping with the medico-centric bias of compliance research, the dominant perspective of this area of study has been largely that of clinical practice. Problems of adherence have been accorded greater attention in medicine than in public health, because the latter is more concerned with prevention than with treatment. However, there are a few exceptions to this general rule. Public health authorities have long been concerned about chronic conditions and communicable diseases that require sustained therapeutic regimens to effectively control them. Among the chronic diseases that have been targeted for improved management are hypertension and diabetes, whereas communicable diseases of concern have been sexually transmitted diseases and tuberculosis (TB). In the following section, we take a closer look at the history of and current issues in TB control, a problem once considered a worry of the past. Midcentury optimism about the elimination of infectious diseases, thanks to an ever-expanding arsenal of antibiotic drugs, has been replaced with a more sober realization that infectious diseases will always be part of the human condition, with the most marginal social groups suffering the brunt of it. Moreover, we now recognize the alarming development of drug-resistant disease strains, a problem directly exacerbated by incomplete treatment of persons with the disease. The story of TB is instructive on all these issues.

⫸ **Focus:** TB Control ⫷

During the 18th and 19th centuries, TB was the leading cause of young adult mortality; it killed people slowly, available treatments were not very effective, and its victims were shunned and stigmatized within their communities. "Consumption" affected all classes of society, but then, as now, the poor and disadvantaged segments were disproportionately burdened with this disease. The discovery of microorganisms at the end of the 19th century, along with the development of effective antibiotic drugs, revolutionized the treatment of infectious diseases, such as TB, in industrial countries. In the 1940s, the new drug streptomycin was found to be particularly effective against *Mycobacterium tuberculosis,* the agent responsible for TB.

In 1900, the mortality rate from TB in the United States and Europe was more than 200 (per 100,000 population). Like other infectious diseases, incidence rates declined in the early part of the 20th century in response to improved health conditions and better nutrition. Following the introduction of streptomycin therapy, incidence rates declined further after 1950, reaching a low of 9.1 (per 100,000 population) during the early 1980s (Wilson, 1990, cited in Morisky & Cabrera, 1997). Since the mid-1980s, however, new cases of TB have increased dramatically worldwide. The World Health Organization (WHO, 2008) reports that by 2006, globally there were more than 9 million new cases of TB occurring each year, with close to 2 million deaths annually from the disease. About half a million cases of drug-resistant TB cases were also reported. The resurgence of TB has been attributed to several factors: its association with immunosuppression in HIV-infected persons; the emergence of drug-resistant strains of the bacillus; a deteriorating public health infrastructure; increased immigration from high-prevalence countries; and conditions associated with higher rates of homelessness and drug abuse in disadvantaged populations.

Despite the multifaceted nature of the "reemergence" of TB, however, many discussions of the problem tend to focus on issues of "noncompliance" within the active patient population. The weight given to this issue is reflected in the fact that "directly observed therapy" (DOT) has been accepted as the standard regimen for the treatment of TB patients considered to be at high risk for not maintaining or completing the typical 6-month course of multiple-drug therapy. DOT involves daily or biweekly doses of medication, a demanding schedule for any person.

Research on adherence or completion of TB treatment has identified a number of contributing factors (Munroe et al., 2007). Morisky and Cabrera (1997) apply a psychosocial model of behavior that organizes the factors into three categories: cognitive, environmental, and reinforcing. The types of cognitive factors that have been investigated reflect the early influence of the health belief model on research in this area. As noted earlier in this chapter, the health belief model was originally developed to guide research on behavior related to TB control, although the primary focus was screening behavior, not treatment. Not surprisingly, the cognitive factors investigated in research on compliance with TB treatment included knowledge about the disease, perceptions of severity and personal susceptibility, and the costs and benefits of treatment.

A wide range of environmental factors, both physical and social, have been linked with adherence to TB regimens. Among these are availability and accessibility of care, including location and facilities, physician competency, follow-up and referral systems, and both direct and hidden costs. It is also important to note aspects of the sociocultural environment, such as how TB fits into the health culture of the group affected (Rubel & Garro, 1992) and the degree of stigmatization from the health care system, family, and community (Hunt, Jordan, Irwin, & Browner, 1989). Because of its insidious transmission to close associates and its high prevalence among people who are poor and socially marginal, TB has long been viewed with dread and disdain by society. This is evident in the low status traditionally accorded to people who work in TB treatment programs. It also underlies the public perception that TB is no longer a serious health problem, because the populations that continue to be affected lack power and influence (people living in developing countries, the poor, immigrants, drug abusers, HIV/AIDS patients, the homeless, prisoners).

Thus far, we have addressed negative influences, or "barriers," to compliance with TB treatment. Determinants of successful therapy have also received attention. Such positive or reinforcing factors, according to Morisky and Cabrera's (1997) psychosocial model, include material, social, and organizational resources. There is considerable evidence that a successful treatment program must provide tangible incentives, such as food, cash, transportation vouchers, and other forms of direct compensation (Fujiwara, Larkin, & Frieden, 1997). Likewise, as is true for all types of sick-role behavior, a strong supportive network of family, friends, health care providers, and links to community services is important. In particular, the quality of patient-provider interaction, including communication of respect and caring, as well as attention to patients' basic welfare needs, is fundamental to the therapeutic process.

Because of the lengthy and frequent treatment involved in TB control, regimen failure tends to be high, which poses risks to the patient, close contacts, and the wider community. One of the most serious risks is the emergence of drug-resistant strains of TB; a high rate of such resistant strains in a community usually reflects an inadequate, or poorly functioning, local TB control program. The adoption of DOT as the standard regimen for TB treatment imposes strict standards of service, delivery, and organization within a program. It also requires a great deal more resources and political support than has characterized TB control in developed countries for much of the 20th century. The history of the New York City TB control program is instructive in this regard.

As in many major cities of the United States, the New York City Department of Health had a robust TB control program in the first half of the 20th century, but public funding, cutbacks, and a deteriorating public health infrastructure eroded the program (among others) during the 1970s and 1980s. The surge in new cases of TB observed in the mid- to late 1980s, and continuing through the 1990s and beyond, sparked a vigorous response from national, state, and local health agencies. In 1992, the city health department initiated a large-scale control program emphasizing DOT, with both clinic-based and outreach components. In the outreach program, community health workers visit patients at home, work, a local hangout, or some agreed-on secluded location and "observe" firsthand the patient taking the medication. In the clinic-based version of DOT, observation of treatment by the staff takes place at the clinic. While many programs reserve DOT for patients judged to be at risk for noncompliance (homeless, drug user, HIV infected, or having a previous history of noncompliance with TB treatment), New York City made DOT the standard procedure for management of all patients. Local commitment to such an intensive program was backed by a city ordinance that allowed mandatory treatment of infected persons and detention of individuals who could not be properly supervised to ensure that they follow treatment. These individuals were kept in a locked hospital ward for the course of their treatment. Between 1992 and 1995, the New York City program had reduced the number of TB cases by 34% and the number of multidrug-resistant cases by 75%, and it was commended by the WHO (Fujiwara et al., 1997).

Despite the success of DOT and other coercive measures, some critics reject the framing of the issue in terms of patient adherence altogether, arguing that locating the problem within the patient population diverts attention from the root cause of the resurgence of TB—widespread "structural violence" against the poor and the disenfranchised (Farmer, 1997, 1999). Critics fault the public health establishment for ignoring the fundamental social conditions that conspire to inflict disease scourges, TB being just one of many, on the world's poor. In the terminology of the Causal Continuum presented in Chapter 3, defining the problem in terms of adherence directs the focus to very proximate behavioral factors related to the sick role, while the critical perspective emphasizes more distal social structural influences.

CONCLUSION

The three main areas of health-related behavior (health behavior, illness behavior, and disease management behavior) correspond approximately to the fields of primary, secondary, and tertiary prevention in public health. Research on health-related behavior provides useful information for assessing population needs for health education and services and for planning and evaluating health programs. Understanding the factors that influence health behavior, for example, helps design interventions to promote lifestyle change and prevent the onset of disease. Determining what influences people to participate in screening programs can help identify ways to increase early detection of health problems. Research on help seeking and illness management can inform disease control initiatives, as well as provide insights into approaches to reduce treatment delay, improve management of chronic conditions, and increase adherence to prescribed therapy.

In the same way that the occurrence of disease can be analyzed in terms of distal, intermediate, and proximate determinants, health-related behavior is also influenced by multilevel factors, including social structure, cultural context, the organization of services, and individual characteristics. This chapter provides a general overview of research findings for health-related behavior. More in-depth discussions of behavioral components of particular health problems are presented in subsequent chapters.

REFERENCES

Abildso, C. G., Zizzi, S., Abildso, L. C., Steele, J. C., & Gordon, P. M. (2007). Built environment and psychosocial factors associated with trail proximity and use. *American Journal of Health Behavior, 21*(4), 374–383.

Aday, L. A., & Andersen, R. M. (1974). A framework for the study of access to medical care. *Health Services Research, 9,* 208–220.

Aday, L. A., & Awe, W. C. (1997). Health services utilization models. In D. S. Gochman (Ed.), *Handbook of health behavior research* (Vol. 1, pp. 153–172). New York: Plenum.

Andersen, R. (1968). *Behavioral model of families' use of health services.* Chicago: University of Chicago, Center for Health Administration Studies.

Andersen, R. (1995). Revisiting the behavioral model and access to medical care: Does it matter? *Journal of Health and Social Behavior, 36,* 1–10.

Anderson, G. (2007). Patient decision-making for clinical genetics. *Nursing Inquiry, 14*(1), 13–22.

Becker, M. H., & Maiman, L. A. (1975). Sociobehavioral determinants of compliance with health and medical care recommendations. *Medical Care, 13*(1), 10–24.

Becker, M. H., & Maiman, L. A. (1980). Strategies for enhancing patient compliance. *Journal of Community Health, 6*(2), 113–135.

Booth-Kewley, S., & Vickers, R. R. (1994). Associations between major domains of personality and health behavior. *Journal of Personality, 62,* 281–298.

Bowman, D. (2008) *Stress in the work place.* Retrieved May 2, 2008, from www.ttgconsultants.com/articles/stressworkplace.html

Breen, N., & Meissner, H. I. (2005). Toward a system of cancer screening in the United States: Trends and opportunities. *Annual Review of Public Health, 26,* 561–582.

Cameron, L., Leventhal, E. A., & Leventhal, H. (1995). Seeking medical care in response to symptoms and life stress. *Psychosomatic Medicine, 57*(1), 37–47.

Chrisman, N. J. (1977). The help-seeking process: An approach to the natural history of illness. *Culture, Medicine and Psychiatry, 1*(4), 351–377.

Clark, N. M. (2003). Management of chronic disease by patients. *Annual Review of Public Health, 24,* 289–313.

De Jonge, P., Latour, C., & Huyse, F. J. (2003). Implementing psychiatric interventions on a medical ward: Effects on patients' quality of life and length of hospital stay. *Psychosomatic Medicine, 6,* 997–1002.

Diefenbach, M. A., & Hamrick, N. (2003). Self-regulation and genetic testing: Theory, practical considerations and interventions. In L. D. Cameron & H. Levanthal (Eds.), *The regulation of health and illness behavior* (pp. 314–331). New York: Routledge.

DiMatteo, M. R. (2004). Social support and patient adherence: A meta-analysis. *Health Psychology 23,* 207–218.

DiMatteo, M. R., Giordani, P. J., Lepper, H. S., & Croghan, T. W. (2002). Patient adherence and medical treatment outcomes: A meta-analysis. *Medical Care 40,* 794–811.

Farmer, P. (1997). Social scientists and the new tuberculosis. *Social Science & Medicine, 43*(3), 347–358.

Farmer, P. (1999). *Infections and inequality.* San Francisco: University of California Press.

Fujiwara, P. I., Larkin, C., & Frieden, T. R. (1997). Directly observed therapy in New York City: History, implementation, results, and challenges. *Clinics in Chest Medicine, 18*(1), 135–148.

Gallacher, J. E., Sweetnam, P. M., Yarnell, J. W. G., Elwood, P. C., & Stansfield, S. A. (2003). Is Type A behavior really a trigger for coronary heart disease events? *Psychosomatic Medicine, 65,* 338–349.

Gochman, D. S. (1997). *Handbook of health behavior research.* New York: Plenum.

Goldstein, M. S. (2000). The growing acceptance of complementary and alternative medicine. In C. E. Bird, P. Conrad, & A. M. Fremont (Eds.), *Handbook of medical sociology* (5th ed., pp. 284–297). Upper Saddle River, NJ: Prentice Hall.

Good, M. D., & Good, B. J. (2000). Clinical narratives and the study of contemporary doctor-patient relationships. In G. L. Albrecht, R. Fitzpatrick., & S. C. Scrimshaw (Eds.), *Social studies in health & medicine* (pp. 243–258). London: Sage.

Griffith, S. (1990). A review of the factors associated with patient compliance and the taking of prescribed medicines. *British Journal of General Practice, 40*(332), 114–116.

Haug, M. R., Musil, C. M., Warner, C. D., & Morris, D. I. (1998). Interpreting bodily changes as illness: A longitudinal study of older adults. *Social Science & Medicine, 46*(12), 1553–1567.

Hunt, L. M., Jordan, B., Irwin, S., & Browner, C. H. (1989). Compliance and the patient's perspective: Controlling symptoms in everyday life. *Culture, Medicine and Psychiatry, 13,* 215–334.

Hunt, L. M., Valenzuela, M. A., & Pugh, J. A. (1998). Porque me toco a mi? Mexican-American diabetes patients' causal stories and their relationship to treatment. *Social Science & Medicine, 46,* 959–969.

Jackson, C., Henriksen, L., & Foshee, V. A. (1998). The authoritative parenting style index: Predicting health risk behaviors among children and adolescents. *Health Education & Behavior, 25,* 319–337.

Jenkins, C. D. (1988). Epidemiology of cardiovascular diseases. *Journal of Consulting and Clinical Psychology, 56*(3), 324–332.

King, K. B. (1997). Psychologic and social aspects of cardiovascular disease. *Annals of Behavioral Medicine, 19*(3), 264–270.

Kleinman, A. (1988). *The illness narratives: Suffering, healing and the human condition.* New York: Basic Books.

Kolker, A. (1996). Thrown overboard: The human costs of health care rationing. In C. Ellis & A. P. Bochner (Eds.), *Composing ethnography: Alternative forms of qualitative writing* (pp. 132–159). Walnut Creek, CA: Sage.

Koss-Chioino, J. D., & Hefner, P. (Eds.). (2006). *Spiritual transformation and healing: Anthropological, theological, neuroscientific, and clinical perspectives.* Lanham, MD: AltaMira Press.

Kotarba, J. A., & Seidel, J. V. (1984). Managing the problem pain patient: Compliance or social control. *Social Science & Medicine, 19,* 1393–1400.

Lee, M. M., Lin, S. S., Wrensch, M. R., Adler, S. R., & Eisenberg, D. (2000). Alternative therapies used by women with breast cancer in four ethnic populations. *Journal of the National Cancer Institute, 92,* 42–47.

Leventhal, H., Brissette, I., & Leventhal, E. A. (2003). The common-sense model of self-regulation of health and illness. In L. D. Cameron & H. Levanthal (Eds.), *The self-regulation of health and illness* (pp. 42–65). London: Routledge.

Lewis, F., & Daltroy, L. (1990). How causal explanations influence health behavior: Attribution theory. In K. Glanz, F. Lewis, & B. Rimer (Eds.), *Health behavior and health education: Theory, research, and practice* (pp. 92–114). San Francisco: Jossey-Bass.

Marquez, D. X., & McAuley, E. (2006). Social cognitive correlates of leisure time physical activity among Latinos. *Journal of Behavioral Medicine, 29*(3), 281–289.

Mechanic, D. (1978). *Medical sociology: A comprehensive text* (2nd ed.). New York: Free Press.

Morisky, D. E., & Cabrera, D. M. (1997). Compliance with antituberculosis regimens and the role of behavioral interventions. In D. S. Gochman (Ed.), *Handbook of health behavior research* (Vol. 2, pp. 269–284). New York: Plenum Press.

Munroe, S. A., Lewin, S. A., Smith, H. J., Engle, M. E., Fretheim, A., & Volmink, J. (2007). Patient adherence to tuberculosis treatment: A systematic review of qualitative research. *Public Library of Science Medicine, 4*(7), 1230–1245.

National Cancer Institute. (2008). *SEER-Medicare: Cancer testing covered by Medicare.* Retrieved May 1, 2008, from http://healthservices.cancer.gov/seermedicare/considerations/testing.html

Pescosolido, B. A. (1992). Beyond rational choice: The social dynamics of how people seek help. *American Journal of Sociology, 97*(4), 1096–1138.

Petrie, K. J., & Wessely, S. (2002). Modern worries, new technology, and medicine. *British Journal of Medicine, 324,* 690–691.

Prokop, C. K., Bradley, L. A., Burish, T. G., Anderson, F. O., & Fox, J. E. (1991). *Health psychology: Clinical methods and research.* New York: Macmillan.

Radley, A. (1994). *The social psychology of health and disease.* London: Sage.

Rimer, R. (2002). Perspectives on intrapersonal theories of health behavior. In K. Glanz, B. K. Rimer, & F. M. Lewis (Eds.), *Health behavior and health education: Theory, research and practice* (3rd ed., pp. 144–160). San Francisco: Jossey-Bass.

Romanucci-Ross, L. (1969). The hierarchy of resort in curative practices: The admiralty islands, Melanesia. *Journal of Health and Social Behavior, 10,* 201–209.

Rubel, A. J., & Garro, L. C. (1992). Social and cultural factors in the successful control of tuberculosis. *Public Health Reports, 107*(6), 626–636.

Sallis, J. F., & Owen, N. (1999). *Physical activity and behavioral medicine.* Thousand Oaks, CA: Sage.

Schou, I., Ekeberg, O., & Ruland, C. M. (2005). The mediating role of appraisal and coping in the relationship between optimism-pessimism and quality of life. *Psycho-Oncology, 14,* 718–727.

Stanton, A. L., Revenson, T. A., & Tennen, H. (2007). Health psychology: Psychological adjustment to chronic disease. *Annual Review of Psychology, 58,* 565–592.

Suchman, E. (1965). Stages of illness and medical care. *Journal of Health and Human Behavior, 6,* 114–128.

Svarstad, B. (1987). Physician-patient communication and patient conformity with medical advice. In L. H. Aiken & D. Mechanic (Eds.), *Applications of social science to clinical medicine and health policy* (pp. 438–459). New Brunswick, NJ: Rutgers University Press.

Taylor, S. (2006). *Health psychology* (6th ed.). Boston: McGraw-Hill.

Trost, S. G., Owen, N., Bauman, A. E., Sallis, J. F., & Brown, W. (2002). Correlates of adults' participation in physical activity: Review and update. *Medicine and Science in Sports Exercise, 34*(12), 1996–2001.

Trostle, J. A. (1997). The history and meaning of patient compliance as an ideology. In D. S. Gochman (Ed.), *Handbook of health behavior* (Vol. 2, pp. 109–124). New York: Plenum.

Turk, D. C., & Meichenbaum, D. (1991). Adherence to self-care regimens: The patient's perspective. In R. H. Rozensky, J. J. Sweet, & Tovian, S. M. (Eds.), *Handbook of clinical psychology in medical settings* (pp. 249–266). New York: Plenum Press.

Weller, S. C., Ruebush, T. R., & Klein, R. E. (1997). Predicting treatment-seeking behavior in Guatemala: A comparison of the health services research and decision-theoretic approaches. *Medical Anthropology Quarterly, 11*(2), 224–245.

Williams, J. K., Skirton, H., & Masny, A. (2006). Ethics, policy and educational issues in genetic testing. *Nursing Scholarship, 38*(2), 119–125.

World Health Organization. (2008). *Global tuberculosis control: Surveillance, planning, financing* (WHO/HTM/TB/2008.393). Geneva: Author. Retrieved April 20, 2008, from www.who.int/tb/publications/global_report/2008/en/index.html

Young, J. C. (1981). *Medical choice in a Mexican village.* New Brunswick, NJ: Rutgers University Press.

6

The Social Environment and Health

Jeannine Coreil

The social environment constitutes an important component of the human ecosystem and frames our understanding of health and illness. Simply stated, the social environment is made up of all the human groups, social systems, and institutional settings that we belong to and interact with in our lives. It includes both the microlevel environment, such as family, work groups, friends, and community organizations, as well as the macrolevel environment, such as professional associations, government agencies, social institutions, and society at large. Concepts and theory related to the social environment are strongly based in sociology and social psychology, the disciplines that study the relationship between the individual and larger social systems, as well as relationships among social entities.

Broadly conceptualized, the social environment encompasses the entire spectrum of proximate to distal factors influencing health and cross-cuts multiple levels of the ecosystem (Berkman & Glass, 2000). At the interpersonal level, constructs such as social influence, social support, and role models have been studied in relation to health. Family systems and peer groups figure importantly at this level of analysis. At the organizational level, work settings, schools, churches, and health care systems represent important components of the social environment. The impact of community-level factors, such as ethnicity and social class, are discussed in other chapters. Chapter 14 discusses community-based interventions to promote health, such as mobilizing community participation through coalitions. The relationship between social capital and population health is discussed later in this chapter. At the societal level, social structure, gender roles, government policies, cultural patterns, and educational systems influence health problems. These macrolevel social environmental factors are addressed in Chapters 3 and 8.

In this chapter, we look at selected aspects of the social environment, including social support, with a special focus on illness support groups, social capital, family systems, and gender roles and the ways in which these domains can affect both the illness process and coping responses.

INTERPERSONAL LEVEL: SOCIAL SUPPORT

Social support can be defined as aid and assistance exchanged through social relationships and interpersonal transactions (Heaney & Israel, 2002). Like stress, social support can have both positive and negative dimensions. While most research on social support has focused on its health-enhancing effects, there is a downside to too much support. For example, being enmeshed in a very dense network of social ties, such as is characteristic of people with deep bonds with the extended family, can generate undesirable social pressures (Rook, 1992). In such situations, social obligations to participate in activities and provide support may outweigh the benefits gained from social integration. However, the vast majority of studies of social support investigate positive aspects.

The literature on social support typically distinguishes four different types: (1) *emotional* (expressions of empathy, love, trust, and caring), (2) *instrumental* (tangible aid and service), (3) *informational* (advice, suggestions, and information), and (4) *appraisal* (information that is useful for self-evaluation). Some researchers also have differentiated between direct and indirect social support and between formal and informal social support (Pearlin & Aneshensel, 1987).

One of the earliest influential studies examined the relationship between the level of supportive relationships a woman had during pregnancy and the frequency of complications she experienced during labor and delivery. In that study, Nuckolls and his colleagues (1972) found that fewer supportive relationships, coupled with high stress, led to greater pregnancy complications. Other research on the positive benefits of social support has focused on the positive attributes of being married. The positive effects of marriage are striking: Married people have lower morbidity and mortality at all ages and for both genders and exhibit higher levels of mental health than their unmarried counterparts. However, there is some question regarding the directionality of the relationship between marital status and health. Much of the research relies on cross-sectional studies, in which it is unclear whether mentally healthy people are more likely to marry (the *social selection* hypothesis) or whether marriage itself leads to better health status (the *social causation* hypothesis).

Because of the limitations of cross-sectional studies, investigators have turned to prospective studies to measure the effects of social support on health outcomes. In a well-known study, Berkman and Syme (1979) interviewed 2,229 men and 2,496 women aged 30 to 69 years living in Almeda County, California, in 1965. Four measures of social support were taken: (1) marital status, (2) contacts with family and friends, (3) church membership, and (4) other formal and informal affiliations. Over the succeeding 9 years, each of the measures of social support independently predicted mortality at follow-up, with marital status and family contact having the strongest effects. A decade later, House, Robbins, and Metzner (1982) replicated and extended this study in Tecumseh, Michigan. These researchers conducted interviews as well as physical exams on 1,322 men and 1,432 women aged 35 to 69. Three measures of social support were (1) intimate social relationships, (2) formal group affiliation, and (3) leisure activities with social network members. Over a follow-up period of 10 to 12 years, significant health benefits of social support were found.

Other replication studies in the United States and Europe confirm the above findings linking social support to positive health outcomes. Furthermore, the evidence shows that the physical health impact of social support is nonspecific; that is, overall morbidity and mortality are enhanced but not the risk of particular medical conditions (Berkman & Glass, 2000). Also, rather than a dose-response type of effect, social support appears to have a curvilinear relationship to health, especially for men living in small communities. At very low levels, lack of support has a strong negative effect on health. At moderate levels, it has a protective effect, but this impact decreases at higher levels.

Interestingly, the strength of the relationship between social support and health seems to vary across different types of communities. Its effects appear to be strongest and most linear for men and women who live in urban areas. In small communities, on the other hand, the association is weaker for women and nonlinear for men, as noted above. Some observers suggest that this gender difference is probably due to the smaller variance and the fewer numbers of women experiencing the lowest levels of support in small communities (Thoits, 1995).

Overall, there is a notable gender pattern in the research findings for social support and health. The association with health benefits is much stronger among men than among women (Williams, 2003). This is consistent with studies of marriage and death of a spouse, where being married is more beneficial for men and being widowed is more detrimental for men than for women. Also, men tend to remarry sooner than women following divorce or the death of a spouse. One explanation for this gender difference is that women benefit more from relationships with female friends and relatives and are less dependent than men on the support derived from marriage. Alternatively, older single men may be socially and demographically in greater demand than their female counterparts, making remarriage easier for them.

Despite the emergence of a rich literature documenting the nature of the association between social support and health, we still lack a good understanding of the biopsychosocial processes that mediate this association, and we know very little about the macrosocial processes that give rise to various social relationships and supports (Berkman, Glass, Brissette, & Seaman, 2000). For example, it is likely that large-scale social changes, such as women entering the workforce in record numbers, the insidious persistence of racial discrimination, and the increasing social isolation of urban environments, contribute to the underlying phenomenon captured by individual measures of social support. A better understanding of the intermediate pathways of effect would give us a better handle on potential interventions to circumvent negative consequences.

Some of the hypotheses that have been advanced regarding the micro- and macrolevel effects for social support on health include biological, psychological, and behavioral mechanisms. At the biological level, it has been suggested that social support reduces cardiovascular and other arousal, thereby triggering the relaxation response that is conducive to adaptation. At the psychological level, social support is suggested to enhance cognitive appraisal of external stress, as when a potential stressor is perceived as nonthreatening. Finally, behavioral explanations posit that social support is associated with a healthier lifestyle, through both direct and indirect regulation of health behavior.

INTERPERSONAL LEVEL: FAMILY SYSTEMS

Family systems can be defined as small, dynamic, semiclosed groups composed of members who have mutual obligations to provide a broad range of emotional and material support. Families have structure, functions, assigned roles, modes of interacting, resources, group culture, and a history that forms part of the developmental or life cycle of the group. Structurally, families are often categorized as nuclear, extended, or attenuated—that is, having more or less members than the basic nuclear core of parents and children. Many of the functions performed by families are societal processes that must be achieved to ensure the survival of the species: reproduction; socialization of children; social control; and provision of food, clothing, shelter, security, social support, and identity. In some societies, families also function as units of economic production, such as in agricultural populations. Contemporary families tend to be viewed more as consumption units, although interest in the household production of health (i.e., investments toward health goals) has grown in recent years.

Many aspects of health status are closely linked to the family environment in which people live. To illustrate some of these, we draw on findings from a study of health and U.S. families conducted by the National Center for Health Statistics (Collins & LeClere, 1996). As previously noted, married persons enjoy many health benefits that unmarried people do not. For example, married men and women of all ages are less likely to be limited in activity due to illness than single, separated, divorced, or widowed individuals. Moreover, middle-aged adults who live alone have higher rates of doctor visits, acute conditions, and short- and long-term disability. It has been suggested that persons living with a spouse are likely to have better health profiles because of lifestyle differences, such as better eating habits and having someone to share a problem with, and because of higher income. The confounding of family composition with income can be problematic. Children living with a single parent or adult report a higher prevalence of activity limitation, disability, and hospitalization and are more likely to be in fair or poor health than children living with two parents. However, children living in the poorest families also report a higher level of activity limitation, poor or fair health, and hospitalization than those in families with higher incomes. Thus, it is difficult to disentangle family structure from economic factors in studies of health impacts.

COMMUNITY LEVEL: SOCIAL CAPITAL

Over the past two decades, interest among scholars has grown in understanding the relationship between social capital and health. As noted in Chapter 4, research on social capital and health grew out of a renewed interest in the influence of neighborhoods and communities on health conditions. *Social capital* is a structural quality of collectivities and "refers to the institutions, relationships, and norms that shape the quality and quantity of social interactions" within a focal community (World Bank, 2004). Communities that are strong in social participation, shared norms, mutual trust, and reciprocity are considered to have high levels of social capital. Such communities are strengthened by greater cohesiveness and collective efforts of coordination and cooperation for mutual benefit (Putnam, 2000). The ability of collectivities to mobilize for action to solve shared problems is sometimes referred to as collective efficacy.

Research on a wide range of public health problems has documented a positive relationship between social capital, and health and well-being. One state-level study found a relationship between social cohesion and trust, on the one hand, and overall age-adjusted mortality rates, on the other (Kawachi, Kennedy, Lochner, & Prothrow-Smith, 1997). Lower levels of trust were associated with higher mortality rates for the major causes of death, including coronary heart disease, cerebrovascular disease, malignant neoplasms, and unintentional injury, as well as infant mortality. Another state-level study found a relationship between social capital and individual self-rated health, controlling for individual risk factors such as smoking, obesity, income, and lack of access to health care (Kawachi, Kennedy, & Glass, 1999). Other studies have found associations between social capital and particular health problems, including mental distress (Campbell, Cornish, & McLean, 2004), violence (Galea, Karpati, & Kennedy, 2002), STI/AIDS (Holtgrave & Crosby, 2003), and adolescent birth rates (Gold, Kennedy, Connell, & Kawachi, 2002).

Across disciplines and research topics, as well as outside the field of health, quite a bit of variation exists in how social capital is conceptualized and measured (Baum & Ziersch, 2003). Social epidemiologic research has emphasized the broader construct of social cohesion—that is, social norms that enable cooperation, reciprocity, and mutual trust (Kawachi & Berkman, 2000). Political scientists have given greater attention to participation in civil society, such as membership in voluntary associations, church groups, sports clubs, and the like, as well as public service and volunteer work, in the creation of social capital (Putnam, 2000). In the education arena, researchers have focused on the role of families and schools in generating social capital through the educational achievement of children (Coleman, 1988). Sociological research has emphasized neighborhood social networks and collective efficacy, especially the ability of local residents to actively engage in social control actions (Sampson, 2003).

Research on social capital and health fits into the broader study of the social environment of communities, much of it influenced by sociological theories of urban ecology and social disorganization (Robert, 1999). The focus of this research is to identify the community-level effects of local environments on the well-being of residents, independent of individual-level risk factors. Many studies in this area have been conducted in high-poverty urban neighborhoods, with the aim of discerning how disadvantaged settings affect individual life chances and quality of life over and above individual socioeconomic position. Poor neighborhoods are associated with ethnic diversity, high rates of residential mobility, social disorganization, and high rates of crime and delinquency. It has been suggested that fear of traveling safely in a community can affect health through social isolation, stress, lack of physical activity, and limited access to services (Robert, 1999).

Some poor communities do have strong *social cohesion*, in which residents interact primarily with others in their neighborhood and have high levels of trust and reciprocity within the group, yet this apparent social capital does not always translate into favorable outcomes. Wilson (1996) proposed a theory to account for this discrepancy. He argued that many poor communities fail to mobilize action for the common good because in these settings the dense social ties do not lead to collective efficacy. In these settings, people have strong within-group relationships but few ties with the mainstream society outside, which would provide access to resources. They also often perceive low levels of control over the local environment, such as crime, safety, the built environment, and services, including its influence on their children. The lack of ties with institutions in the wider community is sometimes referred to as the absence of *bridging capital* in the social capital literature, in contrast to *bonding capital*, which refers to within-group ties (Putnam, 2000). According to this distinction, poor, dangerous neighborhoods might score high in bonding capital but low in bridging capital, and the latter may account for the unfavorable outcomes. There is a growing consensus that bonding capital must precede bridging capital for a community to achieve collective efficacy.

Public health practitioners are beginning to incorporate the concept of social capital in designing interventions, particularly in working with socially and economically disadvantaged communities. The aim of such interventions is to develop or use social capital in such a way that it furthers the goals of health programs. Examples of possible strategies to develop social capital include strengthening coalitions, community networks, participation in voluntary associations, volunteer activities, intergenerational ties, and political participation.

COMMUNITY LEVEL: SUPPORT GROUPS

One of the most remarkable phenomena of recent times is the rapid proliferation of health-related self-help groups in Western society, especially in the United States. There are literally thousands of different kinds of support groups for every imaginable life problem, more than 2,000, in fact, for illness conditions alone. There exist mutual aid entities for every disease recognized by the World Health Association, even the rarest and the most obscure. For example, ever hear of the Arachnoiditis Information and Support Network? No, it is not for people afraid of spiders; it is a self-help group for people affected by a condition that destroys the pia mater of the brain. In addition to groups that meet face-to-face, there has also been an explosion of electronic mutual interest groups that meet through the Internet and in cyberspace. Generally speaking, support group participants tend to be female, white, well-educated professionals, although this sociodemographic profile varies with type of group (Kessler, Mickelson, & Zhao, 1997). For example, men predominate in Alcoholics Anonymous (AA) but are rarely seen at Weight Watchers. There are more support groups for women's health issues, such as breast cancer, than for men's health problems, such as prostate cancer.

Some writers make distinctions between self-help, mutual aid, and support groups. The term *self-help* covers the efforts of both individuals and groups to help themselves, although it is used more often in the context of peer-led group behavior. *Mutual aid*, on the other hand, has the broadest reference and includes people helping others in a variety of domains, such as fund-raising and political advocacy as well as social support. The term *support group* is the most commonly used term to denote groups whose primary functions are supportive communication through group dynamics. Some organizations reserve the term *support group* for professionally led groups, while others use the label for peer-led groups or for any kind of self-help group regardless of leadership.

Despite the ubiquitousness and popularity of health-related support groups, surprisingly little scholarly research has been conducted in this area (Riessman & Carroll, 1995). Research from members' own perspectives consistently shows that the most important benefit experienced by participants is the social support provided through interaction with others similarly affected by a health problem (Levine, 1988). Health care professionals' interest in support groups, in contrast, has tended to focus on the role that such groups can play in facilitating therapeutic goals, including adherence to medical regimens.

Self-help groups offer a unique setting for examining aspects of the broader social environment of health because they are like microcosms that frame larger, more complex social systems (Luke, Roberts, & Rappaport, 1993). The groups encompass not only the individual participants present but also the family systems of which they are a part, as well as their linkages to the health care system, gender structures, and other social institutions. They also represent an excellent example of community-based health resources that operate outside the expert-dominated "official" health services sector.

Probably the earliest, and certainly the most influential, health-related support group is AA. Established in 1935, AA has inspired an array of behavioral disorder self-help groups, all based on the "12-step" model of spiritual self-awareness, behavior change, reconciliation with significant others, and sharing the lessons learned with other members. Like many support groups, AA and other 12-step groups also stress the importance of regular participation in group meetings. Likewise, Weight Watchers, the most influential and widespread weight control support group, emphasizes the necessity of meeting attendance for long-term success with the "program." Another early prototype mutual aid group was the Paralyzed Veterans Association, founded in 1946. Still active today, this group exemplifies the advocacy-oriented organization that conducts fund-raising and lobbies for legislative action and social policy.

Self-help groups have become particularly strong in the area of health-related problems. There are a number of reasons for this. In the late 20th century, we came to recognize the limits of scientific medicine in solving our health problems. At the same time, interest in alternative medicine and approaches grew and gained credibility. There was a backlash to the rampant commercialization of health care in an attempt to preserve the humanistic dimensions of care for the sick. All this fit in with the growing consumer movement that stressed empowerment of lay persons to take control of their own health care. It was also the time when we realized that there would never be enough health care resources to meet all society's needs, that some kind of economizing would be needed. Support groups offer a low-cost alternative to expensive, high-tech medicine. Increased focus on "prevention" as a more cost-effective approach gained attention. Finally, the Women's Movement influenced the health scene through its promotion of "consciousness-raising groups," self-care, and patient rights.

Health-related support groups help millions of people around the world, yet very little attention has been given to this topic in the research or policy literature. Moreover, the benefits of support groups are ignored in economic analyses of disability and quality of life. What factors might account for this? Powell (1994) cites the "culture of professional privilege" as underlying the widespread disregard for support groups. Support groups represent a competing power base within the medical community. Professionals tend to regard peer-led support groups with skepticism, suspicion, and sometimes outright antagonism. One survey found that 90% of professionals think that their colleagues believe there are "serious risks" involved in joining a support group (Chesler, 1990). The perceived risks include misinformation, bad advice, and interference with recommended treatment regimens. Research conducted by professionals on the benefits of support groups has tended to impose an outsider's definition of success, such as "compliance with treatment," instead of members' own definitions, such as adopting a new "meaning" for their illness experience. There are also pragmatic reasons for the paucity of research on support groups. Funding agencies are interested primarily in research on client use of professional services because they are part of the business of selling these services to customers; peer-led support groups do not have market value.

Research on the components of "support" that participants find through self-help groups has identified several common dimensions (Levine & Perkins, 1987). The groups promote a psychological sense of community and an ideology that serves as a philosophical antidote to the problems members face. Often this ideology is incorporated into "sacred writings," such as AA's "Big Book." The meetings provide an opportunity for confession, catharsis, and mutual criticism. Observing other role models and hearing their stories offer coping strategies for day-to-day living. Participants expand their social networks through ties with other members.

If we apply some of the concepts of social support discussed earlier in this chapter, we can say that self-help groups provide many different kinds of support to members: emotional, instrumental, informational, and appraisal. Participants receive empathy, practical assistance, and advice and find a new way of thinking about their illnesses. These forms of support are typically experienced through informal and indirect means. Participation leads to changes in feelings, attitudes, and behavior as a result of the member's internalizing and using a socially shared ideology that offers a useful interpretation of the person's situation (Levine & Perkins, 1987).

SOCIETAL LEVEL: SOCIAL ROLES, SOCIAL STRUCTURE, AND SOCIAL CONSTRUCTION

A great deal of writing about the social environment has been based on the concept of *social roles*—that is, the behavioral norms and expectations associated with a defined status or position in the social structure. For example, people fulfill multiple roles in their lives, including that of spouse, parent, employee, club member, and citizen, each role influencing their personal health situation in distinct ways. The kind of influence one's role may have on health has been conceptualized in various ways, such as the notion of health risks associated with a role or how role demands affect help seeking and the recovery process. Mothers' competing roles in child care and employment have been studied as a possible barrier to seeking health care for their children. In the sociomedical sciences, there has been considerable research on the roles of health care providers and patients, as well as the role of family members in medical care. Studies of role strain in nurses, for instance, examine the multiple demands on the job for efficiency, caring, and technical expertise. In recent years, however, interest in role theory as an explanatory framework for the social environment has waned somewhat. Attention has shifted to *social construction* and *political economy* as theoretical frameworks for social relations.

Cross-cultural and historical studies provide insights into the social construction of gender. Through comparisons across different social settings and time periods, insights can be gained about how much of what we think of as "gender" is basic human nature and how much is culturally constructed and therefore flexible. For example, Margaret Mead's early work on sex and temperament challenged Western notions of sex-based differences in personality characteristics such as nurturance and aggression, and subsequent cross-cultural studies documented substantial variation in gender roles (Schlegel & Barry, 1991). Evolutionary perspectives on gender relations have also challenged assumptions about sex roles; for example, foraging societies are known to be more egalitarian than more complex societies regarding the division of labor between men and women. Historical research on different time periods provides insights into how men's and women's life circumstances affected their health status, such as the effects of war and military duty on the lives and health of men (Leavitt, 1984).

Political-economic research in health emphasizes the social structural relations that underlie unequal access to power and wealth in a society (Fee & Krieger, 1994). For example, a political-economic explanation of gender differences in health might highlight the effects of gender discrimination in education and employment or the exploitation of female sexuality in advertising and commercial marketing (Doyal, 1995).

Theory of Gender and Power

One political-economic theory that incorporates multiple social ecological levels is the theory of gender and power (Wingood & DeClemente, 2002). Originally developed by Robert Connell (1987), the theory is a social structural model that examines three major structures that characterize social relations between men and women. The three structures consist of the sexual division of labor, the sexual division of power, and the structure of social norms and affective attachments. Each structure can be viewed as operating at the societal, institutional, and individual levels of risk factors, including behavioral and biological factors.

Wingood and DiClemente (2002) illustrate the application of the model to HIV risk among women in the United States. The sexual division of labor allocates men and women to certain occupations, which creates inequities in the earning potential of women. This, in turn, increases women's risk of living in poverty, being unemployed or underemployed, and working in high-demand/low-control environments. The sexual division of power focuses on unequal power relations between men and women, leading to risks for women, such as those stemming from male abuse of authority and control in intimate relationships. For example, women often have limited control over sexual behavior, such as the use of condoms, because of unequal negotiating power in their relationships with male partners. They also may be vulnerable to physical violence, exposed to sexually oriented media, and placed at risk in sexual relationships with a high-risk partner. The structure of social norms and affective attachments highlights the way societal norms dictate appropriate sexual behavior for women and shapes women's perceptions of themselves and others. It may lead to the enforcement of strict gender roles and stereotypical beliefs, such as the idea that women's sexuality should be limited to procreation. These factors may in turn be linked to limited knowledge of HIV prevention or beliefs unsupportive of safer sex. Although space does not permit a detailed examination of the ways in which the theory can be translated into preventive interventions, it is worth noting that such interventions incorporate multilevel components that address risks in all three structures of gender and power.

Gender Differences in Health

Earlier approaches to gender focused on *sex differences* and *sex roles* primarily from the standpoint of individual characteristics and behavior. Sex roles were defined in terms of individual psychology, incorporating concepts such as identity, personality, and socialization. It was assumed that much of the sex role distinctions found in a society derived ultimately from biological sex differences and reproductive-role functions, although the social elaboration of the patterns was not necessarily considered to be determined by biology. This notion of sex roles has been increasingly replaced by the perspective of gender as a *social institution*—that is, a complex, organized system with associated ideology and structure—that permeates many aspects of human social life (Lorber, 1997). This perspective views gender as socially constructed, that is, given meaning and substance through social relations (Schofield, Connell, Walker, Wood, & Butland, 2000). Our images and expectations of what "male" and "female" signify are produced through everyday interactions as well as social structural processes (e.g., what the "church" and the educational system say and do). Like other domains of culture such as kinship, religion, and technology, gender affects the lives of individuals, families, and other social institutions. Gender ideology shapes the way we think about the world, and gender stratification reflects the hierarchical order of privilege and power one gender exercises over the other (Doyal, 1995). For example, gender ideology assigns certain characteristics to women, such as emotionality, which may result in differential diagnosis of men and women exhibiting similar psychiatric symptoms. Gender stratification, on the other hand, is reflected in the fact that occupations dominated primarily by women have less prestige and lower salaries than those associated with males.

The terms *sex* and *gender* have come to be used to refer to the biological and social aspects of maleness and femaleness, respectively. Thus, sex differences include anatomical, physiological, hormonal, and reproductive processes, while gender refers to socially defined attributes. A rephrasing of the old nature-nurture question, then, would be, "Is it sex or gender, or both?" This age-old question is still very much alive in the field of gender studies. For example, take the phenomenon of the mortality gap. Around the world, women live longer than men in every society, a pattern that first emerged in the 20th century. In Western industrialized countries, there is an average of 6 to 7 years' difference between male and female life expectancy. The magnitude of the longevity gap varies among countries: In Russia, it is 13 years (72 vs. 59); in the United States, the gap is 5 years (80 vs. 75); and in Nigeria, it is only 1 year (47 vs. 46) (Yin, 2007).

Various hypotheses put forth to explain the differential longevity between women and men have emphasized biological factors (Collins, 1993). First, there is the fertility hypothesis. As we have seen, in foraging and agricultural societies, women typically spend most of their lives either pregnant or lactating, which requires a certain physiological robustness. In industrial societies, lower fertility makes fewer biological demands on women's lives, so they live longer. Also, lower maternal mortality in modern times contributes to overall gains in female life expectancy. A second hypothesis points to the importance of hormones. This theory begins with the fact that male sex hormones provide a favorable environment for the production of low-density lipoproteins, which increase the risk of heart disease, while female hormones boost the production of high-density lipoproteins, which are protective against coronary disease. Add to this men's less healthy lifestyle (improper diet, alcohol, tobacco), and you have a coronary-disease-prone gender group. Finally, it has been suggested that chromosomes may hold the key; that is, men may be genetically programmed to live at a faster pace, and therefore have shorter lives, than women. However, biological explanations are also influenced by social construction processes in that the selection of particular physiological and genetic characteristics for explanatory emphasis tends to validate existing cultural beliefs about gender (Fausto-Sterling, 2000).

Greater understanding of gender effects in some cases has called into question whether some apparent epidemiologic differences are, in fact, real. The case of depression is a good illustration. The relative contribution of biological and social factors to women's higher rate of clinical depression has been debated for some time (American Psychological Association, 2002). As medical understanding of the disease has moved increasingly toward a chemical-imbalance model, with treatment focused on medication, biological explanations of sex differences have gained favor. At the same time, political-economic studies of gender have demonstrated how the health consequences of gender stratification and social disadvantage cannot be ignored in the social production of illness, including depression. Women's depression may be directly related to their disadvantaged position relative to men in society. This is consistent with the view that depression is higher across all groups that experience social discrimination, including the poor and uneducated, who struggle to make a living. Women's systematic exclusion from the power structures of industrial society probably contributes significantly to their depression. However, there is also the view that the prevalence of depression may be more similar across the sexes than we think, because it is simply expressed differently in men and women. Men tend to express emotional problems to a greater degree through aggressive behavior, antisocial activity, and substance abuse, which accounts for the higher rate of violent crime and chemical addiction among men. Additionally, women are socialized to talk about their feelings more openly than men and in conversation are more inclined to reveal feelings of sadness and other negative affects. Such gender differences may mask a large amount of depression in men that goes undiagnosed.

Gender politics shapes the social construction of public health problems in various ways. The significance accorded to particular problems, as reflected in media attention, research funding, targeted programs, and the like, can be influenced by the way advocacy groups frame the issue. For instance, breast and prostate cancer have similar morbidity and mortality in the United States; there are roughly 200,000 new cases per year and about 40,000 deaths annually. Yet for many years, breast cancer has enjoyed a much higher profile in the public eye than prostate cancer. More programs and financial support for research and treatment of breast cancer exist, and it is common to see stories in the media about celebrities and public figures who faced this disease. In contrast, advocacy groups for prostate cancer have faced perplexing obstacles in getting the public interested in their cause. Screening for prostate cancer lags far behind early detection of breast cancer, insurance coverage for routine testing remains controversial, and comparatively little money goes into research. This can be partly explained by the lack of clarity and consensus regarding appropriate treatment for prostate cancer. However, some analysts also attribute the imbalance to our cultural preoccupation with the female body as a sex object, others to the greater organization around women's health issues because of the Women's Movement. Following the lead of women activists, men's organizations are beginning to organize politically to lobby for greater support for prostate cancer and other health problems specific to men.

It fits with the broader gender culture of Western nations that women's health issues are portrayed in a sympathetic light, while men's health issues are often socially constructed to reflect the prevailing negative stereotypes of men and their behavior. Feminists have portrayed the female condition in terms of women being victims of discrimination and subjugation, a narrative that fits with contemporary problems such as domestic violence and depression. Men's health issues, on the other hand, have been described in terms of the just consequences of unhealthy male behavior—their bad habits, such as smoking, drinking, eating fatty food, getting into fights, driving too fast, or indulging in "couch potato" laziness. Headlines such as "Men's Health: Their Own Worst Enemies" (Williamson, 1995) place responsibility on the men themselves for their ills. This interpretation is consistent with gender ideology that describes men as autonomous agents actively controlling their lives and health, even to the extreme of taking excessive risks and acting recklessly. Women, in contrast, are portrayed as passive subjects, often as victims, living out their lives at the mercy of outside influences. As men's health issues begin to receive increased attention, undoubtedly there will be greater awareness of the social pressures that influence men's health.

Gender-focused research on the health care system has addressed a variety of issues related to occupational roles, professional socialization, communication in medical settings, and gender hierarchies in the health labor force. The latter topic, for example, has been addressed from a political-economic perspective by examining the patterns of gender segregation and the corresponding inequalities in income, status, and power. Although women make up 75% of the health labor force, they are concentrated in the lower-status occupations within the health care hierarchy. Only 2% of all female health workers earn the higher levels of income realized by 46% of all male health workers. Also, women who enter traditionally male-dominated technical curative fields earn on average less than half of what men do (Butter, Carpenter, Kay, & Simmons, 1994). Gender bias in the wage gap is partly explained by the fact that "women's work" tends to be devalued in a male-dominated patriarchal society.

⋙ **Focus:** Men's Health ⋙

As an area of specialized study and policy formulation, men's health, compared with women's health, is in an early stage of development (Sabo, 2005; Sabo & Gordon, 1995). One reason for this lag is that for a long time, gender and health research was largely confined to women's health issues. The formative literature on men's health tends to emphasize epidemiologic and sociological perspectives on the observed contrasts between men's and women's health issues. For example, gender differences in overall mortality and in the specific causes of mortality are often highlighted. Males across societies at different stages of development share a common pattern of dying at higher rates than their female counterparts, although the excess mortality observed among males is even more pronounced in industrialized countries (see Table 6.1). In market economies, the ratio of male to female mortality is greater than 2:1, while in developing countries the relative risk of death ranges from 1.17 to 1.39 for men. Much of this differential stems from the fact that men suffer from serious heart disease much more frequently than women. However, among people who get heart attacks, women die more often than men, possibly in part because coronary events are often treated more aggressively in men.

Explanations for male health disadvantages often invoke sociological explanations, such as role expectations and occupational pressures. Scholarly writers still cite as relevant Brannon's early (1976) description of four aspects of Western male identity: (1) "no sissy stuff," (2) "the big wheel," (3) "the sturdy oak," and (4) "give 'em hell." Possible health effects of these idealizations of male identity might include (1) their lack of preventive behaviors and greater risk taking (no sissy stuff), (2) injury-related competitiveness and stress-related frustration (the big wheel), (3) denial of symptoms and delay in seeking treatment (the sturdy oak), and (4) a high rate of male-to-male violence, heavy drinking, and fast driving (give 'em hell).

Male gender identity, and notions of "masculinity" in particular, have been given greater attention in men's health studies generally, compared with the corresponding emphasis on "femininity" in women's health. Courtenay (2000) proposes that health-related beliefs and behavior, like other social practices of men and women, can be seen

TABLE 6.1 Male/Female (M/F) Mortality Ratio (Age: 15–60 years) for Industrial and Developing Countries

	M/F Mortality Ratio
Industrialized countries	
Market	2.31
Nonmarket	1.93
Developing world	
Asia	1.17
Latin America/Caribbean	1.52
Middle East/North Africa	1.17
Sub-Saharan Africa	1.19

SOURCE: Murray, C. J. L., Yang, G., & Qiao, X. (1992). Adult Mortality: Patterns and Causes. In R. G. A. Feachem, T. Kjellstrom, M. Over, and M. A. Phillips (Eds.), *The Health of Adults in the Developing World* (pp. 23–222). New York: Oxford University Press.

as ways of demonstrating masculinity and femininity. In other words, men and women use health behaviors in everyday life as part of a more complex construction of gender identity. For example, men's "denial and disregard for physical discomfort, risk and health care needs are all ways of demonstrating difference from women, who are presumed to embody these 'feminine' characteristics" (Courtenay, 2000, p. 1390).

Men who hold traditional beliefs on masculinity have been shown to engage in greater health risk behavior than men who have less traditional beliefs about masculinity (Courtenay, 2003). The use of steroids among male body builders, despite its serious health risks, has been linked to psychological attempts to achieve the masculine ideal of large size, strength, power, mastery of self and others, and bravery in the face of pain (Klein, 1995; Morrison, Morrison, & Hopkins, 2003). Male patients' responses to reproductive health problems, such as testicular cancer, also focus on self-image and masculinity as key influences (Gordon, 1995). Similarly, the differential health risks of African American males, including higher rates of homicide, suicide, drug use, HIV/AIDS, and other sexually transmitted diseases, has been explained with reference to black men's pursuit of the masculine mystique (Staples, 1995). In addition, patterns of high-risk sexual behavior among gay and bisexual men have been linked to masculine sexual scripts that encourage sexual conquest and the pursuit of danger and excitement in sexual encounters (Levine & Kimmel, 1998). Like many health-related issues, it is important to keep in mind the interconnections between gender and other social factors, including sexuality, race, and social class.

Perhaps because women's health issues have been so politicized, men's health issues also tend to trigger political redefinitions of the problem, often in terms of gender equality and discrimination. For example, when the male impotence drug Viagra burst onto the health scene, its rapid consumer demand and the ensuing debate about insurance coverage sparked pointed criticism from feminist camps that have long fought to get medical coverage of contraceptive pills by insurance companies. That the male sexual function, which some interpreted as "pleasure," was considered a legitimate medical concern but the need to practice birth control was not struck many people as a blatant sexist double standard.

In the practice arena of men's health, the focus has been on health promotion and lifestyle change, that is, getting men to live healthier lives and reduce specific risks such as substance abuse and cigarette smoking. In Britain, where the field of men's health is generally considered by scholars to be more evolved than elsewhere, the men's health and wellness clinic model has gained acceptance (Griffiths, 1996; Piper, 1997; Williamson, 1995), but specialized men's clinics are rare in the United States. Most writers support the position that men's health practice should be broadly defined to include psychosocial as well as physical dimensions of health (Rees & Jones, 1995; Robertson, 1995), including the less common issues for men, such as sexual assault (Rentoul & Appleboom, 1997).

CONCLUSION

In this chapter, we focus attention on selected aspects of the social environment that affect health, namely gender, social support, social capital, and family systems. Many other topics could be addressed under this rubric; indeed, in a sense, the entire book relates to the social environment in one way or another. Thus, the chapter amplifies certain dimensions of the social ecology of health organizing framework, from the microlevel of the family to intermediate systems, such as social capital and support groups, to macrolevel societal structures, such as gender roles. It reviews both theoretical frameworks and approaches to intervention that emphasize the role of the social environment in shaping individuals and protecting them from health risks.

REFERENCES

American Psychological Association. (2002, April). *Summit on women and depression: Proceedings and recommendations* (Conference Report). Washington, DC: Author. Retrieved May 4, 2008, from www.apa.org/pi/wpo/women&depression.pdf

Baum, F., & Ziersch, A. M. (2003). Social capital. *Journal of Epidemiology and Community Health, 57,* 320–323.

Berkman, L. F., & Glass, T. (2000). Social integration, social networks, social support, and health. In L. F. Berkman & I. Kawachi (Eds.), *Social Epidemiology* (pp. 137–173). Oxford, UK: Oxford University Press.

Berkman, L. F., Glass, T., Brissette, I., & Seeman, T. E. (2000). From social integration to health: Durkheim in the new millennium. *Social Science & Medicine, 51,* 843–857.

Berkman, L. F., & Syme, S. L. (1979). Social networks, host resistance, and mortality: A 9 year follow-up study of Alameda County residents. *American Journal of Epidemiology, 109,* 186–204.

Brannon, R. (1976). The male sex role: Our culture's blueprint of manhood, and what it's done for us lately. In D. David & R. Brannon (Eds.), *The forty-nine percent majority.* Reading, MA: Addison-Wesley.

Butter, I. H., Carpenter, E. S., Kay, B. J., & Simmons, R. S. (1994). Gender hierarchies in the health labor force. In E. Fee & N. Krieger (Eds.), *Women's health, politics, and power: Essays on sex/gender, medicine, and public health.* Amityville, NY: Baywood.

Campbell, C., Cornish, F., & McLean, C. (2004). Social capital, participation and the perpetuation of health inequalities: Obstacles to African-Caribbean participation in "partnerships" to improve mental health. *Ethnicity and Health, 9*(3), 305–327.

Chesler, M. A. (1990). The "dangers" of self-help groups: Understanding and challenging professionals' views. In T. J. Powell (Ed.), *Working with self-help* (pp. 119–139). Silver Spring, MD: NASW Press.

Coleman, J. S. (1988). Social capital in the creation of human capital. *American Journal of Sociology, 94*(Suppl.), S95–S120.

Collins, J. G., & LeClere, F. B. (1996). Health and selected socioeconomic characteristics of the family: United States, 1988–1990. *Vital Health Statistics, 10*(195), 1–85. Washington, DC: National Center for Health Statistics.

Collins, R. (1993). Why do women live longer than men? *New Scientist, 140*(1896), 45.

Connell, R. W. (1987). *Gender and power.* Stanford, CA: Stanford University Press.

Courtenay, W. H. (2000). Constructions of masculinity and their influence on men's well-being: A theory of gender and health. *Social Science & Medicine, 50*(10), 1385–1401.

Courtenay, W. H. (2003). Key determinants of the health and well-being of men and boys. *International Journal of Men's Health, 2*(1), 1–30.

Doyal, L. (1995). *What makes women sick: Gender and the political economy of health.* New Brunswick, NJ: Rutgers University Press.

Fausto-Sterling, A. (2000). *Sexing the body: Gender politics and the construction of sexuality.* New York: Basic Books.

Fee, E., & Krieger, N. (Eds.). (1994). *Women's health, politics, and power: Essays on sex/gender, medicine and public health.* Amityville, NY: Baywood.

Galea, S., Karpati, A., & Kennedy, B. (2002). Social capital and violence in the United States, 1974–1993. *Social Science & Medicine, 55*(8), 1373–1383.

Gold, R., Kennedy, B., Connell, F., & Kawachi, I. (2002). Teen births, income inequality, and social capital: Developing an understanding of the causal pathway. *Health & Place, 8*(2), 77–83.

Gordon, D. F. (1995). Testicular cancer and masculinity. In D. Sabo & D. F. Gordon (Eds.), *Men's health and illness: Gender, power and the body* (pp. 246–265). Thousand Oaks, CA: Sage.

Griffiths, S. (1996). Men's health. *British Medical Journal, 312,* 69–70.

Heaney, C. A., & Israel, B. A. (2002). Social networks and social support. In K. Glanz, F. M. Lewis, & B. K. Rimer (Eds.), *Health behavior and health education: Theory, research, and practice* (3rd ed., pp. 189–209). San Francisco: Jossey-Bass.

Holtgrave, D. R., & Crosby, R. A. (2003). Social capital, poverty, and income inequality as predictors of gonorrhea, syphilis, chlamydia and AIDS case rates in the United States. *Sexually Transmitted Infections, 79*(1), 62–64.

House, J. S., Robbins, C., & Metzner, H. M. (1982). The association of social relationships and activities with mortality: Prospective evidence from the Tecumseh Community Health Study. *American Journal of Epidemiology, 116,* 123–140.

Kawachi, I., & Berkman, L. (2000). Social cohesion, social capital, and health. In L. Berkman & I. Kawachi (Eds.), *Social epidemiology* (pp. 174–190). New York: Oxford University Press.

Kawachi, I., Kennedy, B. P., & Glass, R. (1999). Social capital and self-rated health: A contextual analysis. *American Journal of Public Health, 89,* 1187–1193.

Kawachi, I., Kennedy, B. P., Lochner, K., & Prothrow-Smith, D. (1997). Social capital, income inequality, and mortality. *American Journal of Public Health, 87,* 1491–1498.

Kessler, R. C., Mickelson, K. D., & Zhao, S. (1997). Patterns and correlates of self-help group membership in the United States. *Social Policy* (Spring), 27–46.

Klein, A. M. (1995). *Life's too short to die small.* Thousand Oaks, CA: Sage.

Leavitt, J. W. (Ed.). (1984). *Women and health in America: Historical readings.* Madison: University of Wisconsin Press.

Levine, M. (1988). An analysis of mutual assistance. *American Journal of Community Psychology, 16*(2), 167–188.

Levine, M., & Perkins, D. V. (1987). *Principles of community psychology: Perspectives and applications.* New York: Oxford University Press.

Levine, M. P., & Kimmel, M. S. (1998). *Gay macho: The life and death of the homosexual clone.* New York: New York University Press.

Lorber, J. (1997). *Gender and the social construction of illness.* Thousand Oaks, CA: Sage.

Luke, D. A., Roberts, L., & Rappaport, J. (1993). Individual, group context, and individual-group fit predictors of self-help group attendance. *Journal of Applied Behavioral Science, 29*(2), 216–238.

Morrison, T. G., Morrison, M. A., & Hopkins, C. (2003). Striving for bodily perfection? An exploration of the drive for muscularity in Canadian men. *Psychology of Men & Masculinity, 4*(2), 111–120.

Murray, C. J. L., Yang, G., & Qiao, X. (1992). Adult mortality: Patterns and causes. In R. G. A. Feachem, T. Kjellstrom, M. Over, & M. A. Phillips (Eds.), *The health of adults in the developing world* (pp. 23–222). New York: Oxford University Press.

Nuckolls, K., Cassel, J., & Kaplan, B. (1972). Psychosocial assets, life crisis and the prognosis of pregnancy. *American Journal of Epidemiology, 95,* 431–441.

Pearlin, L. I., & Aneshensel, C. S. (1987). Coping and social supports: Their functions and applications. In L. Aiken & D. Mechanic (Eds.), *Applications of social science to clinical medicine and health policy* (pp. 417–437). New Brunswick, NJ: Rutgers University Press.

Piper, S. (1997). The limitations of well men clinics for health education. *Nursing Standard, 11*(30), 47–49.

Powell, T. J. (1994). *Understanding the self-help organization: Frameworks and findings.* Thousand Oaks, CA: Sage.

Putnam, R. D. (2000). *Bowling alone: The collapse and revival of American community.* New York: Simon & Schuster.

Rees, C., & Jones, M. (1995). Exploring men's health in a men-only group. *Nursing Standard, 9*(43), 38–40.

Rentoul, L., & Appleboom, N. (1997). Understanding the psychological impact of rape and serious sexual assault of men: A literature review. *Journal of Psychiatric and Mental Health Nursing, 4,* 267–274.

Riessman, F., & Carroll, D. (1995). *Redefining self-help: Policy and practice.* San Francisco: Jossey-Bass.

Robert, S. A. (1999). Socioeconomic position and health: The independent contribution of community socioeconomic context. *Annual Review of Sociology, 25,* 489–516.

Robertson, S. (1995). Men's health promotion in the U.K.: A hidden problem. *British Journal of Nursing, 4*(7), 382–401.

Rook, K. (1992). Detrimental aspects of social relationships: Taking stock of an emerging literature. In H. O. F. Veiel & U. Baumann (Eds.), *The meaning and measurement of social support* (pp. 157–169). New York: Hemisphere.

Sabo, D. (2005). The studies of masculinities and men's health. In M. S. Kimmel, J. Hearn, & R. W. Connell (Eds.), *Handbook of studies on men and masculinities.* Thousand Oaks, CA: Sage.

Sabo, D., & Gordon, D. F. (Eds.). (1995). *Men's health and illness: Gender, power and the body.* Thousand Oaks, CA: Sage.

Sampson, R. J. (2003). Neighborhood-level context and health: Lessons from sociology. In I. Kawachi & L. F. Berkman (Eds.), *Neighborhoods and health* (pp. 132–146). New York: Oxford University Press.

Schlegel, A., & Barry, H., III. (1991). *Adolescence: An anthropological inquiry.* New York: Free Press.

Schofield, T., Connell, R. W., Walker, L., Wood, J. F., & Butland, D. L. (2000). Understanding men's health and illness: A gender-relations approach to policy, research, and practice. *Journal of American College Health, 48*(6), 247–256.

Staples, R. (1995). *Health among African-American males.* Thousand Oaks, CA: Sage.

Thoits, P. A. (1995). Stress, coping, and social support processes: Where are we? What next? *Journal of Health and Social Behavior, 35*(Extra issue), 53–79.

Williams, D. R. (2003). The health of men: Structured inequalities and opportunities. *American Journal of Public Health, 93,* 724–731.

Williamson, P. (1995). Men's health: Their own worst enemies. *Nursing Times, 91*(48), 24–26.

Wilson, W. J. (1996). *When work disappears.* New York: Knopf.

Wingood, G. M., & DiClemente, R. J. (2002). The theory of gender and power: A social structural theory for guiding public health interventions. In R. J. DiClemente, R. Crosby, & M. C. Kegler (Eds.), *Emerging theories in health promotion practice and research* (pp. 313–346). San Francisco: Jossey-Bass.

World Bank. (2004). *Social capital for development.* Retrieved December 13, 2006, from www.world bank.org/poverty/scapital/index.htm

Yin, S. (2007). *Gender disparities in health and mortality* (Population Reference Bureau). Retrieved May 4, 2008, from www.prb.org/Articles/2007/genderdisparities.aspx?p=1

PART III

Sociocultural Context of Health

The chapters in this section focus on system-level responses to illness, including collective behavior in the control of deviance, the cultural dimensions of health care, and the social construction of public health approaches to health disparities and cultural diversity.

Chapter 7 examines social reactions to disease from the standpoint of illness as a form of deviance, collective behavior in times of crisis, the illness labeling process, and the impact of stigmatized conditions. Processes of medicalization illustrate forms of collective behavior with consequences for individuals and institutions, including the pervasive "at-risk" role. A case study of stigma and tuberculosis highlights the key issues presented in the chapter.

Taking a cross-cultural perspective on health culture, Chapter 8 overviews cultural concepts of illness and care, including cultural models and the organizational cultures of medicine and public health. Frameworks are presented for studying different healing systems and their component sectors. Cultural models of illness are defined and illustrated with examples from research on breast cancer in different ethnic groups. Organizational culture concepts are defined and applied to medicine and public health, and a case study of cultural values in public health departments is presented.

Chapter 9 takes a critical approach to the current discourse on health disparities, diversity, and cultural competence. The concept of race in epidemiologic research is explored in light of current debates regarding the meaning, relevance, and consequence of framing health disparities along racial lines. Approaches to cultural competence likewise are scrutinized for underlying assumptions and unbalanced attention to patient culture. The social construction of cultural diversity in public health is explored and illustrated through an example focused on Haitians in South Florida.

CHAPTER

7

Social Reactions to Disease

Jeannine Coreil

In the preceding chapters, the focus has been on how social factors influence the prevention and control of disease. This chapter takes a different view and examines social *reactions to* disease and health problems. It looks at the process of social reaction in terms of *social control* and *collective behavior*. One of the basic functions of society is to regulate human behavior by keeping people in conformance with the prevailing social norms. This is done through various mechanisms of social control, such as taboos, laws, policies, incarceration, ostracism, social influence, and gossip. There is always a certain degree of variation from acceptable behavior, but too much deviance is a threat to the stability and harmony of the group. Also, some societies and historical periods are more tolerant of divergent lifestyles and conduct than others, while some are noted for their rigid enforcement of correct behavior.

Medical sociologists make a distinction between normative and situational deviance (Pfuhl & Henry, 1993). *Normative deviance* occurs by choice and includes behavior considered immoral, unlawful, or irresponsible. For example, engaging in behaviors known to be bad for one's health, such as smoking, or taking health-related risks, such as riding a motorcycle without a helmet, often leads to censure and blame if it causes health problems. Circumstances that are out of one's control, on the other hand, are considered *situational deviance,* and the affected individuals are not held responsible for it. Victims of misfortune, accidents, and many illnesses are examples of the latter form of deviance. This distinction is relevant for understanding social reactions to disease, because health problems attributed to normative deviance are often stigmatized and treated differently than those attributed to situational deviance, in which the affected persons are not held responsible.

Social control can take various forms, ranging from highly institutionalized to very subtle and informal means. Legislative bodies pass laws designed to deter activities considered harmful to individuals and groups. Age restrictions on the purchase of alcohol and cigarettes would be an example of such laws. Law enforcement and the criminal justice system are very formal institutions with the primary purpose of controlling illegal behavior and enforcing punishment for serious crimes. Government and other bureaucratic regulations as well as social and political policies also serve to shape the behavior of individuals and organizations in deliberate ways. Religious institutions play an important role in upholding moral and ethical standards by condemning certain acts as sinful as well as by reinforcing approved values and ideals. In fact, most social institutions, such as churches, schools, and the media, play a part in the control of deviance. The less visible forms of influence include social ostracism, stigma, and gossip.

Illness, regardless of perceived cause, affects the community in which it occurs. When people get sick, they are unable to function normally and may have to neglect their usual responsibilities. They miss work and cannot take care of personal and familial duties. Others must fill in for them until they get well. If too many people get sick at the same time, it can cause undue strain on the system. For example, employers become concerned if workers take too many sick days as it affects productivity, and multiple illnesses within families can be devastating for the group. In public health, there is concern for protecting the health of communities by controlling the transmission of communicable diseases (see discussion of tuberculosis [TB] control, Chapter 5). The extreme case is an epidemic crisis, where large numbers of people are debilitated or perish within single communities, sometimes leading to a breakdown in the basic functions of everyday life. Thus, the impact of individual or group illness can affect the internal stability of a community by resulting in shifting social norms or the development of new mechanisms for control.

SOCIAL CONTROL OF DEVIANCE

Being Sick Versus at Risk

In the 1950s, the sociologist Talcott Parsons (1951) developed the notion of illness as deviance through his delineation of the *sick role*. Like all social roles, the sick role has attendant rights and duties, which are recognized by society. The classic view of the sick role was based on American health culture during the 1950s and 1960s and was primarily oriented to social expectations in acute illness episodes. It is less applicable to chronic conditions such as hypertension and diabetes, from which people do not "recover" but must be managed over many years. The original model of the sick role included the following aspects. Becoming ill is considered outside a person's control, therefore the sick person is blameless and deserving of sympathy and special privileges. Because of the physical debilitation of illness, the sick person is exempt from the usual responsibilities, and certain indulgences are allowed. For example, we expect sick people to be more dependent, demanding, and self-centered than a well person. However, illness is thought to be undesirable, so the sick person should want to get well and relinquish the role as quickly as possible. To do this, the sick person is expected to seek professional treatment when needed and to comply with prescribed therapy. Refusal to follow doctor's orders can jeopardize one's claims to the privileges of the sick role.

The potential for abuse of the sick role is always there; people can use illness as an excuse for avoiding their obligations (e.g., missing work, skipping school, or canceling an engagement). To counteract this misuse, institutions employ control mechanisms, such as requiring a note from one's doctor to miss work or, in the case of schools, a parent's written verification of illness. Likewise, someone who appears to be exaggerating his or her debilitation or carrying on too long may be accused of malingering, and the person's claims to the sick role may be questioned. In Parson's (1951) view, doctors play a gatekeeper role by exercising authority to legitimize or deny claims to the sick role. However, the changing nature of health problems and medical care management has attenuated the central role of physicians in the illness process.

There have been many criticisms of the sick role concept since its original formulation (Gallagher, 1979; Segall, 1997). As noted above, it is most applicable to acute illnesses that are time limited and treatable with curative therapy. Chronic illnesses and disability do not fit the model very well. People with long-term conditions can control their illnesses with medication or lifestyle modifications, but they do not "get well" in the sense conveyed by a temporary sick role. In some cases, the role is lifelong, and the affected person must adapt and learn to live with the affliction. Moreover, the social construction of many chronic illnesses does in fact place blame on some individuals for their condition. People who engage in unhealthy behaviors are held accountable for the consequences. For example, we make judgments about people who choose to smoke because of the enormous costs incurred by society for their care and the lost productivity associated with smoking-related conditions. Sexually transmitted diseases (STD) are stigmatized because we view risky sexual behavior as irresponsible and in some cases immoral. Also, we tend to attribute greater personal responsibility to illnesses with a large psychosocial component, such as heart disease. In other words, illness has become increasingly viewed as normative deviance as opposed to its traditional conceptualization as situational deviance.

It has also come to be recognized that help seeking is rarely determined exclusively by individual choice; social and economic factors, such as access to care and financing arrangements, play a large role in the use of services. Another weakness of the model is that it does not adequately address the inherent rewards of "secondary gain"; that is, in many cases people like being sick and do not want to relinquish the role. Finally, the Parsonian formulation of the sick role is overly "medicocentric" in that it accentuates the physician's role in treatment and ignores the broader spectrum of activities and influences in illness. For example, self-care and alternative therapy at the individual level and health care reform and corporate capitalism at the macrolevel also play a role. Reformulations of the sick role clearly differentiate it from the "patient role" (Segall, 1997).

The transformation of the sick role in developed nations from situational to normative deviance and the complications of economic factors in help seeking have important implications for public health. With its emphasis on chronic disease prevention and concern for access to care, public health has contributed to the emergence of a new deviant role, the "at risk role." The at risk role has broadened in recent years to include persons identified with genetic risk factors for disease. Unlike the sick role, individuals at risk may not enjoy special privileges or support from the health care system or social environment and may remain in the role for an indefinite time span. People who choose to engage in unhealthy behaviors are considered at risk for various conditions, and they constitute the "target populations" of planned public health interventions. Numerous institutions of surveillance and monitoring have arisen to identify these risk groups.

Various health status and risk factor surveys are periodically conducted by government agencies to monitor the health and lifestyles of target groups. These data are disseminated through reports and press releases that inform the public about how the nation is doing regarding achieving health goals. In addition, through the dissemination of "expert knowledge" and media representations of the "healthy body," individuals internalize ideals of body image and functioning, and through self-monitoring, regulation, and discipline (e.g., weighing oneself daily, perpetual dieting), they strive to attain socially approved states of being (Lupton, 1995). Armstrong (1993, p. 407) describes a "vast network of observation and caution" throughout society, which sustains a level of anxiety and vigilance about the complexity of disease causation. Furthermore, environmental and technological risks have been generalized to the point that everyone, regardless of social position, is considered at risk for something (Petersen & Lupton, 1996).

CASE STUDY   HIV/AIDS as Normative Deviance

Societal reactions to the HIV/AIDS epidemic in the United States offer an instructive example of the public health consequences of a disease viewed as normative deviance. Because the risk behaviors associated with HIV infection are perceived as basically immoral or illegal (e.g., homosexual relations, injection drug use, multiple sex partners, prostitution), the general public has tended to cast blame on victims of the epidemic (Rushing, 1995). As noted in Chapter 1, social reactions to HIV-infected individuals have become much more tolerant and sympathetic since the beginning of the epidemic, but the condition remains stigmatized. In the early days, instead of being absolved of responsibility, infected individuals were viewed as social outcasts, condemned for their own bad behavior. Moreover, prevention programs have been severely hampered by society's reluctance to support education aimed at groups that engage in risky behaviors. Promoting safer sex practices among gay persons and hygienic drug use among injection drug users is often politically unacceptable because many people consider such efforts tacit approval of immoral conduct. To allow taxpayer funds to pay for programs aimed at homosexual behavior is considered by some segments of the public as tantamount to condoning a sinful lifestyle. Consequently, despite the fact that gay men and injection drug users represent the largest risk groups for AIDS in the United States, historically, federal and state-funded prevention programs ironically targeted heterosexual transmission only and scarcely mentioned those groups most in danger of infection.

Not only have prevention efforts been affected by the moral construction of HIV/AIDS, but the victims themselves have also suffered the consequences of stigma, both within their support systems and from the medical establishment. People with AIDS have often experienced rejection by family, friends, and the community; faced employment discrimination; and encountered obstacles to receiving sympathetic and appropriate treatment. This can lead to internalized stigma, as discussed further below.

What's in a Name?

Another way in which society controls deviance is by assigning labels to certain categories of individuals and behavior (Waxler, 1981). The labels, in turn, may lead to special privileges, stigmatizing reactions, marginalization, or other controlling measures. Labeling signals the need for some kind of special or different treatment by society. Terms such as *homeless, disabled, problem patient,* and *indigent* set apart those so labeled as different and in need of special attention. Thus, the social consequences of labeling can be positive or negative.

According to *labeling theory,* once a label is assigned to a person, others tend to perceive him or her through a lens colored by the stereotype associated with the deviant characteristic. For example, the behavior of someone labeled as "mentally ill" is likely to be perceived differently than that of a "normal" person, even if there are no actual differences in the behavior itself (Rosenhan, 1973). Likewise, a "problem child" often gets treated differently than other children. It is not uncommon for labels to have a lifelong impact, with the person's social identity becoming closely meshed with the category. People "become the label," and society treats the person accordingly. Physical disabilities are particularly powerful influences on identity in this way.

The social consequences of verbal labeling parallel the older physical practice of "marking" deviant individuals to indicate their stigmatized or privileged status. In colonial America, thieves and other criminals were branded on the right palms to permanently identify them with their transgressions. To reveal repeat offenders, the accused were asked to raise their right hands in court, which is the origin of the "swearing in" practiced today. African slaves were branded to signify their status as owned property and were denied basic human rights. In the 20th century, European Jews under Nazi rule were required to wear the Star of David on their chests, and later in the concentration camps, they were tattooed with serial numbers to signify an inferior status.

Sometimes labeling can lead to *secondary deviance* when the individual's self-concept or a group's identity subsequently becomes altered. Often the labeled persons' life and self-image become organized around the fact of their "differentness" (Lemert, 1967). Examples of this phenomenon include the recovering alcoholic, whose life is focused around the principles of Alcoholics Anonymous; the physically challenged person, whose handicap becomes the focal point of interaction with others; the mentally ill person, whose diagnosis tends to dominate his or her identity; and gay, lesbian, bisexual, or transgender persons, whose sexual orientation assumes central importance in how others relate to them and how they view themselves.

In a number of cases, labels originally intended to benefit a deviant group have in reality had a mixed impact. For example, the federal legislation mandating public education for "handicapped" children ("special needs" is the more current label) was enacted to ensure special education in public schools for children with disabilities. Some observers have argued that such programs have also led to stigmatization within the school system and have questioned whether the benefits outweigh the costs. Other examples of well-intentioned labels with negative repercussions include posttraumatic stress syndrome, attention deficit disorder, addiction, and premenstrual syndrome (PMS). In the latter case, for instance, the recognition of PMS as a legitimate medical condition with psychological features was initially welcomed by feminists, only to backfire in some respects when it was subsequently used to reinforce negative stereotypes of women as emotionally unstable.

Medicalization

Medicalization is the process by which nonmedical problems become defined and treated as medical conditions (Conrad, 1992). Issues that formerly were considered social problems, family concerns, or even normal life experiences have become increasingly viewed as illness diagnoses, subject to labeling and management by health professionals. For example, compulsive behaviors, childbirth, developmental changes, eating disorders, and even death itself have moved into the realm of medical pathology, with associated treatment protocols. First noted and criticized in the psychiatric field, the scope of medicalization appears to have no bounds, and concerned observers worry about the negative consequences of what the social critic Ivan Illich (1976) calls the "medicalization of life."

More recently, the mapping of the human genome and the proliferation of research focused on identifying genetic bases and markers for specific diseases have accelerated what Lippman (1991) calls *geneticization,* or the expansion of genetic explanations for human health and behavior. "This development has reinforced a genetic essentialism, where the DNA is seen as the essence of life and its problems" (Conrad, 2000, p. 329). Geneticization expands the concept of "at-risk" individuals to include persons carrying a genetic trait for a disease, creating new categories of deviance as well as having the potential for discrimination in health insurance, employment, and other life domains.

Like other processes of labeling, medicalization is a form of social control that casts the experience or behavior in question within the framework of deviance from some idealized "normal" state. We need look no further than the vast field of addictions therapy to see how many behavior patterns have come under the rubric of compulsive disorders: gambling, drinking, overspending, promiscuity, child abuse, and excessive cleanliness. All these used to be viewed as criminal behavior or moral failings, matters best handled by the legal system or one's spiritual advisor. The line between social problems and medical conditions has become progressively blurred. So pervasive is this transformation that some observers make the claim that medicine has replaced religion as the dominant moral ideology and social control institution of contemporary society.

Critics argue that the appropriation of life problems by medicine represents yet another aspect of medical imperialism, part of the insidious process of dominance, monopolization, and surveillance that places everyone under the watchful eye of the medical system. This gaze includes public health institutions as well, as seen in the redefinition of "bad habits" such as smoking, speeding, and unprotected sex as threats to the health of the nation. Medicalization individualizes problems; that is, it transforms socially rooted conditions into personal pathologies. Moreover, it decontextualizes social problems from their multifaceted background, reducing a complex systemic process to a clinical diagnosis. On the other hand, some aspects of medicalization have been hailed as welcome progress from the archaic notions of sin and depravity. Certainly, the more humane treatment of the mentally ill represents an improvement over the confinement of the "insane" in deplorable "lunatic asylums" in earlier centuries. Also, in many cases, medicalization has led to destigmatization, as we have seen with physical disability, infertility, and learning disorders.

Hygienization

Within public health, a parallel process of medicalization has taken place, with more and more issues being defined as "public health problems." Concerns now reach far beyond the traditional bounds of sanitation and hygiene, disease control, and protecting the health of vulnerable populations. In the video "This is Public Health," one narrator comments that "everything around you is public health" (Association of Schools of Public Health, 2008). Now, public health encompasses a myriad array of interests, from injury prevention, noise pollution, and disaster management to domestic violence, chronic sleep deprivation, and genital mutilation. To a large extent, social problems generally have been conflated with public health issues, and a process analogous to medicalization is taking place that might be called *hygienization* (from the Greek term for "health practices"), or even "public health-ification" (Meyer, 2000, p. 1190). Through hygienization, any phenomena concerned with the well-being of large groups of people can be labeled as conditions with public health significance, or often enough public health "emergencies" or "crises" that are "reaching epidemic proportions."

One of the consequences of hygienization is that public health has taken on an agenda that has become unwieldy and controversial with effective solutions difficult to attain. In an essay that argues that public health has become its own worst enemy, Sommer (1995) writes,

> We have claimed as "public health problems" violence, drug abuse, teen pregnancy, and homelessness, all of which are deeply rooted in societal determinants. Yes, we can and should research these problems. Yes, they impact on health. But no, we do not as yet have the technical understanding and tools, or the political support, to do much about them. (p. 658)

Other critics of public healthification have called attention to the consequences of evaluating social problems by their health consequences—in other words, viewing something as problematic primarily because it is health related. Doing this tends to redefine the problem as existing at the individual level, where clinical variables are measured, and not at the structural level of social and economic causes. Meyer (2000) uses the case of homelessness to illustrate this process of redefinition and its consequences. In recasting homelessness as a public health problem, the focus of research and practice shifted from a concern for the health problems associated with being homeless to looking at "risk factors" for homelessness itself. The new research takes a social epidemiologic approach and has identified the risk factors related to sociodemographic characteristics, mental illness and substance use, and dysfunctional family history. The health-related problems of homeless people—poor nutrition, infectious diseases, lack of access to health care, personal safety—declined in emphasis within the literature as homelessness was transformed into a public health problem (Meyer, 2000).

Incomplete Medicalization and Demedicalization

In certain arenas, we find *incomplete medicalization,* where competing definitions of a phenomenon vie for legitimation. For example, in the field of family violence, competing views of spouse abuse define it variously as a sociomedical problem, a criminal issue, and a feminist cause rooted in patriarchy (see Chapter 20). These different constructions have important implications for treatment and control, that is, whether the proper authority for management should be social workers, medical professionals, law enforcement officials, and the courts or structural change within the gender order. The women's movement has consistently worked against the tendency to medicalize women's lives, particularly in the area of reproduction. Likewise, mental health professionals have lobbied against the narrow definition of psychopathology as chemical imbalance to be treated exclusively with drugs. Finally, *demedicalization* also occurs when conditions formerly considered pathological are redefined otherwise. For example, masturbation and homosexuality used to be considered psychiatric conditions, complete with official diagnoses in standard reference books. Both have been eliminated as recognized conditions and are no longer listed in psychiatric handbooks. To a lesser extent, pregnancy and childbirth have also been demedicalized in response to consumer demands that natural life events such as birth and death be humanized and recontexualized in a larger holistic view.

However, it should be noted that demedicalization does not necessarily imply normalization. Homosexuality may no longer be considered a psychiatric disorder, but large segments of society continue to view the behavior as immoral. Likewise, many disabilities have been demedicalized, but persons with disabilities may still be treated differently than "abled" people in their life worlds. The disability community has taken vocal positions on the proper framework for understanding and dealing with persons who are "differently abled." In particular, the thrust of advocacy has been to replace the medical model of disability with a social model that emphasizes the failure of society to accommodate a diversity of abilities in its members (Sussman, 1994).

COLLECTIVE BEHAVIOR

In Chapter 8, we discuss some of the features of the culture of public health, such as its values relating to serving the poor and disadvantaged, which contribute to its somewhat lower prestige and salaries compared with the private medical sector. There are other factors as well related to social deviance that influence the image of public health. This has to do with the fact that the kinds of problems, groups, and behaviors that dominate the public health agenda are heavily weighted toward stigmatized issues and marginalized groups. The public health system deals with some of the most disreputable behaviors (e.g., smoking during pregnancy, drug abuse, violence, drunk driving, environmental pollution) and discredited groups in society (e.g., indigent patients, child molesters, homeless families, pregnant teenagers, the senile elderly). These associations naturally affect the position of public health in the social hierarchy.

Public health is also very involved with the collective response of society to medical problems perceived as threats to the well-being of the community. For example, adolescent pregnancy has been viewed quite variably in the United States during different time periods. In the colonial era, it was considered normative and desirable and did not receive much public attention through the 19th century, but in the 20th century, teen pregnancy came to be identified as a serious social problem warranting vigorous public health control, despite the fact that the rate of adolescent childbearing has decreased steadily since 1920 (Nathanson, 1991). Similarly, we can mention the problematizing of single-parent families, the aging of the population, and other issues that provide interesting perspectives on societal response to perceived deviance. The magnitude and severity of societal response to deviance reflects the degree of perceived danger posed by the problem.

A contemporary example can be taken from the arena of drug dependency. The large number of "cocaine babies" born to crack-addicted mothers in recent years has triggered stringent public health and legal measures to curb the problem in the United States. This issue conjoined several forms of social deviance and medicalized problems, compounded by adverse effects on innocent victims. It involves addiction, itself a large arena of stigmatized behavior and multisectoral societal control. It involves women's reproductive health, a generally medicalized domain, because women at risk for drug use can be screened during prenatal care. Finally, it involves adverse infant outcomes, with long-term demands on social services, hence its public health implications.

Sometimes, efforts to control public health problems through legal measures can have repercussions that conflict with therapeutic goals. For example, women may be reluctant to report spousal abuse because such disclosure within the legal system may place them at risk of having their children taken away from an unsafe environment. Similarly, drug-using pregnant women may avoid seeking prenatal care in areas where drug screening may lead to incarceration or losing one's infant to state care.

Whiteford (1996) reported on the repercussions of such a situation in Florida. In 1987, Florida was the first state to pass a statute that allowed authorities to incarcerate pregnant women who tested positive for illegal drugs and to take custody of their infants after birth. Although the rationale for jailing the pregnant women was to protect the health of the fetus, few incarceration facilities provided prenatal care or addiction treatment. Moreover, jailed women were separated from their other children, putting the welfare of the latter in jeopardy. Consequently, the statute had the undesirable consequence of keeping needy women out of prenatal care. Although drug use among pregnant women cuts across all social classes, it is primarily women from impoverished families or minority groups who seek care at public clinics who are most likely to be "caught." Private providers of obstetrical care rarely screen their patients for drug use. Applying a political-economic analysis to the problem, Whiteford (1996) concluded that "laws that jail pregnant women for their addictions are less about protecting the unborn than they are about punishing women for being poor, pregnant and addicted in a society that denigrates each of those conditions" (p. 249).

An extreme example of collective response to disease threat is societal reactions to serious epidemics. *Collective behavior* refers to evolving, noninstitutionalized responses as opposed to institutionalized, day-to-day behavior (e.g., riots and mobs are forms of collective behavior). In such situations, irrational behavior is not uncommon because people respond to social definitions of the problem that may have little basis in reality. The usual, everyday institutionalized means of coping often prove inadequate, so people turn to desperate means. During the global pandemics of the Middle Ages, for example, all the extreme forms of collective behavior were evident, including massive migration, desertion, persecution, punitive quarantines, ostracism of the sick, scapegoating, and conspiracy theories.

During epidemics, society tends to respond by constructing a moral interpretive framework for the crisis and by placing blame on the victims for their misfortune (Lindenbaum, 2001). Very often, the source of the problem is attributed to foreigners and stigmatized groups. Members of any group against which the dominant population holds suspicion and hostility are frequent targets for blame. Issues of class and racial conflict often surface in the design of measures to control contagion. Indeed, it is the fear of contagion that propels much of the action geared to protect upright citizens from the unsavory sources of infection. The following case study of the Black Death illustrates these points.

CASE STUDY   The Black Death

Also known as the Great Plague, the Black Death epidemic during the 14th century was one of the worst disasters in human history. About one third of the world's population perished from this highly contagious bacterial infection. Although we know now that plague was spread by fleas, at the time, its cause and transmission were a mystery; none of the learned people of the time could offer a plausible explanation. Consequently, doomsday interpretations abounded, and most people believed that the disaster signaled the end of the world. The dominant theory about the cause of the epidemic was that God had sent his wrath upon the world to punish people for their sinful ways. Because of the massive toll, the breakdown in social order was extreme, with almost complete chaos and anarchy in many places.

Avoidance and desertion of sufferers was common. There was a mass exodus from communities, and riots and lawlessness prevailed. People engaged in self-flagellation as a means of expiation for sins believed to be causing this calamity. Most significant for this discussion was that certain groups were singled out as scapegoats for the epidemic. Noblemen, deformed people, suspected witches, and even physicians were accused of spreading the disease, but

Jews received the largest share of the blame, reflecting preexisting social divisions in Europe. During a reign of terror, they were lynched and burned by the thousands across Europe (Rushing, 1995). The fact that Jews became the primary targets is not surprising given their long-standing status as the enemy of flourishing Christianity and their social distance from gentiles. Strict rules prevented contact between gentiles and Jews in the form of marriage, commerce, and domestic service.

Stigma and Disease

Scholars have long recognized the psychosocial impact of disease-related stigma on the lives of persons affected by stigmatized conditions. However, in recent years, this area of research has experienced significant growth in theoretical and methodologic development (Link & Phelan, 2001; National Institutes of Health, 2001; Yang et al., 2007). It is an important area of investigation for public health because, as noted previously, many of the health problems addressed by the public health establishment are highly stigmatized and the consequences of stigma create serious barriers for prevention and disease control.

In his classic book, Goffman (1963) defined *stigma* as a characteristic of individuals who experience "spoiled identity" because of a discrediting trait or life circumstance. He identified three general types of stigma: those arising from physical abnormalities, those related to character defects, and those attributed to marginalized social groups. Although he did not use the current terminology of social construction, his conceptualization of stigma incorporated the notion of contextual relativity; that is, a characteristic alone does not create stigma. It is the actual or anticipated social reaction to something as discrediting that produces stigma. In turn, stigma may negatively affect social relationships and lead to discrimination or other undesirable consequences.

The processes through which stigma affects individuals and situations are complex and dynamic. Social scientists have begun to describe these processes in terms of constructs, domains, and levels of effect. Weiss, Ramakrishna, and Somma (2006) define *health-related stigma* as follows:

> A social process, experienced or anticipated, characterized by exclusion, rejection, blame, or devaluation that results from experience, perception, or reasonable anticipation of an adverse social judgment about a person or group. This judgment is based on an enduring feature of identity conferred by a health problem or health-related condition, and the judgment is in some essential way medically unwarranted. (p. 280)

Others have identified different types of health-related stigmas (van Brakel, 2006). *Perceived or felt stigma* refers to the cognitive dimensions of anticipated or experienced stigma on the part on the affected person. *Internalized stigma* refers to an individual's emotional experience of feeling shame, embarrassment, or low self-esteem as a consequence of the stigma experience. *Stigma enactment,* or enacted stigma, refers to intolerant attitudes and overt discrimination on the part of others, the community, or the health care system. *Structural stigma* refers to institutional policies and practices that unintentionally reinforce negative stereotypes and stigma, such as providing HIV, STD, and TB testing in segregated clinics, which causes clients' diagnoses to be revealed by their seeking services there (Coreil, Lauzardo, Mayard, Hamilton, & Simpson, 2007). Finally, *courtesy stigma* refers to the discrediting of people closely associated with stigmatized individuals, such as family members and close associates (Goffman, 1963). The latter type is analogous to the secondary stigma that reflects onto social service and public health workers who deal with stigmatized clients.

Perceived and internalized stigma operate at the intrapersonal level of the ecosocial system. Discredited individuals are often aware of the negative attitudes held by others and observe behavior indicative of such prejudicial views. Their perceived stigma leads them to expect negative social consequences in their interactions with others and with organizations. They may avoid contact with the health care system to protect themselves from distressing encounters, leading to delays in seeking treatment. They may withdraw from social situations where their condition might be exposed, leading to isolation and loneliness. Internalized stigma may cause feelings of anxiety, sadness, guilt, shame, and embarrassment, which negatively affect the quality of life and the ability to pursue life goals. Fear of involuntary disclosure of their diseased status may lead to poor treatment adherence, such as when people avoid taking medication in front of others or give false addresses so that outreach workers cannot find their homes to check on them.

At the interpersonal level, stigma can disrupt family relations, interfere with friendships, and lead to social avoidance. Persons with HIV and TB may hide their conditions from spouses for fear of rejection and abandonment. Diagnosis of a stigmatized condition may lead to interpersonal violence, verbal abuse, ridicule, teasing, ostracism, and homelessness. Persons with stigmatized conditions may be mistreated, denied food, and forced to take on onerous work within the household. Friends may shun an affected person out of irrational fear that, somehow, the maligned condition will "rub off" on them. Persons with a disfigurement are often judged as bad or somehow responsible for causing their misfortune. They may have difficulty finding a marriage partner or being accepted in desirable social circles. Illness management may be impaired by the withdrawal of family support and refusal to care for the sick member. Some patients with stigmatized conditions report that health care providers show their repulsion or treat them in a demeaning fashion.

Within the larger social environment of communities, organizations, and society, stigma may have economic, educational, and social status impacts. It may diminish one's ability to secure or retain employment, attract business clients, or be accepted in the workplace. It can interfere with educational opportunities and lead to exclusion from religious and civic groups. The health care system itself may enact stigma through discriminatory practices and policies that reflect moral judgments. Patterns of resource allocation for programs and services often reflect the neglectful and derogatory attitudes held by the majority toward stigmatized conditions. It is no surprise that public funding for problems such as mental illness, homelessness, drug addiction, and STD historically has been quite modest.

Like other social factors affecting disease, reducing stigma poses a challenge in public health. Individual counseling with the affected persons can address perceived and internalized stigma, but changing the social context of prejudice is more complex. In general, public attitudes toward diseases change as improved knowledge and understanding diffuse in the population and as better treatment and control mechanisms become available. As noted in Chapter 1, the development of effective antiretroviral drugs contributed to stigma reduction for HIV/AIDS-affected persons. Advocacy initiatives to promote positive images of persons affected by stigmatized conditions have proved effective, such as the use of well-known public figures to speak about their personal illness experiences. An oft-cited example was the former U.S. first lady Betty Ford candidly speaking out about her struggles with alcoholism, and the many high-profile women who have spoken publicly about surviving breast cancer. Other approaches to stigma reduction include planned media campaigns, community awareness events, legislation to protect the rights of affected individuals, training of health care providers to encourage empathy and sensitivity, involving families and communities in support programs, and organizing support groups for affected individuals. A good discussion of various stigma control strategies in relation to levels of the social ecological model is found in Heijnders and Van der Meij (2006).

CASE STUDY   Stigma and Tuberculosis

The study of TB and its relationship to social stigma offers instructive lessons in societal reactions to disease (Macq, Solis, & Martinez, 2006). Numerous books have been written on the social history of TB, documenting the changing social construction of this persistent human affliction. For example, Barnes (1995) chronicles the transformation of TB in 19th-century France from the early romantic idea that consumptive women had heightened sensibilities to the harsher view that TB was a menace spread by the unhealthy behavior habits of the poor. In the 20th century, improved social conditions in urban areas and the availability of antibiotic drugs dramatically reduced TB prevalence, along with the social stigma associated with it. However, as the 20th century came to a close, decline in public health funding and infrastructure worldwide and the reemergence of TB as a coinfection with HIV/AIDS led to restigmatization of TB within societies.

In developing countries, where TB has remained a leading cause of mortality since the 19th century and earlier, the disease continues to be stigmatized because of its association with poverty and discrimination and because of the threat of contagion for people who may be exposed to the disease. Although the availability of effective antibiotic therapy has undoubtedly lowered the degree of TB stigma associated with disease communicability, exaggerated notions of transmissibility and fear of the disease continue to produce stigmatizing effects. In a four-country study of TB conducted in Bangladesh, India, Malawi, and Colombia, Weiss, Auer, Somma, and Abouihia (2006) found a substantial degree of stigma associated with the disease across sites, as well as shared perceptions of fear about contagion from the disease, despite the availability of adequate treatment. In all sites, the character of TB stigma was shaped by exaggerated concern about transmission of the disease to others and consequently reluctance to disclose the disease to significant others. Other findings of the four-country study highlight the local, site-specific aspects of TB stigma. For example, in Malawi, where HIV is hyperendemic, TB-related stigma was closely linked to HIV/AIDS. Because HIV/AIDS is strongly associated with male promiscuity in that setting, TB has taken on some of the same attributions of sexual misconduct. In Bangladesh, women scored higher than men on an overall stigma index and on specific items related to the experience of social exclusion. Finally, in India, stigma was clearly associated with the use of government clinics, which the investigators attributed to the invasion of patient privacy by home visits from health workers and related concerns about loss of confidentiality.

Recommendations for stigma reduction strategies based on the four-country study note the importance of balancing the real need for disease control measures to contain infection, such as the use of masks and short-term isolation, with the need to reduce unfounded concerns about communicability. Public health education should clearly distinguish between appropriate precautions to prevent the spread of infection and exaggerated beliefs about the risk of exposure, with the aim of reducing stigma indirectly.

CONCLUSION

This chapter examined various forms of societal reaction to health problems from the perspective of the sociology of deviance. Within the book's overarching framework, social control of illness can be viewed as part of the macrolevel response of the social environment. As we saw, the more extreme forms of collective behavior in response to threatening situations included irrational behavior, as in the case of deadly epidemics, along with moral sanctions against "sinful" transgressions. Intertwined with such responses are the social processes of labeling, stigmatization, medicalization, and hygienization.

Although the classic Parsonian delineation of the sick role has limited utility for contemporary chronic diseases linked to normative deviance, it nevertheless has an enduring relevance in the general sense that we can identify the consistent ways in which society sets limits on acceptable behavior for sick persons.

The study of collective behavior is important for public health because societal reactions to disease and epidemics have profound repercussions for communities, target groups, and affected individuals. The case of the Black Death illustrates many of the common social reactions to severe health threats. Less dramatic, but equally important, are the various manifestations of social stigma associated with particular diseases. Conceptual and methodologic development of the stigma concept has led to important insights into the process by which individuals and classes of people experience and respond to social exclusion. Strategies for stigma reduction include interventions at all levels of the social ecosystem.

REFERENCES

Armstrong, D. (1993). Public health spaces and the fabrication of identity. *Sociology, 27*(3), 393–410.

Association of Schools of Public Health. (2008). This is public health [Video recording]. Retrieved April 6, 2008, from www.thisispublichealth.org

Barnes, D. S. (1995). *The making of a social disease: Tuberculosis in nineteenth-century France.* Berkeley: University of California Press.

Conrad, P. (1992). Medicalization and social control. *Annual Review of Sociology, 18,* 209–232.

Conrad, P. (2000). Medicalization, genetics and human problems. In C. E. Bird, P. Conrad, & M. Fremont (Eds.), *Handbook of medical sociology* (5th ed., pp. 322–333). Upper Saddle River, NJ: Prentice Hall.

Coreil, J., Lauzardo, M., Mayard, G., Hamilton, E., & Simpson, K. (2007, March 26–30). *Cultural models of tuberculosis in Haitian populations* [Presentation]. Tampa, FL: Society for Applied Anthropology.

Gallagher, E. B. (1979). Lines of reconstruction and extension in the Parsonian sociology of illness. In E. G. Jaco (Ed.), *Patients, physicians and illness: A sourcebook in behavioral science and health* (3rd ed., pp. 162–183). New York: Free Press.

Goffman, E. (1963). *Stigma: Notes on the management of spoiled identity.* Englewood Cliffs, NJ: Prentice Hall.

Heijnders, M., & Van der Meij, S. (2006). The fight against stigma: An overview of stigma-reduction strategies and interventions. *Psychology, Health & Medicine, 11*(3), 353–363.

Illich, I. (1976). *Medical nemesis: The expropriation of health.* New York: Pantheon.

Lemert, E. M. (1967). *Human deviance, social problems, and social control.* Englewood Cliffs, NJ: Prentice Hall.

Lindenbaum, S. (2001). Kuru, prions, and human affairs: Thinking about epidemics. *Annual Review of Anthropology, 30,* 363–385.

Link, B. G., & Phelan, J. C. (2001). Conceptualizing stigma. *Annual Review of Sociology, 27,* 363–385.

Lippman, A. (1991). Prenatal genetic testing and screening: Constructing needs and reinforcing tendencies. *American Journal of Law and Society, 17,* 15–50.

Lupton, D. (1995). *The imperative of health: Public health and the regulated body.* London: Sage.

Macq, J., Solis, A., & Martinez, G. (2006). Assessing the stigma of tuberculosis. *Psychology, Health & Medicine, 11*(3), 346–352.

Meyer, I. H. (2000). Social issues as public health: Promise and peril. *American Journal of Public Health, 90*(8), 1189–1191.

Nathanson, C. A. (1991). *Dangerous passage: The social control of sexuality in women's adolescence.* Philadelphia: Temple University Press.

National Institutes of Health. (2001, May 5–7). Background papers presented at the Conference on Stigma and Global Health: Developing a Research Agenda, Bethesda, MD. Retrieved February 28, 2008, from www.stigmaconference.nih.gov/papers.html

Parsons, T. (1951). *The social system.* Glencoe, IL: Free Press.

Petersen, A., & Lupton, D. (1996). *The new public health: Health and self in the age of risk.* London: Sage.

Pfuhl, E. H., & Henry, S. (1993). *The deviance process* (3rd ed.). New York: Aldine.

Rosenhan, D. L. (1973). On being sane in insane places. *Science (New Series), 179*(70), 250–258.

Rushing, W. A. (1995). *The AIDS epidemic: Social dimensions of an infectious disease.* Boulder, CO: Westview Press.

Segall, A. (1997). Sick role concepts and health behavior. In D. S. Gochman (Ed.), *Handbook of health behavior* (Vol. 1, pp. 289–301). New York: Plenum.

Sommer, A. (1995). W(h)ither public health? *Public Health Reports, 110,* 657–661.

Sussman, J. (1994). Disability, stigma and deviance. *Social Science & Medicine, 38*(1), 15–22.

van Brakel, W. H. (2006). Measuring health-related stigma: A literature review. *Psychology, Health, and Medicine, 11*(3), 307–334.

Waxler, N. E. (1981). The social labeling perspective on illness and medical practice. In L. Eisenberg & A. Kleinman (Eds.), *The relevance of social science for medicine* (pp. 283–306). Dordrecht, the Netherlands: Reidel.

Weiss, M., Ramakrishna, J., & Somma, D. (2006). Health-related stigma: Rethinking concepts and interventions. *Psychology, Health, and Medicine, 11*(3), 277–287.

Weiss, M. G., Auer, C. T., Somma, D. B,. & Abouihia, A. (2006). *Gender and tuberculosis: Cross-site analysis and implications of a multi-country study in Bangladesh, India, Malawi and Colombia* (UNICEF/UNDP/World Bank/WHO, Special Program for Research and Training in Tropical Diseases (TDR), Social, Economic, and Behavioural Research Series, Report No. 3). Retrieved on May 3, 2008, from www.who.int/tdr/publications/publications/sebrep3.htm

Whiteford, L. M. (1996). Political economy, gender, and the social production of health. In C. F. Sargent & C. C. Brettell (Eds.), *Gender and health: An international perspective* (pp. 244–259). Upper Saddle River, NJ: Prentice Hall.

Yang, L. H., Kleinman, A., Link, B., Phelan, J. C., Lee, S., & Good, B. (2007). Culture and stigma: Adding moral experience to stigma theory. *Social Science & Medicine, 11*(3), 1524–1535.

CHAPTER

8

Comparative Health Cultures

Jeannine Coreil

In Chapter 4, we defined the concept of culture as a set of interrelated beliefs and behaviors shared by a social group that persists through time and is transmitted through processes of socialization. Although it is possible to study cultural systems as a whole, such as American culture in general, it is more common for scholars to study smaller subsystems such as ethnic culture, organizational culture, or cultural domains sligion, economics, or health. Table 8.1 shows examples of cultural concepts at the organizational, community, and societal levels.

Empirical research and program development usually focus on *cultural domains* associated with a particular health problem, such as theories of disease causation, illness behavior, dietary patterns, alternative medicine, and consumer values. The comparative study of health cultures can be defined as the cross-cultural study of preventive and therapeutic systems, both past and present. Anthropologists use the term *health culture* to describe the complex system of beliefs, practices, and social arrangements related to the management of illness (Weidman, 1988). The goal of this field of inquiry is to better understand how human

TABLE 8.1 Cultural Concepts at the Organizational, Community, and Societal Levels

Ecological Level	Cultural Concepts
Organizational	Organizational culture, group culture, family culture
Community	Ethnic culture, school culture, urban subcultures
Society	Western culture, culture of medicine, regional culture

populations anticipate and respond to illness. Thus, the focus is on prevention as well as the process of evaluating the signs and symptoms of sickness, and the actions that people take once illness is recognized. The theoretical perspective underlying the approach taken in this chapter is social constructionism, which assumes that people interpret or assign meaning to their experiences based on a worldview shared within the social milieus in which they live. Like other life experiences, illness is socially constructed by individuals and their reference groups through processes such as symptom recognition, illness labeling, and patterned help-seeking responses.

KEY CONCEPTS

Drawing largely from the field of medical anthropology, a broad range of topics have been covered in the cross-cultural study of health cultures. An important part of the literature can be described as the study of *ethnomedicine,* the domain of cultural systems dealing with knowledge, beliefs, treatment practices, and values related to illness. Another segment focuses on the organization and structure of health care systems, including not only the various practitioner roles but also the complexity of social and political structures that connect providers and receivers of care. The systems in question may range from very simple to extremely complex in scope and degree of differentiation. Efforts to encompass the range of complexity have included the development of various frameworks for classifying health systems. For example, some of the basic typologies found in the literature include Western and non-Western systems, modern and traditional therapy, orthodox and unorthodox traditions, and mainstream versus complementary or alternative practices. One problem with classification systems, however, is that they can never sort out the diversity of content into neat categories. This is because the real world rarely fits our neat conceptual schemes and there is ongoing change both within and across health systems. Like all natural systems, health systems are constantly in flux, responding to internal and external forces and adapting to evolving circumstances. Consequently, change processes in health systems represent another area of focused study.

The ethnomedical literature applies various typologies for categorizing different kinds of illness, along with their etiology, prevention, progression, and treatment. For example, Murdock's (1980) fivefold typology differentiates among "natural" causes of ill health, including infection, stress, organic deterioration, accident, and human aggression. Others have identified various "supernatural" forces behind ill health, such as sorcery, witchcraft, divine punishment, the evil eye, magical fright, and breach of taboo. Combining both natural and supernatural causes in a simple typology, Foster (1976) proposed a dichotomy between what he calls "naturalistic" and "personalistic" etiology, the latter including willful intent on the part of human or spiritual agents. Still others have chosen to differentiate between "ultimate" and "proximate" causes of disease, similar to the Causal Continuum presented in Chapter 3. Ultimate causes include abstract teleological concepts such as God's will or natural (evolutionary) selection, as well as sociological constructs such as the political, economic, or gender order of society. Proximate causes typically encompass specific medical diagnoses, biological processes, or pathogenic agents.

Not only do all human groups respond in an organized way when someone becomes ill, they also take deliberate action to maintain good health and prevent the onset of disease (Colson, 1971). In preindustrial societies, preventive efforts might include eating healthy foods, ingesting fortifying teas and herbal preparations, avoiding exposure to extremes of temperature, practicing ritual activities, and observing behavioral taboos. Indeed, some folk preventive measures were quite sophisticated and disease specific, such as variolation, the ancient practice of inoculating individuals with infectious material from sick persons, which evolved into modern immunization practices.

In recent years, there has been a growing interest in indigenous therapies of various forms, but most notably in the area of herbal remedies as a source of new drugs for diseases that affect large numbers of people. About one quarter of pharmaceutical drugs currently on the market are derived from plants, including many used as traditional herbal remedies for centuries. For example, the common aspirin, made from a compound extracted from the bark of willow trees, is a remedy shared with many Native American groups. For centuries, the plant foxglove has been used to combat circulatory conditions, including its derivative digitalis, a drug used to treat heart failure. Some of the newer cancer-fighting drugs also derive from plant sources—such as vincristine and vinblastine, used to treat leukemia and Hodgkin's disease, which are extracted from the common rosy periwinkle, a plant native to Madagascar and part of the local pharmacopoeia. One of the most widely used antimalarial drugs, quinine, derived from the bark of the cinchona tree of South America, was first introduced to the developed world by the Jivaro tribe in the early 17th century. A more recent herbal remedy from China, wormwood, has spurred interest for its ability to control some forms of drug-resistant malaria.

Contrary to popular myth, the oldest profession was not prostitution but healing. Even in the most simple societies where division of labor was based largely on age and gender, role specialization was found in the activities of healing the sick. The earliest healers were magicoreligious practitioners called *shamans,* respected community leaders who specialized in the management of all kinds of human misfortune, both spiritual and natural. The healing arts were tightly integrated with religious practices. As societies became more complex, other specialized secular healer roles emerged, such as the *traditional birth attendant, herbalist,* and *bonesetter.* For centuries, *physicians* were the primary medical professional, providing general care for all kinds of illness, and since the 19th century, *nurses* have become increasingly important in staffing health institutions. Over time, highly bureaucratic medical systems have evolved, along with many different occupational categories, to handle the increasingly specialized management of illness. Today, we have literally hundreds of distinct practitioner categories in the health field, from highly specialized medical fields to a plethora of nursing specialties, to a diverse array of allied health practitioners. Also part of this array is a complex spectrum of mental health, social welfare, and public health professionals. Clearly, the trend is toward ever-increasing role specialization, a phenomenon related to the growing fragmentation of health care.

Everywhere, when someone becomes ill, there are patterned and organized responses to the event based on the assessment of the particular episode. The response is very focused and tailored to the particular kind of illness the sick individual is suspected to have. In other words, there is rarely an all-purpose sick care response. The concerned caretaking group attempts to determine the nature of the illness, its causes, what sequella are likely to occur, what treatments and help-seeking actions are warranted, and what the likely outcome will be for the patient and significant others. Taken as a whole, this series of actions produces an *explanatory model* (Kleinman, 1980) for the illness. Explanatory models of illness are socially constructed for specific episodes, but they share many aspects with more general cultural models of illness categories. For example, if someone develops a runny nose and watery eyes, he or she may decide that the symptoms are caused by a simple cold and act according to a personal explanatory model of the common cold. On the other hand, sudden loss of consciousness in some societies is immediately suspected to indicate supernatural etiology, setting into motion appropriate care for spiritual disorders.

Medical systems, like other domains of culture, express core values within the larger cultural system. For example, Western biomedicine embodies the core values of Western culture, which have traditionally been identified as individualism, mastery over nature, future time orientation, "doing" activity orientation, and internal locus of control (Stein, 1990). These values underlie aspects of Western medicine, such as the focus on the individual patient, the conquest mentality toward disease, and faith in the healing power of applied technology. In Chapter 7, we discussed the sick role in Western society, which prescribes that appropriate steps be taken to treat illness; this can be linked to the action orientation of the larger culture. Moreover, patients are expected to behave in a manner that shows concern and planning for the future, such as keeping appointments, getting regular checkups, and living healthy lives to prevent illness. We expect all this because people also are supposed to be in control of their lives and responsible for their own health, not acquiescent to external forces—sometimes to the point of "blaming the victim." These values are also touched on in the section on the culture of public health.

Although Western medicine has become the dominant cosmopolitan system of care throughout the world, a great deal of medical pluralism remains, and this is not likely to change. One way of conceptualizing the heterogeneity that characterizes the medical arena across cultures is to apply a tripartite structure of popular, professional, and folk sectors (Kleinman, 1980). According to this scheme, the *popular sector* of medicine is the largest and most frequently used resource. It consists of self-care, over-the-counter medication, family care, advice from friends and neighbors, peer support groups, and other sources of help from lay persons. The *professional sector*, on the other hand, includes organized systems of bureaucratic medicine practiced by individuals who have undergone formal training and who are bound by government regulation (e.g., licensure). Professionals differ from folk healers in that they learn a codified body of knowledge and must conform to established, peer-controlled standards of practice. In contrast, individuals who fall within the *folk sector* of medical care learn their trade informally, usually through an apprenticeship, operate independently of bureaucratic regulation, and are not expected to conform to any set standards. Examples of folk sector practitioners in European and North American countries include traditional midwives, energy channelers, root doctors, and spiritualist healers.

In postmodern industrial societies, pluralistic medical systems are often described in terms of an *orthodox* or "dominative" medical system and *heterodox* traditions that include "complementary" and "alternative" medicine (Baer, 2004). The distinction here is primarily political-economic; that is, what is defined as orthodox has more to do with legitimation and control of the medical marketplace and less to do with normative use or even professionalism. For example, a 1993 study of alternative medicine use in the United States included chiropractors in its scope of inquiry (Eisenberg et al., 1993) despite the widespread public acceptance of chiropractic as a valued professional form of care that is typically covered by health insurance. In most instances, insurance coverage can serve as an indicator of what is considered orthodox care; but in this case, chiropractors remain marginalized politically from the powerful and monopolistic medical profession. Other forms of alternative medicine, such as massage and relaxation therapy, are treated as orthodox and covered by insurance only if they are prescribed by a physician, again reflecting the political-economic nature of the legitimation process.

Also referred to as *lay referral systems* or *hierarchy of resort*, the concept of therapeutic networks encompasses the process of seeking help from different sources and the patterned sequence and regularity of the various components involved (Helman, 2007). People do not respond to illness in an ad hoc, trial-and-error approach. They use past experience, accumulated knowledge, contemporary advice, and referral to develop a strategy for obtaining the best results for the means available. Therapeutic networks become patterned within health cultures, and their basic outlines can be discerned through research. For example, in the vast majority of illnesses, people do not immediately seek professional care following the first symptom; they watch and evaluate what happens and seek informal advice from family and friends. The decision to consult a medical specialist may be based on recommendations from someone they know and trust who has experienced a similar problem. Once in the system, a patient may "shop around" among providers until he or she is satisfied with the diagnosis and/or care received. Often, the therapeutic network will be profoundly influenced by the perceived nature of the illness. For example, if supernatural etiology is suspected, this may dictate involvement of a magicoreligious healer right away. In another instance, an illness may at first appear to be caused by natural forces, and a Western practitioner might be consulted; then, only after repeated failures to obtain a cure will a traditional healer be consulted.

CULTURAL MODELS OF ILLNESS

Cultural models are schemas that represent the shared understanding of phenomena within a domain. They consist of interrelated sets of elements forming a mental template for understanding and responding to life situations (Coreil, Wilke, & Pintado, 2004). People draw on such models to inform everyday experience and to solve problems (D'Andrade, 1995). Shared cultural models arise from the common experiences and problems faced by members of defined groups and the responses to those problems that become routine over time (Strauss & Quinn, 1997). For example, the immunologic model of disease posits that individual health is maintained through a strong immune system that fights off infectious and allergenic agents that are constantly present in the environment. Illness occurs when the immune system fails to ward off these threats. Therefore, one should take precautions to maintain a healthy immune system in order to avoid getting sick. Alternatively, the psychosocial model of disability assumes that notions of impairment are culturally variable and shaped by the social context in which the physical disability occurs (see Chapter 7). Some members of disability communities contend that it is society that should change to be more accepting and accommodating to people who are differently abled. Researchers have investigated cultural models of illness for a variety of health problems, including temporomandibular joint disorder (Garro, 1994), hypertension (Dressler & Bindon, 2000; Dressler, Bindon, & Neggers, 1998), cervical cancer (Chavez, Hubbell, & Mishra, 1999), and breast cancer (Mathews, 2000), among others.

Three types of illness models that have been studied include etiologic/pathophysiologic models (causes and biological processes involved in the development of disease/illness), treatment models (e.g., antibiotic therapy or behavioral regimens), and psychosocial impact models (e.g., social support viewed as both a buffer against illness and an important aspect of recovery). Particular attention has been accorded to etiologic models of illness, because how people respond to illness is closely related to perceived causes. Help-seeking, treatment behavior, and self-management of sickness, for example, are influenced by our mental template of what the problem means (e.g., severity, etiology, prognosis) as well as a cognitive schema for how to respond (e.g., seek professional attention vs. "watch and wait"). For example, a study of hypertension among African American women in New Orleans found that adherence to prescribed antihypertensive medication varied significantly by the cultural model of the illness held by patients (Heurtin-Roberts & Reisin, 1992). In the study population, two different lay models of illness were identified, one called "high blood" or "high blood pressure," similar to the biomedical model of hypertension, and another called "high-pertension," which differed from the biomedical model. "High-pertension" was considered a nervous disorder related to stress, worry, anger, and having an excitable, tense personality. Women who attributed their illnesses to the latter condition were significantly less likely to follow the prescribed medication regimen than women who thought they had "high blood."

Etiologic models can be loosely categorized into "scientific" and "popular" domains. In contemporary Western biomedicine, several etiologic models are recognized, including genetic/congenital, germs/pathogens, immunologic, environmental, psychosocial, and public health models. Current-day popular models, on the other hand, which overlap to some extent with scientific models, include lifestyle (e.g., diet), naturalistic (e.g., food additives), emotions and stress (e.g., job strain), and moralistic models (e.g., punishment for bad behavior). Popular models of breast cancer, for example, encompass all these common etiologic explanations. Beliefs about causality include dietary factors, especially fat consumption; toxic chemicals in the environment; the stressful pace of life; and, in some populations, sexual misconduct.

CASE STUDY   Cultural Models of Breast Cancer

A number of researchers have investigated cultural models of breast cancer among a variety of ethnic groups in the United States. The anthropologist Holly Mathews and her colleagues (Matthews, Lannin, & Mitchell, 1994) found that among African American women in rural North Carolina, the indigenous model of breast cancer was based on both general and specific illness models in this population. The model drew on the general blood paradigm of illness etiology that is widely distributed in populations of African origin. Bad or contaminated blood was thought to contribute to the pathophysiology of breast cancer in the study population. In addition, a more specific plant metaphor was used to describe the disease, in which breast cancer was thought to originate with a "seed" that remains dormant until disturbed through biopsy, invasive surgery, and exposure to air. It then can begin to move and grow, establish roots, take the form of "knots," and respond to surgical "pruning" like a trimmed bush (i.e., it grows back thicker). These folk models of breast cancer were linked in some women to delayed help seeking and reluctance to undergo biopsies and lumpectomies.

Distinctive models of breast cancer have also been found among Latinas. Using cultural consensus analysis, Chavez et al. (1999) identified two models of breast cancer in the Los Angeles, California, area. The first model, which the researchers describe as the biomedical model, includes three types of causality: family history, reproductive behavior, and environmental pollution. Both Anglo women and physicians in the study subscribed to this model. A different model, labeled the Latina model, was identified among first-generation Latin American immigrants. This model attributed breast cancer to physical injury to the breast, breast-feeding, and immoral sexual behavior. Because of the moral overtones, breast cancer was stigmatized in the immigrant community, and some women felt ashamed to disclose their diagnosis. Interestingly, second- and third-generation Chicano women who had been living in the United States for many years subscribed to a bicultural model of breast cancer that integrated aspects of both the biomedical and the Latina models.

In a study of cultural models of breast cancer in the Tampa Bay area (Coreil et al., 2004), the researchers, interviewing Euro-American members of breast cancer support groups, identified five core elements of the shared model of the illness and recovery from its consequences: (1) the recovery narrative, (2) group metaphors, (3) perceived benefits, (4) group processes, and (5) contested domains. The *recovery narrative* refers to the ideology espoused by the group regarding what is considered a desirable illness recovery experience. In the breast cancer community, the recovery narrative is often discussed in terms of "survivorship," that is, how survivors of breast cancer should approach the long-term challenge of living their lives as fully and successfully as possible. Recovery narratives exist for many health problems. For example, many individuals recovering from addictions follow "12-step" programs modeled on the principles of Alcoholics Anonymous, which are grounded in the idea that addicted individuals have experienced loss of control over their lives and must give up their will to a higher power to begin recovery. The literature on breast cancer identifies recurrent themes underlying the narrative of recovery, including the cult of survivorship, the importance of maintaining a positive attitude, and the use of sports and military metaphors. In addition to underscoring the importance of optimism and positive thinking for successful recovery, the Florida study highlighted the significance of being initiated into a "sisterhood" and viewing the recovery experience as an opportunity for personal growth and fulfillment.

The role of the support groups in transmitting group culture was particularly important. Group processes such as modeling, storytelling, use of humor, social comparison, and helping others were identified by members as mechanisms for learning to effectively cope with the recovery experience. However, group dynamics also revealed contested domains, in which some members held views in conflict with the dominant model. Areas of discord challenged the core tenet of maintaining an unwavering positive attitude and "fighting spirit" and revealed dissatisfaction with the "cheerleading" ethos of the sisterhood. Discomfort was also expressed regarding emotional sharing and giving extensive medical information at meetings. Some of these same themes have been identified in other studies of illness support groups (see Chapter 6).

WESTERN MEDICINE AS AN ETHNOMEDICAL SYSTEM

Early comparative studies of health cultures described non-Western medical systems in terms of how they differed from "modern, scientific medicine," the latter implicitly assumed to represent the standard against which to evaluate all other healing traditions. This somewhat ethnocentric approach has been replaced by a more critical perspective, which views Western medicine as just one among many equally legitimate ethnomedical systems, though acknowledging its global political and geographic dominance (Rhodes, 1996). In keeping with this critical stance, anthropologists and others have offered fairly consistent ethnographic descriptions of the "culture of medicine" as practiced in Europe and North America, including some of the following components. First and foremost, Western medicine is founded on the principles of modern science and, like other scientific traditions, gives primacy to the rational and empirical study of physical phenomena. Only that which can be objectively observed and measured is considered real. Thus, patients' subjective reports of experience and perceptions are accorded much less significance than the physical and chemical data derived from physical examination, laboratory tests, and electronic machines. If something cannot be seen or measured, it doesn't exist, because the primary language of science is mathematics.

Like Western thought, in general, scientific medicine divides the world into two distinct realms, the physical and the mental. Often referred to as mind-body dualism, this separation of phenomena into thought and matter has profoundly shaped our theories of illness and the organization of medical practice. Because of this dichotomous thinking, a separate specialty, psychiatry, has developed to deal with mental illness, and even within this discipline, chemical therapy through medication has dominated treatment patterns. Traditional constructions of illness view what goes on in the mind as independent of bodily processes. Diseases generally tend to be viewed as "entities" within a mechanical body, analogous to foreign enemies invading a physical terrain. The germ theory of disease dominated most of the 20th century, complete with military metaphors of war and defense (e.g., germ-fighting drugs, the war on cancer, one's battle with illness, and campaigns to eliminate threats to health). Furthermore, the locus of treatment in Western medicine is the individual person, with clinical practice organized around patient-centered care. Environmental factors have been given much less attention than what goes on inside the bodies of sick persons. Thus, the war is seen as a series of individual battles with the goal of warding off disease.

Research and practice in Western medicine rely heavily on technological developments, such as those associated with surgery, chemotherapy, radiology, and advanced life support systems (Hahn, 1995). Sometimes called the "cult of technology," this bias toward the use of sophisticated equipment and machines parallels the weaponry of modern warfare. It also underlies the prestige and status associated with those medical specialties that rely heavily on advanced technology. The "high-tech" orientation of Western medicine, and particularly the American version of it (see below), has become a point of much debate and criticisms in recent years. Critics point out the dehumanizing effects of a system that worships technology at the expense of emotional sensitivity and respect for people (Davis-Floyd, 1994).

Another distinctive feature of modern medicine is the "cult of efficiency," the organization of care so as to maximize the economic use of time, personnel, and other resources. Nowhere is this value more evident than in hospital settings, where patients are treated like vessels for sick organs, tightly regimented, and managed and controlled through round-the-clock procedures and routines. The importance of efficiency is also manifested in doctor's offices, where activities are organized to maximize the most productive use of staff time, particularly that of the physician. Across diverse studies of patient experiences in medical settings, recurrent complaints point to deep-seated patient dissatisfaction with what they perceive as being insensitively treated like commodities in a production factory. Not only are patients treated as "goods," but the entire health care system has been transformed into a vast industrial complex. Health and health care have become "big business," leading to increasing commodification and marketing like other products for sale in the marketplace (although more so in the United States than in Europe and Canada).

Finally, as we saw in Chapter 7, Western medicine has demonstrated a tendency to take over more and more areas of life under its purview, a process sometimes described as the "medicalization of life." Vast areas of human welfare formerly considered social, moral, family, or behavioral problems and issues have been labeled illnesses or disorders of some sort, with medical views on proper management replacing traditional wisdom. Bad habits, personal failings, disorderly conduct, and moral transgressions have been given diagnostic, medical labels. Furthermore, many natural bodily processes and changes previously viewed as part of the normal process of human development have likewise been medicalized and brought under the oversight of medical treatment. For example, a range of events related to women's reproductive lives, adolescence, and old age in general have been reconstructed as medical problems to be addressed by professionals.

Within these broad outlines of Western medicine, differences can be observed across national boundaries and sometimes by regions in a single country. For example, medicine as practiced in the United States has been contrasted with medical practice in other industrialized countries on several points. U.S. medicine has been described as "aggressive" and invasive, quick to intervene with the "biggest guns" technology has to offer. For example, the rates for most types of surgery are by far the highest in the United States, and end-stage, life-prolonging treatment is used much more vigorously than in other places. Most antibiotics and other medications are used more extensively, and there is far heavier reliance on high-tech apparatus and tests. Payer (1988) sums up American medicine as aggressively attacking "the virus in the machine," highlighting its approach to the body as a set of parts to be tuned, repaired, or replaced, much like the way we view an automobile.

However, the picture of Western medicine drawn above represents an ideal type and does not take into account the vast heterogeneity of an increasingly complex system. There are many areas of medicine that depart from this stereotypical view. It is partly an issue of semantics, because we use the term *medicine* to include all activities within the health care system, and there are many different professions involved. For example, the field of nursing is widely recognized as oriented to holistic patient care that does not reduce a patient to a diseased organ. Other allied health professions, and certain medical specialties as well, likewise take a more psychosocial view of illness, so it is misleading to think of medicine as a monolithic entity. Even within mainstream, "hardcore" medical practice, however, noteworthy changes have taken place in recent years. There is increasing recognition of the psychogenic origins and social embeddedness of illness and of the need to approach treatment from a holistic perspective that goes beyond the boundary of physical bodies. The walls separating mind and body are eroding as researchers and practitioners demonstrate the integration of thoughts, feelings, and physiology. Alternative and complementary healing are rapidly gaining legitimacy within orthodox medicine, and greater attention is being accorded to the therapeutic environment.

ORGANIZATIONAL CULTURE

Earlier in this chapter, we defined health culture as including the organization of health services. However, in comparison with the volume of research on the cultural beliefs and behavior of patients or clients, very little attention has been given to organizational culture in public health. Curricula for public health students rarely include content focused on understanding organizational behavior, and yet most graduates will find employment within bureaucracies where they will have to learn the culture of the workplace in order to function effectively. This imbalanced attention to client culture mirrors the tendency of anthropologists to "study down" and focus on the disadvantaged and "underdogs." Observers have called attention to the need for "studying up" and focusing our lens on elites, those who wield power and authority in allocating resources and setting policy. Greater understanding of organizational culture is an important step in reversing the overemphasis on client culture as the source of program failure in public health. One of the key challenges of health bureaucracies is being able to transcend their own cultures and become more sensitive to the cultures they serve (Foster, 1987).

Organizational culture can be defined as follows:

A pattern of shared basic assumptions that the group learned as it solved its problems of external adaptation and internal integration, that has worked well enough to be considered valid and, therefore, to be taught to new members as the correct way to perceive, think, and feel in relation to those problems. (Schein, 1992, p. 12)

Like other cultural entities, organizations can be described in terms of ideology, language, core values, rules, practices, rituals, artifacts, and many other features. People who work within organizations learn the group norms, philosophy, patterns of communication, and specialized terminology of the workplace. They "learn the culture" in both conscious and unconscious ways. A distinctive feature of organizations is the emphasis placed on leadership in shaping the culture of the organization. Leaders play a central role in creating and changing the culture of their organizations through processes such as goal setting, modeling, reward structures, resource allocation, policies, and formal statements.

Cultural studies of heath care organizations often focus on ideology and core values, such as those embedded within formal mission and values statements. *Mission statements* identify the purpose of the organization and the goals it strives to achieve. *Value statements* describe the principles that guide the organization in its activities and reflect the fundamental beliefs or truths of the organization. To illustrate these concepts, this section focuses on differences in mission and value statements across three major types of public health organizations, including public sector, private for-profit, and private nonprofit organizations (Orban, 2008). Public sector organizations, such as county and state health departments, often include service-oriented mission statements that emphasize commitment to protecting the health of defined populations. For example, the Citrus County (Florida) Health Department's mission is "to promote and protect the health and safety of all visitors and residents of Citrus County." Private for-profit organizations, on the other hand, tend to emphasize cost-effectiveness and profitability in defining their missions. This characteristic is reflected in the mission statement for the former managed care company Columbia Health Care: "To work with our employees, physicians and volunteers to provide a continuum of quality health care cost-effectively for the well-being of the communities we serve." Private nonprofit organizations, on the other hand, tend to be more similar to public sector organizations in their service orientation, but they often face financial constraints similar to for-profit groups and often reflect specialized interests. For example, the East Pasco Health Center, which is funded through religious groups, describes its mission as "Working together to provide quality and compassionate healthcare in a Christian environment."

The values espoused across health care organizations also reflect core features of organizational culture. Generally speaking, value statements of public and nonprofit organizations emphasize public service principles related to meeting the needs of client groups, including values such as respect, compassion, integrity, high-quality care, and responsible use of resources. In contrast, for-profit organizations, such as health care corporations, tend to emphasize values of profitability, innovation, and leadership in the field. While both for-profit and public sector organizations are concerned with cost, quality of care, and access to services, the order of priority of these components differs across types of organizations, as shown in Table 8.2. These differing priorities shape policies, practices, and decision making within the respective groups. In recent years, widespread privatization of public health

TABLE 8.2   Value Priorities in For-Profit and Public Sector Organizations

For-Profit Sector	Public Sector
Cost	Access
Quality	Quality
Access	Cost

services, such as contracting out basic community services to profit-oriented companies, has led to significant reordering of priorities and culture change within these organizations. We will return to this topic in the following section, which describes the culture of public health.

THE CULTURE OF PUBLIC HEALTH

As with all cultures, public health professionals working in the prevailing U.S. system share certain *implicit assumptions,* and its practitioners take them for granted until someone from outside the group calls attention to them. Many of these cultural orientations are incorporated into this textbook and taught in schools of public health as part of students' enculturation into the profession. Examples of these basic assumptions include the conceptualization of health as a state of complete well-being rather than the mere absence of disease, the belief that disease states are influenced by multiple factors as presented in the social ecology of health model, and the value placed on primary prevention. Public health is firmly rooted in the public sector of society and, therefore, must frame its core issues as affecting the "common good." It must be successful in making claims that something constitutes a serious "public health problem warranting attention and resources." In Chapter 9, we discuss how these core features have played an important part in framing the discourse on "cultural diversity" and "health disparities."

Some of the most important assumptions that guide public health professionals mirror the dominant *value orientations* shared by the broader society. Public health professionals, like most North Americans, believe that it is possible to uncover the objective causes of disease (rationalism) and search for a better understanding of the factors that place people at risk of premature death, disease, and disability. They believe that the world acts according to laws that can be understood, and while change is inevitable, laws can be discovered to predict and direct its course (positivism). They are also optimists—they believe that it is both desirable and possible to improve society. The government is expected to work toward greater equity, and public health professionals typically view themselves as part of a systematic effort to make society a better place to live. Like other health care providers, public health professionals are guided by a strong value placed on "doing" and the expectation that humans can master nature. These orientations are manifest in large-scale efforts to eradicate problems; public health has officially waged "War on Poverty" and "War on Cancer" and mounted a multimillion-dollar campaign—"America Responds to AIDS." Even when their efforts prove to be ineffective, public health professionals continue their fight, believing that increased funding or new tactics will yield the desired results. The view that disease and poverty are intrinsic to life and can never be eradicated is inconceivable.

Much of public health work takes place through agencies, organizations, and programs. As such, most public health practitioners work within health bureaucracies; thus, their work culture is shaped by the general features of these institutions. It is useful therefore to examine some of the characteristics of *bureaucracies as sociocultural systems*. Bureaucracies are organized into hierarchical, integrated, and functional units. The units are variously grouped into programs, services, departments, divisions, branches, and agencies. Each unit has defined goals that are linked to the larger mission of the organization. However, each unit also seeks to preserve its status and power within the organization, and despite lofty mission statements, the primary goal of a bureaucracy is to perpetuate itself and preserve the status quo. Formal policies and practices are couched in terms of client needs, but in practice, the actions of bureaucracies are guided by organizational needs foremost (Foster, 1987).

We tend to think of organizations as providing services to clients "out there" in the community, but in fact, most bureaucracies primarily interact with other agencies. For example, the U.S. Centers for Disease Control and Prevention (CDC) deals mostly with other government agencies and state health offices. State-level health offices interact with district- and county-level health departments. County health departments interface primarily with local clinics and services within their jurisdiction. Clinic management deals with the staff of various programs provided on site or in the community. It is only at the level of specific programs that staff interact directly with clients—the so-called "frontline" workers of public health, such as nurses, social workers, and outreach personnel. In the international arena, multinational organizations such as the World Health Organization interact primarily with national Ministries of Health, which in turn, interface hierarchically with divisions within their respective countries in much the same way as the CDC described above. Essentially, you have bureaucracies working with other bureaucracies, each seeking to maintain its position within the larger system. Yet people who work in bureaucracies have little insight into the cultures of their own organizations and even less understanding of other organizations with whom they interface.

CASE STUDY   "Making a Difference"

Cultural Values in Local and State Health Departments

C. A. Bryant, J. Coreil, L. M. Phillips,
L. K. Buhi, J. Nodarse, and J. W. Corvin

This section presents a new case study of organizational culture within local and state-level public health agencies in the United States. Data are drawn from research conducted for the Texas Food and Nutrition Supplemental Program for Women, Infants, and Children (WIC) (Bryant et al., 1998, 2001), participant observation conducted in a county health department, and 25 semistructured interviews with public health professionals from six states conducted as part of an ongoing collaborative study of the culture of public health by a team of researchers from the University of South Florida.

Almost everywhere, state and local county/city health departments are structured as nonprofit governmental agencies and administered by health professionals and staff who are trained to follow strict ethical codes. Guided by a shared commitment to serve, administrators and staff try to provide assistance to all, while operating within limited resources. Of special concern are disenfranchised populations and those at increased risk of disease, death, and disability. Even when efforts to help these "hard-to-reach" populations fail, public health professionals find it distasteful to shift their efforts to other segments of the population that may be more responsive to their efforts. Not only is it unimaginable to give up trying to reach resistant populations, but because these groups are usually the poorest or neediest, public health professionals feel obliged to allocate the greatest amount of time and resources in an effort to do something to help them.

A recurrent theme in respondents' narratives about their work was the tremendous importance placed on helping others and making a difference in people's lives. Whether this occurred through one-on-one counseling with clients, working on teams, or directing programs, participants repeatedly echoed the phrase *making a difference*. For these public health workers, the impact of their efforts was real, tangible, and rewarding:

> "I feel like if what I do can make a difference in somebody's life, then I've met my purpose."

> "I always wanted to help people. Sounds silly, but that was a lot of it. I was very interested in health, and I wanted to help people and the community was where I wanted to do it."

> "If what I can do by developing some poster or some video or whatever can make a difference in somebody's life then I've done my job. And it's worthwhile."

> "And there is going to be a lot of different barriers. But if you slowly continue to work at it, I think that we all come together and every single day we sit around the table and know that we are making a difference."

Public health professionals' almost religious zeal to "make a difference" is such a dominant value that it may supersede efficiency, cost-effectiveness, and accountability. As in many service cultures, public health administrators may tolerate misdirection and inefficiency in the short run as long as the programs are fulfilling their self-generated mission in the long run (Kotler & Andreasen, 1991, p. 76). Some health departments have recently hired program managers, who are trained in corporate culture, with the expectation that they will evaluate more closely program cost-effectiveness and eliminate waste. But when these administrators try to eliminate programs that have failed to demonstrate their effectiveness, they often encounter widespread resistance and resentment by staff members, who view programs intended to "do good" as the goal rather than just one means for fulfilling their mission.

Public health employees' commitment to the ultimate goal of the programs they work with is evident in job satisfaction studies. In surveys of employees working for the WIC program, for example, the most frequent reason given for working in the program is the desire to make a difference. Even when higher-paying positions become available elsewhere, many employees continue to work for WIC because it gives them an opportunity to help families in need. In fact, the sacrifices employees make in terms of lost wages, longer hours, and stressful work settings make some of them feel superior to those who opt for easier, less meaningful work (Bryant, Davis, Unterberger, & Lindenberger, 1993):

> "The deepest satisfaction I have is the knowledge that women, infants, and children get the necessary food and education, and a feeling of family. And I also enjoy being a help to the nutritionists and clerks because they are MY family."

> "I think one of the things that I feel good about is the fact with all the research that we have to prove that WIC makes a difference, that we know that it's really making a difference in pregnancy outcomes and in the health of mothers and babies."

> "I think (WIC) is an important program because it helps women, infants, and children. It gives them a healthy start, and that is why I think it's important. It's kind of like working for our future, building America's future."

> "I was in a restaurant talking with somebody, and I said, 'I work for this program called WIC,' and this total stranger across the table said, 'I just want you to know I love WIC; it helped me so much,' and you could see that she was quite successful now, but she said, 'There was a time when I needed WIC, and it made all the difference.' Those are the kind of success stories that helps us think why we're doing this job . . . because we do make a difference."

The desire to make an impact can also be a source of frustration for public health professionals. Clients are expected to be needy, humble, and grateful for the assistance provided them, and when they do not meet these expectations, employees are frustrated. When WIC employees were asked what they disliked about their jobs, many responded with distasteful stories about WIC participants who are ostentatious, own expensive goods they cannot afford, or fail to appreciate the help offered:

> "What's the most difficult part? Dealing with participants that act like the world owes them everything."

> "What gets me is when they [clients] come in and say, 'I pay my taxes, I want my milk'."

> "They come in with new clothes, fancy jewelry, and $300 purses. Then they tell you they don't have any income. They get pregnant every 9 months."

At the local level, the culture of public health is also reflected in the physical setting in which its practitioners work. The saying that "poverty rubs off on those who work within its midst" has visible support in the U.S. public health system. Employees typically are required to work in small workspaces separated by partitions rather than private offices with doors. Waiting areas are usually crowded and noisy. And many health departments are located in economically disadvantaged neighborhoods, where needy families can easily access their services. A proposal to house public health services in expensive, spacious buildings with lavishly furnished private offices would probably be rejected by both taxpayers and many public health professionals as incongruous with the organization's self-image. Camaraderie flourishes among employees in most public health departments. Teamwork is highly valued, and knowledge is shared freely. It is rare for individuals to be concerned with getting credit for an innovative idea; when a new program is successful, everyone involved shares a sense of satisfaction. Salaries in public health are typically lower than in the private medical sector. However, many nurses and nutritionists enjoy greater autonomy than their counterparts working in physician-dominated hospitals and private medical practices. Employee attributes that are valued highly include compassion, kindness, thoughtfulness, humility, and dedication, as well as the more typical employee characteristics, such as competence and dependability.

> "I like the interconnectedness of the public health community, and it's really a wonderful feeling to work on this bill with people from a lot of different backgrounds and industries to feel like we are doing something that makes a difference and really matters in improving the health of people's lives."

> "By and large, now having an impact is not as an individual person [but] rather by working as a team."

> "It is important for us to work together and for me to support them [her team]. It has a broader impact than working one-on-one."

Recent changes in the health care market have highlighted the cultural boundaries that separate the public health and private medical sectors. Most public health professionals mistrust profit-motivated organizations, including the managed-care companies with whom they now compete for Medicaid patients. Public health professionals expect the profit motive to override the service mission in these organizations. They claim that medical providers working for private for-profit organizations do not understand the special needs of the poor and worry that the emphasis on efficiency and profit will limit the resources allocated to education and ancillary services (health education, WIC, social services) needed by economically disadvantaged clients:

> "But you know public health, I don't know. But just having that nonprofit mindset . . . I was like, I really want to be in nonprofit. I mean it's a different world. It's a total different world. And I hated being in a for-profit."

Some public health workers claim that private providers are ill-prepared to work across ethnic and class lines, and many resent the private sector's sudden interest in caring for a population that is overlooked when government reimbursement levels are not profitable. They are concerned that if and when managed-care services cease being profitable, poor patients will be pushed back into a public health system that is no longer prepared to serve them. These attitudes reflect the implicit values that unite public health workers as members of a professional culture focused on caretaking of the poor and distinguish them from other health-related organizational cultures.

CONCLUSION

Cultural dimensions of illness, medical care, and public health are important in all societies, both simple and complex. Perspectives in comparative health cultures have changed radically from the early days, when Western scientific medicine was used as the standard for evaluating other healing traditions. A more relativistic view characterizes current frameworks, which recognize the constructed nature of all emic therapeutic concepts, including those of scientific medicine. The study of cultural models of illness provides insights into the ways members of a social group organize the shared knowledge and behavioral norms related to a particular heath problem.

While most ethnomedical research has focused on non-Western healing traditions and folk sector health care in industrial countries, reinforcing the general societal view that "cultural difference" is something "others" had, in this chapter, we emphasize the cultural dimensions of mainstream health institutions. We overview the culture of medicine as described in the scholarly literature, including the distinctively American brand of practice, drawing on the sizeable body of published work in this area. Curiously, almost nothing has been written to date describing the culture of public health per se, although some researchers have addressed the issue indirectly through more narrowly defined questions. Thus, we offer some formative ideas on the culture of public health, with particular emphasis on the worldview of local and state health departments.

REFERENCES

Baer, H. A. (2004). *Toward an integrative medicine: Merging alternative therapy with biomedicine.* Walnut Creek, CA: AltaMira Press.

Bryant, C. A., Davis, M., Unterberger, A., & Lindenberger, J. (1993). *Determinants of prenatal care utilization.* Tampa, FL: Best Start Social Marketing.

Bryant, C. A., Kent, E., Brown, C., Bustillo, M., Blair, C., Lindenberger, J., et al. (1998). A social marketing approach to increase customer satisfaction with the Texas WIC Program. *Marketing Health Care Services, Winter,* 5–17.

Bryant, C. A., Lindenberger, J. H., Brown, C., Kent, E., Schreiber, J. M., Bustillo, M., et al. (2001). A social marketing approach to increasing enrollment in a public health program: Case study of the Texas WIC Program. *Human Organization, 60*(3), 234–246.

Chavez, L. R., Hubbell, F. A., & Mishra, S. I. (1999). Ethnography and breast cancer control among Latinas and Anglo women in Southern California. In R. A. Hahn (Ed.), *Anthropology and public health: Bridging differences in culture and society* (pp. 117–141). New York: Oxford University Press.

Colson, A. C. (1971). *The prevention of illness in a Malay village: An analysis of concepts and behavior* (Developing Nations Monograph Series 2, No. 1). Winton-Salem, NC: Wake Forest University, Overseas Research Center,.

Coreil, J., Wilke, J., & Pintado, I. (2004). Cultural models of illness and recovery in breast cancer support groups. *Qualitative Health Research, 14*(7), 905–923.

D'Andrade, R. (1995). *The development of cognitive anthropology.* New York: Cambridge University Press.

Davis-Floyd, R. E. (1994). The technocratic body: American childbirth as cultural expression. *Social Science & Medicine, 38*(8), 1125–1140.

Dressler, W. W., & Bindon, J. R. (2000). The health consequences of cultural consonance, cultural dimensions of lifestyle, social support and arterial blood presure in an African American community. *American Anthropologist, 102,* 244–260.

Dressler, W. W., Bindon, J. R., & Neggers, Y. H. (1998). Culture, socioeconomic status, and coronary heart disease risk factors in an African American community. *Journal of Behavioral Medicine, 21,* 527–544.

Eisenberg, D. M., Kessler, R. C., Foster, C., Norlock, F. E., Calkins, D. R., & Delbanc, T. L. (1993). Unconventional medicine in the United States: Prevalence, costs and patterns of use. *New England Journal of Medicine, 328*(1), 246–252.

Foster, G. M. (1976). Disease etiologies in non-Western medical systems. *American Anthropologist, 78,* 773–782.

Foster, G. M. (1987). Bureaucratic aspects of international health agencies. *Social Science & Medicine, 25*(9), 1039–1048.

Garro, L. C. (1994). Narrative representations of chronic illness experience: Cultural models of illness, mind, and body in stories concerning the temporomandibular joint (TMJ). *Social Science & Medicine, 38,* 775–788.

Hahn, R. A. (1995). *Sickness and healing: An anthropological perspective.* New Haven, CT: Yale University Press.

Helman, C. G. (2007). *Culture, health and illness* (5th ed.). London, UK: Hodder Arnold.

Heurtin-Roberts, S., & Reisin, E. (1992). The relation of culturally influenced lay models of hypertension to compliance with treatment. *American Journal of Hypertension, 5*(11), 787–792.

Kleinman, A. (1980). *Patients and healers in the context of culture: An exploration of the borderland between anthropology, medicine, and psychiatry.* Berkeley: University of California Press.

Kotler, P., & Andreasen, A. (1991). *Strategic marketing for non-profit organizations* (4th ed.). Englewood Cliffs, NJ: Prentice Hall.

Mathews, H. F. (2000). Negotiating cultural consensus in a breast cancer self-help group. *Medical Anthropology Quarterly, 14,* 394–413.

Mathews, H. F., Lannin, D. R., & Mitchell, J. P. (1994). Coming to terms with advanced breast cancer: Black women's narratives from Eastern North Carolina. *Social Science & Medicine, 38,* 789–800.

Murdock, G. P. (1980). *Theories of illness: A world survey.* Pittsburgh, PA: University of Pittsburgh Press.

Orban, B. (2008). *Mission and values in public health.* Lecture in online course, Principles of Health Policy and Management, College of Public Health, University of South Florida, Tampa.

Payer, L. (1988). *Medicine and culture.* New York: Penguin.

Rhodes, L. A. (1996). Studying biomedicine as a cultural system. In C. F. Sargent & T. M. Johnson (Eds.), *Handbook of medical anthropology* (pp. 165–180). Westport, CT: Greenwood Press.

Schein, E. H. (1992). *Organizational culture and leadership* (2nd ed.). San Francisco: Jossey-Bass.

Stein, H. F. (1990). *American medicine as culture.* Boulder, CO: Westview Press.

Strauss, C., & Quinn, N. (1997). *A cognitive theory of cultural meaning.* Cambridge, UK: Cambridge University Press.

Weidman, H. H. (1988). A transcultural perspective on health behavior. In D. S. Gochman (Ed.), *Health behavior: Emerging research perspectives* (pp. 261–280). New York: Plenum Press.

9

Health Disparities, Diversity, and Cultural Competence

Jeannine Coreil

In Chapter 3, we presented the basic concepts and principles of social epidemiology, focusing on the unequal distribution of disease across social groups defined by commonly used categories such as gender, age, socioeconomic status, race, and ethnicity. Most of the public health literature uses the foregoing terms uncritically, assuming that there exists a widely shared understanding of their meaning and referents. However, in recent years, scholars have challenged established conventions of reporting health trends according to standard demographic indicators, particularly in the use of the terms *race* and *ethnicity*. In this chapter, a more reflexive and critical perspective is taken in examining the discourse on issues of diversity as well as various public health approaches to eliminating health disparities.

THE CONCEPT OF RACE

Throughout the 20th century, the concept of race was extensively used in public health with little critical scrutiny. However, in recent years, the concept and its underlying meaning have been the focus of growing critical analysis (Cooper, 2002; Kittles & Weiss, 2003; Krieger, 2003; LaVeist, 1996, 2000). Traditional use of the race concept is rooted in the notion of biological differences between different racial groups. Thus, the commonplace practice of reporting differences in health status by race presumes that the observed variation reflects the influence of genetic factors in disease patterns. In addition, the standard convention of controlling for race in epidemiologic research is widely viewed as a technique for reducing potential confounding of biological determinants in research findings; yet there is little evidence to support these assumptions. Genetic diversity within traditionally defined racial groups is many times greater than genetic differences between groups. More than 30 years ago, Lewontin (1972) estimated that diversity between individuals in a population accounts for about 85% of total human genetic variation, diversity within a single racial group accounts for 8.3%, and genetic differences between groups accounts for only about 6.3%. Population biologists have long abandoned the notion of discrete "races" of individuals sharing significant genetic makeup. Even within anthropology, the discipline within which the concept of defined races arose in the 19th century, the biological concept of race has been thoroughly discredited (American Anthropological Association, 1998).

Why, then, has the concept of race remained so central in the field of public health? The answers are complex and multifaceted, and the related debates are far from settled. However, it is possible to identify some of the relevant issues. To begin with, public health, like other American institutions, exists within a larger societal context where racial categories have profound social ramifications. For decades, the U.S. Census Bureau has enumerated the population by various racial groupings, such as the current "standard" categories of White, Black, Asian, American Indian or Alaska Native, and Native Hawaiian or other Pacific Islander. However, what is considered a "race" has varied considerably; since 1900, more than 26 different race terms have been used to identify populations in the U.S. Census (American Anthropological Association, 1997). The 1990 census added Ethnic Origin identifiers to separate out cultural subgroups, most importantly, the Hispanic/Latino population, creating a complex combination of racial and ethnic categories. Government health agencies highlight racial differences by reporting disease and mortality rates by racial groups and rarely by socioeconomic status. Renewed interest in health disparities has generated even greater attention to race as a source of health inequalities. A plethora of data have documented racial differences in health status in the United States. But official reports and research articles rarely define what is meant by the term *race* and rarely specify whether a biological or social referent is implied.

In the social sciences, the concept of race is largely viewed as a social construct with minimal biological significance. For the most part, race has been conflated with ethnicity, such that the term *race/ethnicity* is increasingly used to denote sociocultural groupings. Concomitant with the shift to ethnicity as the primary referent, the term *African American* has replaced the more racially oriented term *black*. Observed racial health disparities are now viewed as part of larger societal inequalities in social welfare, stemming from social disadvantage and racism but not from genetic variation. Research has shown that self-reported racism accounts for a significant portion of observed disparities in health status previously attributed to biological differences. For example, studies that control for perceived exposure to discrimination have demonstrated a substantial reduction in black-white differences in hypertension, preterm births, low birth weight, and other negative health outcomes (Krieger, 2003; Paradies, 2006). Evidence supporting this association has also been reported from the United Kingdom. Prospective data from the Whitehall II study found that individuals who perceived that they were often treated unfairly were at higher risk for coronary heart events and impaired health functioning 10 years later (DeVogli, Ferrie, Chandola, Kivimäki, & Marmot, 2007).

The concept of race can no longer be used uncritically in public health. In the absence of a valid biological referent, race can at best be viewed as an emic or folk category, a social construct that incorporates multiple meanings in different contexts. Biology may constitute one component of the folk definition, but it cannot be taken as the defining feature. In line with a constructivist view, the term *ethnoracial* may offer a more appropriate alternative label (Dressler, Oths, & Gravlee, 2005), or perhaps we should discard race altogether and simply use the term *ethnicity*.

Ethnicity is a much broader construct than race or place of origin. It refers to social groups with a shared history, sense of identity, and cultural roots that may or may not exist independent of racial identity. For example, ethnic groups often share a common language, food, music, and customs. In 1997, the American Anthropological Association (AAA) recommended that federal reporting systems consolidate the terms *race* and *ethnicity* into a single term, such as *ethnic origin*s, that is more meaningful to the American people.

HEALTH DISPARITIES

While public health concern for the health conditions of socially disadvantaged groups has roots as far back as the 19th century (see Chapter 1), over the past two decades, increasing attention has been focused on the persistence or even worsening of gaps between the health status of minority groups and the majority population. In the United States, this problem has come to be known by the catchphrase *health disparities*. In particular, the phrase references black-white differences as well as health disadvantages characteristic of other ethnic groups "of color," such as Hispanics, Asians, and Native Americans.

The discourse on health disparities is often traced to a landmark report published in 1985 by a task force commissioned by the Secretary of Health and Human Services and titled *Black and Minority Health: Report of the Secretary's Task Force* (Department of Health and Human Services [DHHS], 1985). The report highlighted the alarming fact that despite steady improvements in health indicators for the U.S. population in general, the gap in mortality and illness rates between African Americans and European Americans had remained relatively stable, signaling that there remained serious challenges to achieving the goal of reducing health inequalities in American society. The following year, the Office of Minority Health was created within DHHS to address health issues affecting racial and ethnic minorities. The persistence of the health gap has been repeatedly documented in subsequent publications, such as the Institute of Medicine's 2003 report, *Unequal Treatment: Confronting Racial and Ethnic Disparities in Health Care* (Smedley, Stith, & Nelson, 2003). This report drew attention in particular to unequal access to health care and the poor quality of services received by minority groups.

A large enterprise has emerged around the topic of health disparities in public health. A plethora of books, reports, journal articles, initiatives, and programs have appeared, spanning the entire spectrum of academic, government, and private sector domains. The broad goals of these diverse undertakings include, first, getting a handle on the phenomenon itself by understanding why disparities exist and, second, translating this knowledge into effective strategies and programs to address the problem.

We will first review some of the major theories that have been proposed to account for health disparities in the United States. Dressler et al. (2005) describe five models that have been proposed to account for observed differences in racial and ethnic minority health status: (1) the racial-genetic model, (2) the health behavior model, (3) the socioeconomic status model, (4) the psychosocial stress model, and (5) the structural-constructivist model.

In the *racial-genetic model,* health disparities are explained in terms of genetic variation across populations. For example, possible genetic explanations have been offered to account for the higher rates of hypertension and low birth weight among African Americans and the higher rates of diabetes among Mexican American populations. A specific example of the theory is the salt retention hypothesis regarding hypertension, which posits that a salt-thrifty gene was selected for among African slaves imported to the New World. It suggests that those who survived water deprivation during the Middle Passage carried a gene enabling greater salt retention, a trait that elevates risk for high blood pressure in current-day populations. The genetic theory is complicated by the fact that it invokes the ongoing debate regarding the viability of treating race as a biological construct as well as by the growth of research on genetic markers for disease in biomedical research.

The *health behavior model* proposes that health disparities can be attributed to differences in the prevalence of specific behavioral risk and protective factors for disease, such as smoking, diet, exercise, and substance abuse. Racial and ethnic differences in tobacco use, for example, have been cited as contributing to differences in chronic disease mortality rates from cancer and heart disease. In recent years, increasing attention to obesity as a risk factor for diabetes and cancer has focused attention on differences in diet and physical activity across different ethnic groups (Kandula, Kersey, & Lurie, 2004).

In the *socioeconomic model,* differences in health status across racial and ethnic groups are attributed to the fact that a disproportionate percentage of minority groups are found within the lower socioeconomic class. It is well established that lower income and lower levels of education and occupational status are correlated with increased risk of morbidity and mortality; because of this correlation, the confounding of social class and race/ethnicity can lead to misleading interpretations of health statistics.

The *psychosocial stress model* seeks to explain health disparities in terms of structural, interpersonal, and psychological stress experienced disproportionately by members of socially disadvantaged groups. In particular, institutional and interpersonal racism have been hypothesized to explain black-white differences in health outcomes. This includes both limited opportunities for economic well-being and perceived discrimination in daily life. In addition, research in this area has investigated the effects of living in high-stress neighborhoods, working in high-stress jobs, experiencing job insecurity and unemployment, and the strain of striving for success amid many obstacles.

Finally, the *structural-constructivist model* of health disparities integrates a dual perspective, focusing on the health implications of racially stratified societies and on the social construction of goals and aspirations within minority groups. It incorporates a constructivist perspective on the concepts of race and ethnicity as part of its theoretical approach. In addition, it emphasizes the reality that "life goals are culturally constructed within communities of color" and "the implications for health when those goals are limited by racial stratification" (Dressler et al., 2005, p. 243).

Using the case of black-white disparities in rates of hypertension, Dressler et al. (2005) apply the five theoretical models in light of available evidence and conclude that two of them, the psychosocial stress model and the structural-constructivist model, offer the strongest potential for explaining observed disparities.

CULTURAL COMPETENCE

In tandem with the expansion of research on health disparities, there has evolved a complementary growth of programs promoting *cultural competence* within the health workforce. Virtually every professional organization, government agency, and service institution (not to mention commercial and educational fields as well) has enthusiastically embraced the need to promote cultural competence among its practitioners through operational policies and training programs. Originally developed within the field of social work, the concept of cultural competence refers to the ability of health care providers to deliver culturally appropriate services to members of different ethnic and linguistic groups. The notion has been expanded to include organizational competence as well, as reflected in the definition adopted by the U.S. Health Resources and Services Administration Bureau of Primary Care (U.S. Bureau of Health Professions, 2008):

> Cultural competence is a set of attitudes, skills, behaviors, and policies that enable organizations and staff to work effectively in cross-cultural situations. It reflects the ability to acquire and use knowledge of the health-related beliefs, attitudes, practices and communication patterns of clients and their families to improve services, strengthen programs, increase community participation, and close the gaps in health status among diverse population groups.

As part of a larger society-wide "diversity" movement, there has been a proliferation of cultural competence training programs in the health field. In most of these programs, the concept of cultural competence is based on one or more developmental models that use a continuum schema to represent the movement of individuals and organizations through stages of increasing proficiency. The most widely used model is based on the seminal work of Cross and colleagues (1989), which identifies six stages of competence development: (1) cultural destructiveness, (2) cultural incapacity, (3) cultural blindness, (4) cultural precompetence, (5) basic cultural competence, and (6) cultural proficiency. The stages are considered dynamic and nonlinear; that is, organizations may be at different stages at various times, due to staff and management turnover, for example, or depending on the cultural groups in question. The first stage describes negative or discriminatory attitudes and practices toward a cultural group, while the second stage refers to lack of the capacity to respond to the needs of a culturally distinct clientele. Cultural blindness describes a perspective of indifference, where the expectation is that everyone will be treated the same way and assimilation is the goal. Unique features of cultures are neither valued nor nurtured. Precompetence can be described as the stage of good intentions and goals regarding fostering diversity, but without a clear plan or ability to achieve the stated goals. Cultural proficiency is reached when the organization has implemented fully integrated systems of resource development, operations and procedures that achieve cultural competence in all functions and goals.

The last part of the definition quoted above, that cultural competence reduces health disparities, has become a widely accepted assumption but has received little scrutiny. In a critical editorial challenging this assumption, Henderson (1993) criticizes the bandwagon of cultural diversity as a "red herring" that serves to reify cultural difference as something "deviant" or "other." In his view, it promotes a lopsided view of culture as essentially a characteristic of marginal or disadvantaged client populations, not something that afflicts dominant mainstream groups. Henderson argues for replacing the diversity lens with a more complex model of "intercultural influence," that is, a process involving mutual interactions among multiple cultural groups, including organizational and occupational cultures in health service settings. In a similar vein, Gregg and Saha (2006) point out the fallacies in promoting cross-cultural medical education programs as a means to reducing health disparities. The authors argue that an inherent mismatch exists between current cultural competence training programs and the goal of reducing disparities. They cite two important reasons for this incongruity. "First, in trying to define cultural boundaries or norms, programs may inadvertently reinforce racial and ethnic biases and stereotypes while doing little to clarify the actual complex sociocultural contexts in which patients live" (p. 542). Second, too often the concepts of health disparities and cultural incompetence are conflated, leading to the dubious assumption that competently delivered care will eliminate existing disparities. These critics and others view the preoccupation with "cultural" differences as a deflection of attention away from the more troubling realities of racism, discrimination, poverty, and shamefully inadequate access to health care.

Models of individual competence development propose stages of awareness and proficiency analogous to those described above for organizations. For example, an early, simple model proposed by Pedersen (2000) from the mental health counseling field identified three basic stages: awareness, knowledge, and skills. From the field of primary care, Borkan and Neher (1991) formulated the model of ethnosensitivity, which positions practitioners along a continuum ranging from fear, superiority, and minimization to relativism, empathy, and integration. From the education field, a similar model proposed by Bennett (1993), the developmental model of intercultural sensitivity (DMIS), depicts the movement of individuals from an ethnocentric to a relativistic view of other cultures. The six stages of this model include denial, defense, minimization, acceptance, adaptation, and integration. Cultural sensitivity training programs aim to promote movement of individuals through the stages toward higher levels of proficiency, with the goal of attaining full integration of cultural knowledge and skills in one's occupational role.

Although the various continua are not intended to be strictly linear, they are somewhat simplistic in presenting a unidirectional framework in which individuals and organizations are expected to become knowledgeable about the culture of the clients served. The frameworks do not address the need for service providers to understand their own individual and organizational cultures. Similarly, the notion of "health literacy" is primarily conceptualized in terms of clients learning basic health information. Research on health literacy focuses on the degree to which individuals have the capacity to obtain, process, and understand the basic health information and services needed to make appropriate health decisions. Little attention is given to the degree to which professionals have the ability to critically evaluate their own cultural backgrounds as well as the organizational practices and assumptions that guide their work (see Chapter 8). It is equally important for practitioners to possess competence and literacy about the dominant social and cultural systems that provide services to clients.

Often the phrase *cultural sensitivity* is used to mean no more than showing basic empathy and sensitivity to patients in general and treating them as individuals in a respectful and caring manner. In a study seeking to identify ways to provide culturally sensitive tuberculosis services to the Haitian population of South Florida, the authors report that one of the most important themes expressed in the focus groups was the cultural preference for a "one-on-one" personalized approach to connect effectively with the Haitian community. Such an approach was described as one based on "respect, consideration, sensitivity and trust" (Coreil, Lauzardo, & Heurtelou, 2004, p. 67). Do we need to discover this basic principle over and over again with different cultural groups? There is nothing specifically "cultural" about treating patients as human beings.

For example, regarding the topic of cultural competence in handling infant deaths, clearly the loss of the child represents one of the most traumatic events a parent can experience, and sensitivity to the family's psychosocial response on the part of health professionals is extremely important. The challenge of dealing with infant death has received attention in the cultural competence literature and policy arena (Bronheim, 2003; Shaefer, 1999); however, how much is competent care in such situations a matter of cultural sensitivity, as opposed to general sensitivity to parents of any cultural background? A publication aimed at raising practitioner awareness of this topic ostensibly makes the case for sensitivity to loss of a child in the Latino family yet states, "There is no single way that Latinos grieve the loss of a loved one or respond to any of life's circumstances" (Shaefer, 1999, p. 4). Nevertheless, several generalizations are presented, including the following:

- After an infant dies, some families experience anger and confusion evoked by conflicts between traditional values and beliefs and those implicit in the health care system. (*Isn't this true for all patients?*)
- In response to prenatal tests that find congenital defects and lead to advisement of termination, parents may not accept the recommendation. (*Isn't abortion a difficult and controversial issue for most ethnic groups and especially predominantly Catholic groups?*)
- Following fetal death, providers may recommend waiting several days for spontaneous labor and delivery to ensue, but some Latinos believe the delay may lead to cancer. (*Aren't there many cancer-related folk beliefs, some very similar to this one, throughout the population?*)
- In case of infant death, Latinos hold a funeral ceremony, with earth burial preferred, while family members dress in black and often say special prayers, such as the 9-day "novena." (*Isn't this common among Catholics from diverse ethnic backgrounds?*)

Galanti (1991a, 1991b) has noted the importance of recognizing the difference between cultural *generalizations,* such as those noted in the above example, and *stereotypes,* or preconceived ideas about a group that often serve as obstacles to seeing individual differences within the group. Generalizations about cultural differences can serve as a starting point for exploring the belief systems and behavioral patterns of individuals, but stereotypes tend to function as end points, preventing us from getting to know others for who they are instead of who we already think they are. Too often, cultural competence translates into a "checklist" mentality of cultural diversity that encourages stereotyping.

THE SOCIAL CONSTRUCTION OF CULTURAL DIVERSITY IN PUBLIC HEALTH

This section analyzes the underpinnings and impact of the social construction of *cultural diversity* in public health as a case example of the influence of disciplinary culture on professional practice (Coreil, 2001). Like other contemporary institutions in the United States, public health has embraced in earnest the need to address issues of cultural diversity in research and practice. Indeed, the word *diversity* has become a touchstone for a broad social agenda associated with equity, justice, access, empowerment, and community. As we observe this agenda unfold across disciplines, it is important to examine the process and consequences of such focused attention. This perspective has been neglected in the discourse on diversity. What is needed is a critical, reflexive stance that examines the consequences of framing issues around the notion of diversity.

Understanding cultural diversity in health care requires a contextual approach that encompasses the multidirectional construction of cultural reality among interacting groups. For example, clients construct the culture of providers as they experience it, just as providers construct the culture of clients. At a different level, researchers reconstruct both cultures to "study" a phenomenon. In the same way that the culture of medicine influences the cultural reality of patients (Good, James, Good, & Becker, 2003), the culture of public health constructs the notion of cultural diversity in client populations. Some aspects of this process are similar to the influence of medicine on patients, but public health has distinctive features that give a unique twist to its cultural diversity discourse. Some of the key features of the culture of public health that shape this domain are examined below.

Location in the Public Domain

First, public health is firmly rooted in the public sector of society and therefore must frame its core issues as affecting the "common good." It must be successful in making claims that something constitutes a serious "public health problem" warranting attention and resources. For example, a frequently observed strategy is to define a problem as reaching "epidemic proportions," thereby appealing to the idea that large numbers of people are threatened. The ability to direct political action and public resources to the problem depends on the success of this framing challenge.

The location of public health within the public domain also means that its work is inherently political. One need only look at election campaigns in the United States to observe the way health issues are routinely channeled to serve the political agenda of candidates and governments. Here, public health contrasts with clinical medicine, which is located primarily in the private sector and therefore is less prone to politicization of issues. The social construction of cultural diversity in health care generally is heavily influenced by local, state, and national politics. Likewise, it is susceptible to the fads and bandwagons of popular culture (e.g., the "needy" groups that get sympathy vary over time).

Because public health programs are supported largely by taxes and charitable donations, advocates must compete for scarce resources. Stewards of the common good must prioritize the needs of society and communities in general and make choices among competing demands. In this context, census groups emerge as very visible target populations that allow the system to appear to "do something for the needy" without implementing a major overhaul of social welfare to meet the needs of all poor and disadvantaged people. Showcasing programs for "special populations" makes our flawed health care system appear more responsive to the needs of citizens than it really is.

Epidemiology as the Core Discipline

In addition to reflecting the political pressures on its public sector domain, the culture of public health reflects aspects of its core discipline, epidemiology, and these likewise shape the construction of cultural diversity. Epidemiologic principles are based on the assumption that illness is unevenly distributed within populations, and therefore the focus of research and practice is the collection of data that segregate people into "risk" groups identified by race, gender, age, and economic status. The collection and analysis of data based on standardized "sociodemographic" factors are deeply embedded in research, surveillance, monitoring, program planning, and other practice arenas, creating over time the reified conception of such groups as essential social categories.

In a related vein, program planning in public health is based on the core assumption that all activities should be "population based," that is, aimed at a defined "target group." Moreover, the preferred target groups are typically those considered "hard to reach," marginalized, and therefore most needy. Practitioners see their mission as helping the most vulnerable and least powerful segments of society, more so than meeting the needs of the mainstream middle class. This focused attention on disenfranchised groups often has the inadvertent consequence of reinforcing marginalization, stereotypes, and discrimination. It is difficult to promote respect for groups that are pitied because they are deviant from an assumed norm.

Core Values

The core values of public health also feed into the construction of diversity. These core values include humanitarianism, universalism, and altruism—the belief in the desirability of helping fellow human beings, the notion that all people should enjoy the benefits of society, and the expectation that these efforts not be motivated by selfish goals. Furthermore, public health practitioners are assumed to be motivated to "make a difference" and "do something helpful," but in return clients are expected to be needy, humble, and grateful (see Chapter 8). Thus, the groups deemed worthy to receive special attention through the diversity lens should maintain attitudes and act appropriately to validate this designated status. Similarly, public health's rationalist and positivist worldview dictates that for every problem, there is a solution. Unwavering optimism propels the myriad battles in the "war on disease." It is assumed that something can and must be done to solve the problems confronting our society.

Basic Assumptions

Finally, underlying the diversity agenda is the basic assumption that greater attention to cultural diversity is a *good* thing and will lead to positive benefits for the defined group. This is not always the case. Too sharp a focus on the needs of the culturally different can reinforce negative stereotypes and sometimes draw unwanted attention. As noted above, cultural competence training can strengthen widely held generalizations about cultural groups. Well-intentioned programs targeted at disadvantaged populations can underscore undesirable features of the group's public image. Advocacy initiatives and media stories related to the health needs of disadvantaged groups may have a decidedly mixed impact on public perceptions of the group. Even the work of researchers who focus their lens on health disparities and cultural diversity can contribute to stereotyping.

Conflation of Diversity With Census Categories

Like other institutions, in many ways, the health field has generated an oversimplified and reductionist construction of cultural diversity based on the standard census labels used to categorize our pluralistic population. These categories are set by directives from the U.S. Office of Management and Budget, which establishes "standard" groupings to be used for administrative purposes by federal agencies (U.S. Office of Management and Budget, 1997). These labels represent sociopolitical constructs that inform policy development, regulation, budgeting, and related bureaucratic operations. The groupings may or may not be significant for health-related purposes, yet public health researchers treat them unquestioningly as if they are.

The one "ethnic" category used in the current census, "Hispanic or Latino," leads to much epidemiologic data being reported as White non-Hispanic, Black non-Hispanic, non-White Hispanic, and so forth. There is little evidence to support the meaningfulness of such artificial categories, and in fact, research indicates that for most Americans, the boundaries between race and ethnicity are blurred (AAA, 1997).

Before the monolithic "White" category emerged in epidemiologic research, it was common to find studies of European-origin ethnic groups, such as Italian Americans, German Americans, Irish Americans, and other groups that have immigrated to the United States. A broader view that encompasses the cultural dimensions of multiple social identities, such as gender culture, occupational culture, and class culture, as well as ethnicity, is needed.

Even within health care settings, provider and organizational culture are also multidimensional. Distinct subcultures are associated with the various professions and functional roles, as well as with social roles outside the organization. In keeping with the medico-centric orientation of the health field, researchers have tended to focus their attention on the dominant subculture of medicine as shaping the dynamics of medical encounters between persons of diverse backgrounds. However, this may not always, or even usually, be the case. For example, in a public health setting, the cultural dynamics of an interaction between a Haitian American female client and a European American male outreach worker will undoubtedly contrast with the dynamics between a Haitian American male client and a European American female doctor. All the terms in these equations are important and have weight, and such interactions are far more complex than can be expressed with a stereotype such as "Haitian client in the public health system."

CASE STUDY   Haitians, Stereotypes, and Tuberculosis

The following examples illustrate some of the pitfalls of well-intentioned public health efforts to address health disparities among culturally diverse groups. Drawing on the author's research on culture and tuberculosis among persons of Haitian origin living in South Florida (Coreil, 2007; Coreil et al., 2004), it highlights this ironic dilemma: Public health action aimed at improving the health of minority groups can inadvertently contribute to the social marginality that leads to health disparities.

In 2001, the Florida Bureau of Tuberculosis and Immigrant Health was concerned by epidemiologic evidence that TB rates were very high in the state's Haitian population. The problem was closely related to HIV co-infection; possibly the highest co-infection rate in the world has been reported for this population. About 60% of Haitians in Florida diagnosed with tuberculosis are HIV positive, and among young men, the co-infection rate is 76% (Lauzardo, Duncan, Szwed, Narita, & Hale, 2001). Based on these data, the Bureau concluded that the real problem was the high rate of undiagnosed HIV. If more Haitians were screened for HIV and then tested for tuberculosis, those who tested positive for latent TB infection would constitute an ideal target group for preventive therapy. Therefore the logical solution seemed to be one of getting more Haitians screened for HIV, then tested for TB.

In many contemporary public health settings, the intervention of choice for culturally different populations is the social marketing campaign, in which qualitative research is used to design messages that promote desirable health behaviors (see Chapter 15). In keeping with this trend, the Bureau approached the author to conduct ethnographic research to help design a campaign to increase HIV and TB screening within the Haitian population. The first concern was how such a program might be affected by the legacy of stigma associated with HIV/AIDS in this population (Farmer, 1992, 1997, 1999). The health planners at the Bureau had not considered this aspect of the situation to be a serious problem but were nevertheless very interested to learn more.

A series of focus groups revealed that Haitians in Florida clearly *did not want a campaign targeted at them for HIV or TB* (Coreil et al., 2004). Such a program would again single out Haitians as poor, sickly, contagious, and a threat to public health. If there were to be an intervention, to be acceptable to Haitians it should be targeted at the entire population, including other ethnic groups.

One of the key issues that emerged from the ethnographic study was confidentiality; more specifically, fears varied considerably with regard to organizational setting and provider occupation. Patients felt that private physician offices were more protected from unwanted disclosure of private health information, while public health clinics were considered vulnerable to loss of confidentiality. The common practice of setting up specialty clinics in public health departments, such as STD or TB clinics, was emphatically rejected, again because of the risk to confidentiality. Also, different health care providers were seen as posing variable risks to loss of privacy. Physicians were trusted the most to keep confidences because people expected them to adhere to a strict professional code of ethics. In contrast, support staff such as auxiliary nurses, receptionists, and lab technicians, who had access to patient records, were not trusted to protect confidentiality because they were unrestrained by the same strictures on conduct. Moreover, these clerical and technical staff tended to reside within the same community as patients and thus were likely to know them or their families personally.

Age cohorts had a significant effect on knowledge about the diseases. Younger people, for example, were much better informed about the difference between latent infection and active TB and showed greater receptivity to the notion of preventive therapy. The implication of this finding is that it may be more beneficial to target age groups in the community rather than particular ethnic groups.

The study also found that part of the problem was misinformation and bad practices within the medical community itself. For example, physicians in community practice were not well informed about how the BCG vaccine, which most people born in Haiti received as infants, affects TB screening in adults. Some physicians incorrectly believed that individuals vaccinated with BCG will skin test positive for life; they therefore assumed that routine TB screening is not useful in this population. These physicians advised people who received the BCG vaccine as children not to be tested for TB because the test results would be misleading. In fact, the BCG vaccine does not cause a false-positive skin test for TB infection beyond 10 years after its administration. Thus, some of the misinformation about tuberculosis screening in this population was attributable not to patients' culture but to advice given to them by their providers.

The ethnographic study concluded that it would not be advisable to target Haitians for HIV and TB screening in isolation from the wider community. The last thing local Haitians wanted was to see public advertisements urging Haitians to get "free HIV and TB screening" at the health department. Furthermore, the study found, the principle of increasing the cultural competence of staff (e.g., by hiring native, Creole-speaking staff) is not uniformly embraced. Although Haitians do prefer seeing Creole-speaking physicians, they clearly prefer that clinics *not* employ Haitian support staff because of the perceived risk of loss of confidentiality. This finding runs counter to much of the literature on cultural diversity in health care, which promotes the premise that cultural similarity between staff and patients improves service delivery.

Political advocacy and media attention can also fuel stereotypes in unexpected ways. In 2003, the author and colleagues began a study of stigma and tuberculosis among Haitians residing in South Florida. The research team consisted of local Haitians trained in social science and public health. Champions of the Haitian population of South Florida had long called attention to the special needs of this population, especially in the realm of health services, and sympathetic officials were vigilant about opportunities to highlight these needs. Likewise, agencies such as the Bureau of Tuberculosis and Immigrant Health, like many government health offices, look for opportunities to enhance public perception of the importance of the work they do, as public awareness helps justify requests for sustained or increased funding (see Chapter 8 for a more detailed discussion of this topic). On World TB Day 2004 (March 24), the bureau issued a press release highlighting the increase in TB cases statewide for the previous year. The statement noted that a large percentage of the new cases were diagnosed among "foreign-born" persons, this being the standard label used by the CDC and other federal agencies to refer to immigrant groups. A follow-up interview by a media source revealed that Haitians made up more than half the TB cases in the foreign-born group. The following day, the author received a call from one of the Haitian researchers on the study. She reported that while driving in her car, she had heard a broadcast on National Public Radio that asserted that tuberculosis rates were on the rise in Florida because of Haitian immigration to the state. She was dismayed that once again her ethnic group was being singled out for unflattering attention on a national stage.

Finally, it is important that researchers be sensitive to the impact of their own professional activities in the area of cultural diversity. The author's own research project had the unfortunate effect of reinforcing the stereotype of Haitians as purveyors of infectious disease. Efforts to recruit study participants were not always welcome, and some questioned why an outsider was coming into their community and talking to everyone about tuberculosis. Moreover, publishing articles and giving presentations on the study at professional meetings reinforces within the scientific community the image of Haitians as a special risk group for infectious diseases, conjuring up old images of AIDS and the 4-Hs (homosexuals, heroin users, hemophiliacs, and Haitians). When making presentations at professional meetings about the study, the author has made it a point to acknowledge that conducting research on a stigmatized disease within a marginalized population itself contributes to the social production of stigma.

Summary

In summary, the social construction of cultural diversity in public health (and other domains) should be examined to better understand the process and consequences of defining problems in these terms. It describes how core features of the culture of public health shape our approaches to diversity and give meaning to basic constructs in this arena. It makes the case for redefining cultural diversity in terms of the complex process of intercultural influence among ethnic, organizational, occupational, and other cultural systems in health care settings. Finally, it calls on researchers to take a critical stance regarding their own contribution to the social construction of health problems by understanding the ways in which their own disciplinary culture influences their scholarly work.

CONCLUSION

In this chapter, current discourse on health disparities, cultural diversity, and cultural competence is examined from a critical perspective to illustrate how the underlying assumptions and practices of public health are often taken for granted. It challenges the meaningfulness of treating race as a biological construct and discusses alternative explanations for health disparities among racial groups. The assumptions underlying cultural diversity and cultural competence practices are likewise scrutinized in light of prevailing discourses on cultural difference. The argument is made for greater attention to the cultural competence and health literacy of professionals' own organizational and occupational cultures. By questioning some of the taken-for-granted principles of diversity and competence and by showing how well-intentioned actions can sometimes have adverse consequences, the chapter challenges us to rethink many issues that have remained largely unexamined. This kind of critical analysis is sometimes referred to as "deconstruction" in social science. The purpose of deconstruction here is not to eliminate attention and concern for health disparities and cultural diversity but to make us more reflexive about how public health problems are framed and acted on. By understanding the influence of our own cultural and institutional contexts on the work that we undertake, we are better equipped to step outside the blinders of conventional wisdom and thus enabled to envision new approaches to eliminating health disparities.

REFERENCES

American Anthropological Association. (1997). *Response to OMB Directive 15, Race and ethnic standards for federal statistics and administrative reporting.* Retrieved May 3, 2008, from www.aaanet.org/gvt/ombdraft.htm

American Anthropological Association. (1998). AAA statement on race. *American Anthropologist, 100,* 712–713.

Bennett, M. J. (1993). Towards a developmental model of intercultural sensitivity. In R. M. Paige (Ed.), *Education for the intercultural experience* (pp. 21–71). Yarmouth, ME: Intercultural Press.

Borkan, J. M., & Neher, J. O. (1991). A developmental model of ethnosensitivity in family practice training. *Family Medicine, 23*(3), 212–217.

Bronheim, S. (2003). *Infusing cultural and linguistic competence into the multiple systems encountered by families following the sudden, unexpected death of an infant* (Policy Brief). Washington, DC: National Center for Cultural Competence, Georgetown University Center for Child and Human Development.

Cooper, R. (2002). A note on the biological concept of race and its application in epidemiologic research. In T. A. LaVeist (Ed.), *Race, ethnicity and health* (pp. 99–114). San Francisco: Jossey-Bass.

Coreil, J. (2001, October 12). *The social construction of cultural diversity in public health.* Paper presented at the Conference on Diversity and Health Care, Russell Sage Foundation, New York.

Coreil, J. (2007, January 23–25). *Disparities, cultural and language competence and quality of care for diverse populations: What is the problem?* Paper presented at the 1st Annual Clinical and Preventive Practice Management Summit, Florida Department of Health, Jacksonville, FL.

Coreil, J., Lauzardo, M., & Heurtelou, M. (2004). Cultural feasibility assessment for tuberculosis prevention among persons of Haitian origin in South Florida. *Journal of Immigrant Health, 6*(2), 63–69.

Cross, T., Bazron, B., Dennis, K., & Isaacs, M. (1989). *Towards a culturally competent system of care* (Vol. 1). Washington, DC: CASSP Technical Assistance Center, Center for Child Health and Mental Health Policy, Georgetown University Child Development Center.

Department of Health and Human Services. (1985). *Black and minority health: Report of the Secretary's task force.* Washington, DC: Author.

DeVogli, R., Ferrie, J. E., Chandola, T., Kivimäki, M., & Marmot, M. G. (2007). Unfairness and health: Evidence from the Whitehall II study. *Journal of Epidemiology and Community Health, 61,* 513–518.

Dressler, W. W., Oths, K. O., & Gravlee, C. C. (2005). Race and ethnicity in public health research: Models to explain health disparities. *Annual Review of Anthropology, 34,* 231–252.

Farmer, P. (1992). *AIDS and accusation: Haiti and the geography of blame.* Berkeley: University of California Press.

Farmer, P. (1997). Social scientists and the new tuberculosis. *Social Science & Medicine, 44*(3), 347–358.

Farmer, P. (1999). *Infections and inequalities.* Berkeley: University of California Press.

Galanti, G. (1991a). Basic concepts. In *Caring for patients from different cultures* (pp. 1–19). Philadelphia: University of Pennsylvania Press.

Galanti, G. (1991b). Conclusions. In *Caring for patients from different cultures* (pp. 187–200). Philadelphia: University of Pennsylvania Press.

Good, M. D., James, C., Good, B., & Becker, A. (2003). *The culture of medicine and racial, ethnic and class disparities in health care.* In Brian D. Smedley, Adrienne Y. Stith, & Alan R. Nelson (Eds.), *Unequal treatment: Confronting racial and ethnic disparities in health care* (pp. 594–625). Washington, DC: National Academies Press. (Background paper commissioned by the Institute of Medicine, Committee on Disparities in Health Care)

Gregg, J., & Saha, S. (2006). Losing culture on the way to competence: The use and misuse of culture in medical education. *Academic Medicine, 81*(6), 542–547.

Henderson, N. (1993). The "cultural diversity" epidemic [Editorial]. *Gerontological Health Newsletter, 4.*

Kandula, N. R., Kersey, M., & Lurie, N. (2004). Assuring the health of immigrants: What the leading health indicators tell us. *Annual Review of Public Health, 25,* 357–376.

Kittles, R. A., & Weiss, K. M. (2003). Race, ancestry, and genes: Implications for defining disease risk. *Annual Review of Genomics and Human Genetics, 4,* 33–67.

Krieger, N. (2003). Does racism harm health? Did child abuse exist before 1982? On explicit questions, critical science, and current controversies: An ecosocial perspective. *American Journal of Public Health, 93,* 194–199.

Lauzardo, M., Duncan, H., Szwed, T., Narita, M., & Hale, Y. (2001). Tuberculosis among individuals of Haitian origin in Florida: Opportunities for intervention. *American Journal of Respiratory and Critical Care Medicine, 163*(5, Part 2), A-100.

LaVeist, T. A. (1996). Why we should continue to study race . . . but do a better job: An essay on race, racism and health. *Ethnicity & Disease, 6,* 21–29.

LaVeist, T. A. (2000). On the study of race, racism, and health: A shift from description to explanation. *International Journal of Health Services, 30*(1), 217–219.

Lewontin, R. C. (1972). Apportionment of human diversity. *Evolutionary Biology, 6,* 381.

Paradies, Y. (2006). A systematic review of self-reported racism and health. *International Journal of Epidemiology, 35,* 888–901.

Pedersen, P. A. (2000). *Handbook for Developing Multicultural Awareness* (3rd ed.). Alexandria, VA: American Counseling Association.

Shaefer, J. (1999, July). *When an infant dies: Cross-cultural expressions of grief and loss* (Bulletin of the National Fetal-Infant Mortality Review Program). Washington, DC: U.S. Department of Health and Human Services, Maternal and Child Health Bureau.

Smedley, S. D., Stith, A. Y., & Nelson, A. R. (2003). *Unequal treatment: Confronting racial and ethnic disparities in health care* (Institute of Medicine report). Washington, DC: National Academies Press.

U.S. Bureau of Health Professions. (2008). *Definitions of cultural competence.* Retrieved February 10, 2008, from http://bhpr.hrsa.gov/diversity/cultcomp.htm

U.S. Office of Management and Budget. (1997). *Revisions to the standards for the classification of federal data on race and ethnicity* (Federal Register notice, October 30, 2007). Retrieved May 3, 2008, from www.whitehouse.gov/omb/fedreg/ombdir15.html

PART IV

Special Populations Through the Life Cycle

The fourth section of the book takes a life span perspective by examining health issues affecting populations at different stages of the life cycle. Age and life stage influence both the kinds of health problems encountered and the ways in which individuals and society respond to the health challenges of the groups affected. These principles are illustrated in the areas of reproductive health, adolescent health, and health of the elderly.

Chapter 10 takes the view that reproductive health issues affect people at all stages of life, especially during the childbearing years when matters of family planning, infertility, and maternal health figure importantly. The problem of unintended childbearing is presented in greater depth to illustrate the important factors at different ecological levels that affect health behavior and outcomes.

A developmental perspective on adolescence frames the discussion of health concerns reviewed in Chapter 11. The social construction of risk and youth figures importantly in this area. The problem of adolescent tobacco use is analyzed in greater depth to show the impact of intrapersonal, interpersonal, family, community, society, and policy factors on smoking and related behaviors as well as approaches to prevention.

In Chapter 12, public health issues of the elderly population are reviewed by first looking at the demographics of an aging society. The most important health issues affecting older persons are discussed, including cardiovascular disease, cancer, and dementia. Planning for the health care needs of the older population presents a major challenge for public health. In addition to medical needs, quality-of-life issues are important areas to be taken care of.

10

Reproductive Health

Wendy L. Hellerstedt

A t the 1994 International Conference on Population and Development in Cairo, 179 countries stressed the need to address reproductive health in order to eliminate poverty, given its fundamental association with economic, social, and environmental development (Fathalla, Sinding, Rosenfield, & Fathalla, 2006). At the 2005 World Summit review of the Millennium Development Goals at the United Nations (UN), world leaders affirmed that reproductive health was a basic right and committed themselves to "achieving universal access to reproductive health by 2015" (UN, 2005). Limiting access to reproductive health services and information, thus, can be seen as a violation of human rights, and the denial of services is a potentially preventable cause of mortality and morbidity. For example, it is estimated that 90% of deaths from unsafe abortions and 20% of maternal deaths could be avoided if women and couples had access to effective and safe contraception (Cleland et al., 2006).

Despite the critical role of reproductive health in population health, evidence-based educational materials, programs, and policies are not universally available even in developed countries. This is because reproductive health is not just a health matter. It is also a sensitive issue because it involves exposures and outcomes that are associated with sexual behavior. While sexual behavior is an intensely private concern, it is also the focus of public discourse, where misinformation and ideology may supersede evidence. This is exemplified by the widespread promotion of, and funding for, abstinence education for youth in the United States: More than $1 billion in federal aid has been spent for state-run abstinence-only programs (Boonstra, 2002). Despite the lack of evidence that abstinence education reduces the risks for pregnancy or sexually transmitted infections (STIs), it continues to be taught, and comprehensive sex education programs continue to decline, in contrast to the general experience in Europe, which has access to comprehensive sex education and much lower rates of adolescent pregnancy and STIs than the United States (Lindberg, Santelli, & Singh, 2006; Singh & Darroch, 2000; Trenholm et al., 2007; Underhill, Montgomery, & Operario, 2007).

Politics and culture are thus strongly linked to reproductive services and messages about sexual behavior. They also reflect, and inform, the environments in which individual behaviors are played out: Social vulnerability, marginalization, gender roles, and power inequities all constrain and limit sexual expression. The physical and built environments also affect reproductive health. For example, endocrine disruption, caused by environmental exposures, may affect male and female fertility and increase the risk of poor birth outcomes (Naz, 2004). Exposure to disasters, natural and human-made, also has profound effects on reproductive health. Soldiers and citizens exposed to war or violent conflict are at high risk for rape, STIs, unintended pregnancy, and poor pregnancy outcome (Al Gasseer, Dresden, Keeney, & Warren, 2004; Jewkes, 2007). Women exposed to natural disasters, such as Hurricane Katrina in the United States, are at risk for unintended pregnancy, STIs, and poor birth outcomes (Kissinger, Schmidt, Sanders, & Liddon, 2007).

Because norms, policies, resources, and physical environments vary geographically, reproductive health conditions—and models to explain them—can vary by country, by regions/states, by cities, and even by neighborhoods. Sometimes, the very nature of a reproductive health condition varies across populations and regions. An example of this is how the "problem" of cesarean deliveries is defined in developed and developing countries. The United States has an excess of cesarean deliveries and has had a goal to reduce the rate of cesarean deliveries for almost 25 years, but it has had little success (about 28% of all births are delivered by cesarean) (Menacker, 2005). Other developed countries have similarly high rates, likely associated with elective cesareans for nonmedical factors (Minkoff & Chervenak, 2003). In sub-Saharan Africa, which has one of the highest rates of the human immunodeficiency virus (HIV) in the world, the "problem" is very different. Cesarean deliveries are medically indicated for HIV-positive women to reduce the risk of mother-to-child transmission. Because women lack access to medical interventions, cesarean delivery rates are lower than 5% in all 42 sub-Saharan African countries except Kenya and lower than 2% in Burkina Faso, Madagascar, Niger, and Zambia (Buekens, Curtis, & Alayón, 2003). Thus, the problem with cesarean deliveries in the developed world is an excess of nonmedically indicated procedures, while in sub-Saharan Africa the problem is that the procedure is not available to women with high-risk pregnancies.

This chapter continues with the World Health Organization's (WHO) definition of reproductive health to stimulate ways of thinking about the topic and to describe a few major reproductive health indicators. It concludes with a discussion of a social ecological model to address a vexing reproductive health problem: adolescent childbearing.

WHAT IS REPRODUCTIVE HEALTH?

Reproductive health is defined by the WHO as follows:

> A state of physical, mental, and social well-being in all matters relating to the reproductive system at all stages of life. Reproductive health implies that people are able to have a satisfying and safe sex

life and that they have the capability to reproduce and the freedom to decide if, when, and how often to do so. Implicit in this is the right of men and women to be informed and to have access to safe, effective, affordable, and acceptable methods of family planning of their choice, and the right to appropriate health-care services that enable women to safely go through pregnancy and childbirth. (WHO, 2005b)

This simple definition contains the following key assumptions about reproductive health.

Reproductive Health Involves Physical, Mental, and Social Well-Being

Reproductive health is not limited to family-planning counseling and testing for STIs. It involves more than biology; it also includes satisfaction and sexual health, which enhance life and personal relations. Reproductive health includes the absence of fear and coercion in sexual matters. Gender-specific stigmas and sexual violence result in poor reproductive health, and combating them is critical. For example, in India, male homosexual acts are illegal, and many homosexual men are shunned by their families, often during adolescence, and they turn to sex work because they have no other options. Because of the social stigma attached to homosexuality and the lack of legal protection, homosexuals in India tend to be exposed to violence from the police and clients and do not generally have easy access to condoms or testing for STIs (Asthana & Oostvogels, 2001). In developed countries, homosexuality is more accepted (although there are striking examples of differential treatment, stigma, and discrimination), and male homosexuals have access to (and, in fact, are targeted for) HIV and STI prevention efforts, screening, and treatment. However, there are many examples of insufficient outreach and knowledge to men who have sex with men (MSM) in developed countries, as researchers continue to discover high-risk and novel sex drug use among MSM that defies safer-sex messages (Schwarcz et al., 2007). Data also show that same-sex activity among women in developed countries may be a marker for adverse reproductive health outcomes, including STIs (Marrazzo, Stine, & Koutsky, 2000; Mercer et al., 2007). This suggests that the stigma associated with same-sex relationships for women may affect their taking precautions and/or seeking health care.

Reproductive Health Is Relevant to People at All Stages of Life

Traditionally, women between the ages of 15 and 44 years are considered to be of reproductive age, reflecting only the years when women are most likely to become pregnant. The WHO definition is extended to everyone, reminding us that children have sexual awareness and that the elderly are sexual beings with reproductive health concerns. Reproductive health is not just about people who have the probability of being involved in a pregnancy.

An extension of the WHO inclusion of all-age individuals is the adoption of a life course approach to study reproductive health, which addresses the entirety of individual lives, from the womb to the grave. The life course is not only about biological aging; it reflects the intermingling of past and present individual and social factors on an individual's reproductive health. Any reproductive outcome (e.g., pregnancy) is associated not only with an individual's current circumstances (e.g., exposure to sexual activity, use of contraceptives) but possibly with his or her past experiences as well. For example, the ability to become pregnant (or cause a pregnancy) is associated with an individual's exposure to STIs, which are the major known cause of infertility, especially if untreated (Cates, Rolfs, & Aral, 2001). Past experiences can also have subtle, and difficult to measure, influences on the risk for pregnancy involvement (e.g., childhood exposure to patriarchal attitudes may influence men's attitudes about using contraceptives). Exposures in utero can also influence pregnancy risk. For example, women and men whose mothers were exposed to diethylstilbestrol when they were pregnant have increased risks for infertility and reproductive cancers (Newbold & Jefferson, 2004). The fetal origins hypothesis is not as well studied for reproductive health as it is for cardiovascular disease (Barker, 2004), but model development is still under way (Gluckman, Hanson, Morton, & Pinal, 2005). It is possible that future research will uncover in utero exposures (e.g., nutrients, environmental exposures, infections) that affect adult risk for infertility and reproductive cancers.

A life course approach also emphasizes that reproductive outcomes overlap and influence one another. As shown in Figure 10.1, the risk for childbearing during adolescence is associated with age at sexual debut (first vaginal intercourse), use of contraceptives, and decisions about pregnancy resolution (Hayes, 1987). Each of these three outcomes, or steps toward childbearing, has unique and shared antecedents. This figure also demonstrates the potential efficacy of preventive and health promotion efforts, at each step, to reduce adolescent childbearing: Increasing age at sexual debut, early introduction of effective and user-friendly contraception to sexually active youth, and access to legal abortion services could each reduce risk for teen childbearing.

Family Planning Is an Important Component of Reproductive Health

The WHO definition states that people should be able to choose when—and if—they have children. Family planning is thus not only about planned births but also about planned periods free of pregnancy. In fact, most people will spend the bulk of their reproductive lives trying to avoid pregnancy involvement: For women in the United States, the average age at first vaginal intercourse is 17 years, the age at first birth is about 26 years, the age at which a woman desires no more children is about 31 years, and the average age at menopause is 50 years (Alan Guttmacher Institute, 2002). A woman will spend about 33 years at risk of pregnancy if she is sexually active from the age of sexual debut to menopause. If she wants to have children, the average women will want to have them over a 6-year period. She will thus spend 27 years trying to *avoid* getting pregnant.

Similar data about age at sexual debut and desired ages at first and last child are reported for men in the United States (Alan Guttmacher Institute, 2002).

FIGURE 10.1   Steps to Adolescent Childbearing and STIs

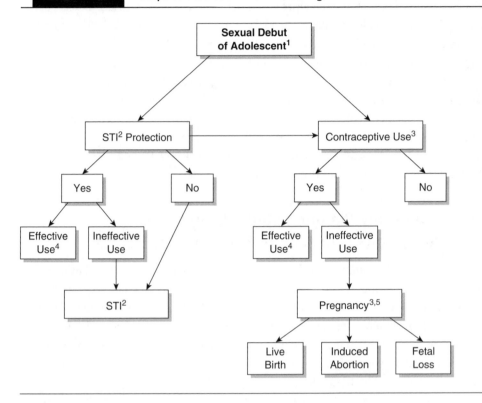

1. *Adolescent* is defined as 10 to 25 years of age; most youth will have had sexual debut by 25 years.
2. STI = sexually transmitted infection.
3. Contraceptive use and pregnancy are only relevant for fertile individuals who engage in heterosexual (penis in vagina) intercourse.
4. Effectiveness is determined by product quality and behavioral compliance (correct use).
5. Pregnancy involvement for males.

A critical, and missing, component of many discussions of family planning is the fact that some people choose to not ever be parents. This notion is so unacceptable, even in developed countries, that "child-free" people may be stigmatized at worst and pitied at best. There are varying estimates of how many adults in the United States are voluntarily and lifelong child-free, but it is likely somewhere near 8% (Lisle, 1996). The rates may be higher in Europe, with estimates as high as 20% in the United Kingdom (Mitchell, 2004).

Men as Well as Women Have Reproductive Health Needs

Rates of STIs are high among young men, especially poor, minority men in their early 20s. There are racial disparities in reproductive health risks globally. In the United States, for example, about 15% of male teens are African Americans, but African American youth (females and males) account for about 55% of HIV infections reported in 2003 (Centers for Disease Control and Prevention [CDC], 2005). Testicular cancer is the most common cancer among men aged 20 to 34. Despite their risk, only about 14% of American men between 15 and 49 years of age have a sexual/reproductive health visit annually (Guttmacher Institute, 2005). The reproductive health status of middle-aged and older men is not frequently studied, but in a recent survey in Australia of men who were older than 40 years, researchers found that 34% of the sample reported at least one reproductive health disorder; the most common disorder was erectile dysfunction, reported by 21% of the men. Less than one half of the sample sought treatment for their disorder (Holden et al., 2005). Sexual health education for men is needed globally and should include guidance to encourage the growth and development of a secure sense of sexual identity, promote the physical and emotional aspects of sexual intimacy, and reassure men about the necessity of reproductive health care visits.

Access to Family-Planning Methods and Safe Birthing Options Is Critical to Reproductive Health

While the WHO definition promotes a medical approach to reproductive health, it also asserts that methods must be acceptable to users, thus acknowledging that access is affected by individual and cultural, as well as macroenvironmental, factors. The definition highlights the relationship of family planning (i.e., having wanted children) to safe pregnancies. Imbedded in this is the realization that the health of future generations begins well before conception: If the parents' health is good before conception, many problems for the offspring can be prevented. Planned pregnancies allow women to recover adequately from previous pregnancies, build social and material resources, and address health problems. In developing countries, these problems may range from STI treatment to resolving inadequate nutrition; in developed countries, the issues are similar and range from preconception STI and substance use treatment to resolving nutritional issues, including obesity.

REPRODUCTIVE HEALTH INDICATORS

Reproductive health surveillance varies by region, and the problems associated with measurement are substantial. Some countries do not have effective surveillance in place, some countries (including the United States) may have difficulty enumerating the experiences of disenfranchised people (e.g., the homeless, historically underserved people), and some measures of interest are extremely difficult to assess, often because they are sensitive or because comprehensive screening is not done (e.g., infertility, abortion, STIs, unintended pregnancy, and childbearing). Assessment issues should always be considered when programs and policies are developed to promote reproductive health because poor assessment can lead to misdirection in terms of identifying populations in need and can make it impossible to evaluate the effectiveness of programs and policies. Assessment—and the development of interventions to improve reproductive health—should always consider both protective and risk factors. Finally, programs and policies that are feasible and acceptable in one setting may not be possible in another setting because of variations in culture, resources, and populations at risk.

Fertility and Infertility

In 2006, there were more than 137 million births in the world (123.5 million of them in developing countries) (Population Reference Bureau, n.d.). Worldwide, fertility has been declining, and contraceptive use has been increasing for decades. The factors that promote fertility are complex. Fertility is often considered in the context of whether family-planning needs are being met. This supposes that couples, and women, can clearly articulate desired family size and that contraceptives are used effectively. Even in developed countries such as the United States, it is estimated that perhaps 50% of all pregnancies are mistimed or unwanted (Finer & Henshaw, 2006), and almost one third of all women will have one or more unintended births (Henshaw, 1998). In the United States, unintended pregnancies and births are strongly associated with socioeconomic status (Finer & Henshaw, 2006; Henshaw, 1998). A study of 41 countries also found that higher fertility and lower contraceptive use were found among the poorer compared with the wealthier segments of society (Gillespie, Ahmed, Tsui, & Radloff, 2007).

Fertility rates are often examined in light of contraceptive prevalence. In developed countries, it is estimated that 78% of women, aged 15 to 49, who are in a sexual union, use some form of contraception (hormonal, barrier, or behavioral). The total fertility rate in developed countries is 1.6 lifetime births per woman. In developing countries, contraceptive use is estimated at 65% for women at risk for pregnancy, and total fertility is 3.0 lifetime births per woman. In the least developed countries, contraceptive use is 32%, and total fertility is 5.4 lifetime births per woman. From 1990 to 2000, contraceptive use increased worldwide and more than doubled in 13 developing countries, all of which started at very low rates. During that same period, fertility fell around the world; it decreased by one birth or more per woman in 40 developing countries (Zlidar et al., 2003).

It is estimated that there may be 80 million involuntarily childless persons in the world. The etiology of infertility is largely unknown, but STIs are the major known cause. The epidemiology of infertility and childlessness (voluntary and involuntary) is not well understood, and cultural norms may contribute to difficulties in collecting evidence and proposing preventive and treatment measures. In many developing countries, infertility is neglected because of lack of resources and because the subject is not discussed: Not having children is unacceptable and is viewed as a personal failure (Runganga, Sundby, & Aggleton, 2001; Widge, 2002). Furthermore, historically, there has been more interest in curbing fertility rates in developing countries than in addressing infertility. Gender roles may also influence how a couple represents childlessness and, thus, can affect surveillance and treatment. Nene, Coyaji, and Apte (2005) interviewed couples who went to a hospital in Pune (India) because they were childless and also because they were experiencing sexual dysfunction. The women were distressed because of their "barrenness," and the men faced emotional pressure because of their sexual dysfunction. The women preferred to accept the stigma of infertility rather than expose the sexual dysfunction of their husbands.

Abortion

Abortion is unique among reproductive health indicators: It is one of the most common reproductive procedures for women, yet data about legal abortions are of variable quality because of its controversial nature. Data about illegal abortions are difficult to find and are often estimated from hospital and clinic reports. Unsafe abortions are almost always those that are illegal. There are about 42 million abortions annually worldwide (about one fifth of all pregnancies). Forty-eight percent of all abortions are unsafe (and not legal), and more than 97% of all unsafe abortions were in developing countries (Sedgh, Henshaw, Singh, Ahman, & Shah, 2007). Overall abortion rates are similar in the developing and developed world, but unsafe abortion is concentrated in the developing countries. Abortion is an important indicator of the unmet need for contraceptives. While data are needed for program and policy planners, a recent examination of legal abortion in 60 countries showed that data are of variable completeness (Sedgh, Henshaw, Singh, Bankole, & Drescher, 2007). Of the 60 countries, 33 had relatively complete counts. Two countries, the Russian Federation and Cuba, recorded more abortions than live births; it was estimated that an average woman would have 1.7 (Russian Federation) and 1.3 (Cuba) abortions in her lifetime. Countries in Eastern Europe have the highest rates of abortion. Many countries in Northern and Western Europe, which have broad access to contraceptives and comprehensive sexual education (Singh & Darroch, 2000), have among the lowest rates of abortion. The rate of abortion in the United States is slightly higher than that of many developed countries, particularly for women above the age of 30 years (Sedgh, Henshaw, Singh, Bankole, et al., 2007).

Abortion has historically been important to population fertility control. In the early stages of fertility decline, in a country or region, increases in abortion almost always precede or accompany increases in contraceptive use. This pattern has been seen in diverse areas such as North Africa (Tunisia, Egypt), Latin America (Venezuela, Columbia, Chile), and Asia (Thailand, India) (Streatfield, 2001). Abortion rates tend to decline when contraceptive use—and effectiveness of use—increases to a substantial level (Marston & Cleland, 2003). This may be the case in China, although data are incomplete: Abortion appears to be declining as the use of IUDs (intrauterine devices) and other contraceptive options is increasing (Sedgh, Henshaw, Singh, Ahman, et al., 2007).

Unwanted pregnancies are not entirely avoidable, but they are affected by the social acceptability and availability of effective contraception. Unwanted pregnancies may also be reduced through policies that guarantee health coverage for contraceptives (Culwell & Feinglass, 2007) and programs that challenge gender inequities and thus reduce sexual violence and improve the sexual negotiation skills of women and couples.

Safe Motherhood

The differential incidence of unsafe motherhood reflects the most profound health disparity between women in developed and developing countries (Cook & Dickens, 2002). There are about 136 million births in the world annually. Approximately 550,000 women between the ages of 15 and 49 years die every year from complications of pregnancy and childbirth; 99% of these deaths occur in developing countries (primarily sub-Saharan Africa and Asia), and most are preventable (Filippi et al., 2006). A woman in sub-Saharan Africa is 175 times more likely to die from a pregnancy-related cause than a woman from a developed country

(WHO/UNFPA/UNICEF/World Bank, 1999). Mortality is the most extreme—and the most uncommon—response to a pregnancy complication. It is estimated that 9.5 million women suffer from pregnancy-related illnesses, 1.4 million come close to death, and 10 to 20 million experience pregnancy-related disabilities (Murray & Lopez, 1998; Say, Pattinson, & Gulmezoglu, 2004; WHO, 2000). Maternal mortality and morbidity are also closely linked to infant and child outcomes. In Nepal, for example, infants who survive the deaths of their mothers are six times more likely to die in the first week of life, 12 times more likely to die between the ages of 8 to 28 days, and 52 times more likely to die between the ages of 4 to 24 weeks compared with infants whose mothers did not die (Katz et al., 2003).

The WHO/UNFPA/UNICEF/World Bank (1999) statement on safe motherhood indicates that while countries around the world vary by maternal health status and resources, there are common elements globally that can affect maternal morbidity and mortality: (1) national policies and legislation, (2) community and family factors, and (3) health care systems. When interpersonal characteristics are also considered, these elements are consistent with a social ecological model of risk, and they provide a framework to assess safe motherhood potential across countries. The following national policies and legislation suggested by the WHO/UNFPA/UNICEF/World Bank are relevant to developed and developing countries.

Family Planning. Planned pregnancies are the most likely to be healthy pregnancies. The risk factors for unsafe motherhood, then, are policies that restrict women's access to family-planning services (e.g., by requiring that she be an adult, be married, have her husband's approval). Protective policies are those that promote couple access to effective, client-oriented, and confidential family-planning services and a wide choice of effective and safe contraceptive methods. Policies are important, but they have to be implemented to be effective. For example, in India, abortion has been legal for decades, but access is limited by the scarcity of low-cost services (Grimes et al., 2006).

Programs for Adolescents and Children. Policies and programs that promote safe motherhood are those that encourage late marriage and childbearing; provide economic and educational opportunities for young people; and allow young people to take responsibility for their sexual health by providing them with health information and services. The statement indicates that "all children, before they reach the age at which they become sexually active, need to be taught the risks of unprotected sex and helped to develop the skills needed to protect themselves from sexual coercion."

Health Care Access. The WHO/UNFPA/UNICEF/World Bank (1999) indicated that safe motherhood is related to: (1) the prevention of pregnancy through family-planning services for women, men, and adolescents, including women postabortion; (2) the prevention of pregnancy complications through the provision of prenatal, obstetric, and postpartum care; and (3) the management of pregnancy complications through the availability of skilled birth attendants and a system of referral for complications. A striking example of differences in the prevalence of pregnancy complications between developing and developed countries is mother-to-child transmission (MTCT) of HIV: About 100 cases occur every year in the United States (CDC, 2007a), while an estimated 420,000 children worldwide were infected with HIV in 2007, most of them in developing countries and most of them through MTCT (WHO, n.d.). Not only are there stark differences between developing and developed countries in family planning, HIV screening, and HIV treatment resources for pregnant women, but in both, there are gender-based cultural factors that affect the ability of women to protect themselves from infection and their willingness to disclose their infections to health care providers (Medley, Garcia-Moreno, McGill, & Maman, 2004).

Sexually Transmitted Infections

STIs are a modern epidemic but not a modern disease: Hippocrates wrote about gonorrhea transmission. There are many types of STIs (e.g., chlamydia, gonorrhea, syphilis, genital warts, hepatitis, HIV), and their symptoms and consequences vary. If untreated, gonorrhea and chlamydia can cause permanent damage to the reproductive system, human papillomavirus (HPV) is associated with cervical cancer, and HIV can be life threatening. Having one STI increases the risk of acquiring another one. Assessing the impact of STIs is difficult, as they can only be counted if several conditions are met: People are screened for them, health providers diagnose them, and reliable surveillance systems exist. In the United States, health care providers are not required to report all STIs to state and national surveillance systems, so incidence and prevalence can only be estimated for STIs such as HPV. Some STIs are curable (e.g., syphilis, gonorrhea, chlamydia, trichomoniasis), and some are not (e.g., HIV, HPV). Incidence (new cases) and prevalence (existing cases) data for the same noncurable STIs can be extremely different, depending on the rate of acquisition and the number of individuals with lifelong infection.

The WHO estimates that 340 million new cases of curable STIs occur every year. The greatest number of infections occur in South and Southeast Asia, sub-Saharan Africa, Latin America, and the Caribbean. Within countries and between countries, STI incidence and prevalence vary, reflecting social, cultural, economic, and religious factors (WHO, 2005a). Women are at greatest risk for STIs and experience more complications than men. Youth are at high risk for STIs worldwide, with more than one fifth to greater than one half of the incidence among people younger than 25 years old (Dehne & Riedner, 2001). Of the 18.9 million new cases of STIs in the United States in 2000, 48% were among 15- to 24-year-olds (Weinstock, Berman, & Cates, 2004). Thus, despite data that suggest increased use of condoms and delayed first age at intercourse (Santelli, Lindberg, Finer, & Singh, 2007), youth still need to improve their knowledge about condoms, their access to condoms, and their sexual negotiation skills.

The incidence of STIs may be increasing. In 2006, in the United States, more than 1 million cases of chlamydia were reported, a record high. After declining throughout the 1990s, the rates of syphilis increased, especially among MSM, whose rates increased 54% from 2001 to 2006. The reported number of STI cases is likely much smaller than the actual number of cases. With chlamydia, for example, fewer than one half of all cases are likely reported (CDC, 2007b). About 25% of women in the United States have HPV; the prevalence is highest in women who are in their early and mid-20s (45%) (Dunne et al., 2007).

According to the WHO (2007), the global prevalence of HIV leveled off in 2007, and the number of new infections fell. In 2007, an estimated 33.2 million people had HIV, 2.5 million became newly infected, and 2.1 million died of AIDS. There were an estimated 1.7 million new HIV infections in sub-Saharan Africa in 2007, a significant reduction since 2001. Sub-Saharan Africa is the most severely affected area, with an estimated 22.5 million people living with HIV, which is 68% of the global total. In Africa, the prevalence of HIV infection is higher among females than males, while in developed countries men often have twice the rate of infection (WHO, 2007).

HIV is not entirely sexually transmitted. Globally, about 11% of new infections are in infants who acquire the virus from their mothers; 10% are from injection drug use; 5% to 10% are associated with sex between men; and 5% to 10% occur in health care settings. Sexual transmission between men and women accounts for the remaining two thirds of the new infections. About one half of the people who acquire HIV become infected before the age of 25 years, and in developing countries, the majority die before the age of 35 (survival is much better in developed countries). By the end of 2005, there were 15.2 million AIDS orphans, defined as children younger than 18 years who have lost one or both parents to AIDS (WHO, 2007).

A 2002 Institute of Medicine report suggested that ecological approaches to health, and to STI prevention, are particularly useful and needed (Institute of Medicine, 2002). For STIs, factors from many levels interactively contribute to risk behavior above and beyond the effects of a single, individual factor (DiClemente, Salazar, Crosby, & Rosenthal, 2005; Mandara, Murray, & Bangi, 2003; Small & Luster, 1994). As with all reproductive health outcomes, the patterns of acquisition, transmission, and course of STIs vary by individual characteristics and access to health-promoting programs and policies. Culture also plays an important role in STI risk, and cultural issues can complicate STI education, screening, and treatment efforts. For example, men whose cultures or religions are intolerant of homosexuality may have high-risk encounters that they keep secret from partners and health care providers. Adolescents who take virginity pledges may be at higher risk for STIs because when they ultimately engage in sexual behavior, they may be less likely than adolescents who did not take pledges to use protection (Brückner & Bearman, 2005). Data show that women who have sex with women may be at higher risk for STIs than others (Marrazzo et al., 2000; Mercer et al., 2007), perhaps because they are reluctant to seek counseling for sexual matters. Many women are not in charge of sexual decision making and are at higher risk for unprotected sexual encounters. Men and women who are involved with illicit substances engage in high-risk sexual behaviors, and some subgroups may engage in highly specific, and dangerous, cobehaviors that put them at risk for STIs (Schwarcz et al., 2007).

UNINTENDED ADOLESCENT CHILDBEARING

There are more than 1 billion 10- to 19-year-olds in the world, and their contributions to the reproductive health of populations are increasing, especially in the developing world (Bayley, 2003). Adolescent pregnancy and childbearing pose huge health risks: Pregnancy is the main cause of death for 15- to 19-year-old girls globally, accounting for about 60,000 deaths per year

(WHO, 1998). Adolescent childbearing inhibits a young woman's economic and educational prospects in developed and developing countries, and it may be a key contributor to poverty among women (WHO, 1998). Men are less well studied, but it is likely that early parenthood is also correlated with diminished socioeconomic prospects for males as well (Alan Guttmacher Institute, 2002; Teti, Lamb, & Elster, 1987). Adolescents are the *only* population subgroup for whom it is generally agreed on, among public health workers, that childbearing should be prevented (i.e., delayed until adulthood).

Rates of adolescent (15–19 years) childbearing vary dramatically worldwide: In developed countries alone, rates vary from 8/1,000 in France to 29/1,000 in the Russian Federation. Japan and most European countries have low rates of adolescent childbearing, with the United States among the few with high rates (41/1,000). In developing countries, the birth rates among 15- to 19-year-olds is high, with rates of more than 100/1,000 adolescents in most of sub-Saharan Africa, parts of Asia (e.g., Afghanistan, India, Bangladesh), and some Latin American countries (e.g., Guatemala, Honduras, Nicaragua) (Bearinger, Sieving, Ferguson, & Sharma, 2007).

In the United States, about 13% of all births are to women younger than 20 years, and it is estimated that about 79% of these births are unintended (e.g., mistimed or unwanted) (Abma, Martinez, Mosher, & Dawson, 2004; Henshaw, 1998). The notion of "intention" is culturally specific, and in developed countries it may relate to an important demographic shift in the definition of "adolescence." The age at which adolescence stops and adulthood begins has been extended by some researchers and organizations to 21 years (e.g., American Academy of Pediatrics) or 24 years (e.g., CDC). Because adolescence is considered a transition period between childhood and adulthood, and thus a period of social dependence, a cultural value in developed countries may be that individuals delay pregnancy and childbearing to later ages. They will thus have a much shorter period of childbearing— and a somewhat shorter period of child rearing—than they have experienced in the past. Thus, the expectations about adolescent childbearing are different from what they were 50 years ago: The highest recorded rate of teen childbearing in the United States was 96/1,000 in 1957 (more than twice as high as the current rate), and about 85% of adolescent mothers were married (compared with 21% in 2004) (Boonstra, 2002). The expectations for delayed motherhood in the United States and other developed countries coincide with important shifts in societal expectations about women completing a high school education, attending college, and finding employment. However, the impact of a macroenvironmental variable, such as improvement in the economic status of women, may vary by subgroups and by reproductive outcome, especially in environments where racism or classism persist (Geronimus, 2003). Quite simply, disenfranchised and impoverished youth may realistically perceive that the costs of early childbearing are not high, given their other options. Variations in the perceived "opportunity costs" of adolescent childbearing in the United States may explain why it is concentrated among the most socially vulnerable youth (Hillis et al., 2004; Klein & Committee on Adolescence, 2005).

There are several considerations in developing a model to describe adolescent unintended childbearing: (1) The antecedents to adolescent childbearing for high-risk teens may be very different from those for low-risk teens. For example, in the United States, the offspring of adolescent mothers are themselves at risk for early childbearing (i.e., high risk). For these children, adolescent parenting may be normative, and their risks for early childbearing will be different from that of a child who was born to adult parents (i.e., a child for whom early childbearing would be nonnormative). (2) It may make sense to examine risks for childbearing, pregnancy, and STIs in an integrated fashion, because reproductive health outcomes cluster within individuals, within communities, and within countries (Kirby & Lepore, 2007; Meade & Ickovics, 2005). (3) Consistent with an integrated approach is the idea that the path to adolescent childbearing has several steps (as shown in Figure 10.1), and the correlates of each step will contribute to the final outcome. (4) Adolescent childbearing is not the same as adult childbearing—its antecedents and consequences are very different.

Complex dynamics influence adolescent decisions about sex and their paths to a variety of reproductive outcomes. In the United States, much of the research about adolescent sexual risk taking and reproductive outcomes has focused on females, probably because they suffer greater consequences than males. Most of the research has also focused on age at sexual debut and contraceptive/condom use rather than on pregnancy and childbearing. Figure 10.2 and the following paragraphs describe some major correlates of sexual behaviors (which over lap between levels of influence) that can lead to adolescent childbearing.

Intrapersonal-Level Factors

Sexual experience (i.e., having ever had intercourse) should be distinguished from sexual activity (usually defined as having experienced a sexual act, usually intercourse, within a given time frame) because sexual activity among youth is sporadic. Sexually experienced youth have long periods of abstinence and are not continuously at risk for pregnancy. In the 2002 National Survey of Family Growth (NSFG), 69% of the 18- to 19-year-old females reported that they were sexually experienced (i.e., had ever had intercourse), but 54% reported that they were sexually active in the 3 months prior to the survey (Abma et al., 2004). Thus, sexually active youth are at the highest risk. Behavior and age often intersect in describing adolescent risk for childbearing. According to the 2002 NSFG data for adolescents, 25% of females and 18% of males used no method of contraception at first intercourse, and the most popular contraceptive at first intercourse was the condom (66% of females and 71% of males reported this method). Use of other forms of contraception increased sharply with older age at first intercourse and with increasing experience with intercourse: 83% of females and 91% of males used some form of contraception (ranging from hormonal methods to withdrawal) at last intercourse (Abma et al., 2004). Compared with adults, female youth have higher failure rates for contraceptives that demand behavioral compliance; data are not available for males (Glei, 1999). The higher failure rates for females may be related to the relatively sporadic nature of intercourse for youth, relationship instability, partner characteristics, less skill in resisting pressures or being able to negotiate about sex or contraceptive use, less knowledge about sexuality and fertility, or immature cognitive development.

There are several demographic and biologic characteristics that correspond to sexual risk taking, and thus childbearing risk: physical maturity, adolescent older age, same-sex

Unintended Childbearing

Behavior
- Substance use
- Early age at first sex
- Contraceptive use
- Abstinence

Biological
- Early puberty
- Age
- Parity

Psychological/Cognitive
- Self-esteem
- Family-planning knowledge
- Pregnancy feelings
- Health literacy

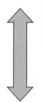

Home
- Income
- Household mobility

Family
- Mother's feelings about contraception
- Family abuse and adverse experiences
- Parental low education
- Lives with parents
- Mother was a teen mom
- Discuss family planning with parents
- Feel connected to parents
- Norms

Peers and Partners
- Discuss family planning
- Age of partner
- Partner's feelings about family planning
- Peer/partner deviance

School
- School achievement
- Sense of safety at school
- School connectedness
- Aspiration to attend college
- Sexual education at school

Extracurricular Events
- Employment
- Involved in sports or service

Neighborhood Quality
(e.g., safety, unemployment, crime, service availability)
- Rural/urban
- Norms

Identified Community or Culture
- Youth
- Race
- Ethnicity
- Gender
- Class

Policy
- Abortion
- Family planning
- Sex education

Health Care and Counseling
- Access
- Acceptability
- Comprehensiveness

attraction, family poverty, African American race, and Hispanic ethnicity (Kirby & Lepore, 2007). Cognitive development and skills, as measured by academic performance and plans for future education, are protective (Kirby & Lepore, 2007). There are several personality traits or psychological correlates of risk that are protective, including feelings connected to school, parents, or a significant adult; having a religious affiliation; and having an internal locus of control (Kirby & Lepore, 2007). Obviously, many of these characteristics cannot be changed by interventions.

Several behaviors, beyond contraceptive use, are risk factors, including substance use and involvement in violent activities; involvement in sports activities may be protective (Kirby & Lepore, 2007). Values and attitudes associated with sexual behavior may be indirectly related to risk for childbearing, whereas pregnancy feelings may be directly related (Kirby & Lepore, 2007). Once an adolescent has had one child, she is at increased risk of having another during adolescence: About 25% of adolescent births are not first births (Ventura & Freedman, 2000).

Interpersonal-Level Factors

Adolescents are less likely to engage in risky sexual behaviors and more likely to engage in protective sexual behaviors if they are able to communicate openly with their parents about sexual health (Miller, Levin, Whitaker, & Xu, 1998; Miller & Whitaker, 2001; Whitaker, Miller, May, & Levin, 1999). Parent-child discussions about specific sexual health behaviors and attitudes that occur before the onset of sexual activity are the most effective way to reduce sexual risk behaviors (Miller et al., 1998) and may indirectly affect risk for adolescent childbearing. High level of parental education, high-quality family interactions (measured by satisfaction), parental disapproval of teen sex, parental acceptance of contraceptive use for teens, and parental supervision are protective for adolescent pregnancy, but the research on childbearing is sparse (Kirby & Lepore, 2007). Hillis et al. (2004) showed increased risk for adolescent pregnancy (they did not examine childbearing) in a retrospective study of adults who reported childhood exposure to someone with substance abuse problems or mental illness; had an incarcerated family member as a child; suffered childhood verbal, physical, or sexual abuse; had divorced parents; and were exposed to intimate-partner violence as a child. Adolescent childbearing may be intergenerational in the United States: The offspring of adolescent parents may be at highest risk of being adolescent parents themselves (Campa & Eckenrode, 2006).

Peer influences can be protective (e.g., positive peer norms, support for condom or contraceptive use) or can enhance risk (e.g., substance use, deviant behaviors, permissive values about sex, and sexually active, pro-childbearing attitudes or behaviors) for pregnancy and contraceptive use, although childbearing has not been studied frequently (Bearman & Brückner, 1999; Cavanagh, 2004; Kirby & Lepore, 2007). Older partner age is one of the few partner characteristics that have been studied relative to risk for childbearing, and the results have been inconsistent (Abma & Sonenstein, 2001; Zavodny, 2001). Zavodny (2001) found that some partner characteristics were protective against pregnancy, including the male partner having a higher level of education than the female and sharing the same religion. In terms of contraceptive use, partner support of contraceptive use may be protective against pregnancy (Murphy & Boggess, 1998), and partner alcohol use may be a risk factor (Kowaleski-Jones & Mott, 1998).

Organizational-Level Factors

School-level sexual health education can reduce the risk of adolescent sexual risk taking (and perhaps childbearing). About one third of adolescents in the United States received no formal sex education in 2002, compared with about 20% in 1995 (Lindberg et al., 2006).

In an article encouraging the incorporation of comprehensive sexual education in schools, Boonstra (2007) stated,

> Since 1996, when a major overhaul of the nation's welfare policy prompted a massive escalation of funding in this area, the federal government . . . has spent well over one billion dollars to promote premarital abstinence . . . through highly restrictive programs that ignore or often actively denigrate the effectiveness of contraceptives and safer-sex behaviors . . . the federal government has been supporting and evaluating single-purpose abstinence promotion programs since the early 1980s, and there is now evidence suggesting that they may be harmful to young people in the long term. Meanwhile, there is still no comparable federal program to support comprehensive approaches that promote delayed sexual activity as well as protective behaviors for when young people do initiate sex, even though such programs have been shown to be effective at accomplishing both. (p. 2)

Data from the national Add-Health survey showed that 7th to 12th graders who made virginity pledges were just as likely to have acquired an STI as nonpledgers when followed up 5 to 6 years later. Of concern is that the pledgers were less likely to use condoms, seek testing, and be treated for STIs (Brückner & Bearman, 2005).

Adolescents in the United States may not be getting contraceptive information when they need it most, and the most socially disenfranchised youth may be at highest risk. A 2002 survey showed that about one half of sexually experienced males and 60% of females had received instruction about birth control methods before they first had sex. Minority and low-income youth were especially disadvantaged: For example, one third of black males had received instruction about birth control prior to first sex, compared with two thirds of their white peers. Adolescents living below 200% of poverty were less likely than higher-income peers to have received birth control education before first sex (Lindberg et al., 2006). Receipt of contraceptive information and contraceptives themselves is critical in reducing adolescent childbearing. Data from a large national survey indicate that most of the decline (86%) in adolescent pregnancy and childbearing in the past decade in the United States was the result of dramatic improvements in contraceptive use; just 14% of the decline was attributed to a decrease in sexual activity (Santelli et al., 2007). In examining the organizational influences, it would appear that school-based comprehensive sexual health education has the potential to promote contraceptive use and, thus, reduce the risk for pregnancy, childbearing, and STIs.

Community-Level Factors

Neighborhood quality may be associated with childbearing risk, although many studies have shown weak or no associations by using census-type variables for neighborhood status (Cubbin, Santelli, Brindis, & Braveman, 2005; Way, Finch, & Cohen, 2006), possibly because they failed to measure neighborhood quality with sufficient precision. Neighborhood quality may interact with other variables to strengthen or weaken risk for early childbearing. Crowder and Teachman (2004), using the Panel Study of Income Dynamics, found that neighborhood disadvantage might be central to explaining the relationship of family dynamics to adolescent pregnancy. Neighborhood quality could also have an impact at a certain threshold (e.g., at extremes of disorganization or poverty) or for a specific group of individuals (e.g., low-income youth).

Of current interest are youth development interventions. These interventions focus on enhancing the assets of adolescents as a mechanism to reduce risk. The programs provide opportunities for adolescents to build skills, including those that allow them to function successfully in social contexts. Service-learning projects can be a component of youth development interventions, and such programs are often palatable to community stakeholders and parents (Gallagher, Stanley, Shearer, & Mosca, 2005). In a review of 73 programs to reduce adolescent sexual risk taking, Kirby (2002) concluded that four types of programs held the most promise: (1) specific sex education curricula; (2) one-on-one counseling in a health clinic; (3) service-learning programs; and (4) intensive, multicomponent youth development programs.

Societal-Level Factors

Because adolescents are not economically or socially independent, they are vulnerable to state and federal legislation about reproductive health. According to Dailard and Richardson (2005),

> The public policy debate over whether teenagers should be allowed to obtain reproductive health services confidentially or required to involve their parents dates back to the 1970s, when teen sexual activity became increasingly visible and teen pregnancy was first deemed a national social problem. Although teenagers did not initiate sexual activity any earlier over the course of that decade . . . the age of marriage was rising. Therefore, pregnancies that would have occurred to teenagers within marriage in previous years increasingly occurred before marriage. At the same time, pregnant teenagers became less likely to marry to "legitimize" their pregnancies and births, and more teens began to terminate their pregnancies following the national legalization of abortion in 1973. (p. 6)

Public policy has long allowed minors access to confidential reproductive health services, without the involvement of their parents. However, access to abortion has been another matter. Most states require parental involvement in a minor's decision to have an abortion. Many states require the consent or notification of only one parent, usually 24 or 48 hours before the procedure; it is common for states to have a medical emergency exception and a judicial bypass procedure through which a minor may receive court approval to obtain an abortion without parental involvement. There is great variation between states in adolescent abortion access. Given that about 85% of the counties in the United States lack an abortion provider, and some parental involvement is required to obtain an abortion, it is thought that some adolescents may be denied access and, thus, will have unintended births (Jones, Zolna, Henshaw, & Finer, 2008).

CONCLUSION

Reproductive health has been described as the cornerstone of population health. It has also been described as a human right. Every woman who dies during childbirth in sub-Saharan Africa and every teenager who has an unwanted pregnancy in urban America reminds us that we may be far away from the goal to ensure reproductive health for everyone in 2015. The goals of reproductive health are quite simple: well-being at all stages of life; a safe and satisfying sex life; the freedom to decide whether, and when, to have children; the right to be informed of reproductive services; and the ability to access appropriate services. The means to attain these simple goals, unfortunately, are complex and demanding. Cultural values may need to be challenged, financial commitments must be made, and political differences must be set aside.

REFERENCES

Abma, J. C., Martinez, G. M., Mosher, W. D., & Dawson, B. S. (2004). *Teenagers in the United States: Sexual activity, contraceptive use, and childbearing, 2002* (Vital Health Statistics Series, No. 23). Hyattsville, MD: National Center for Health Statistics.

Abma, J. C., & Sonenstein, F. L. (2001). *Sexual activity and contraceptive practices among teenagers in the United States, 1988 and 1995* (Vital and Health Statistics Series, No. 23). Hyattsville, MD: National Center for Health Statistics.

Al Gasseer, N., Dresden, E., Keeney, G. B., & Warren, N. (2004). Status of women and infants in complex humanitarian emergencies. *Journal of Midwifery & Women's Health, 49,* 7–13.

Alan Guttmacher Institute. (2002). *In their own right: Addressing the sexual and reproductive health needs of American men.* New York: Author.

Asthana, S., & Oostvogels, R. (2001). The social construction of male 'homosexuality' in India: Implications for HIV transmission and prevention. *Social Science & Medicine, 52,* 707–721.

Barker, D. J. P. (2004). The developmental origins of adult disease. *Journal of the American College of Nutrition, 23,* 588S–595S.

Bayley, O. (2003). Improvement of sexual and reproductive health requires focusing on adolescents. *Lancet, 362,* 830–831.

Bearinger, L. H., Sieving, R. E., Ferguson, J., & Sharma, V. (2007). Global perspectives on the sexual and reproductive health of adolescents: Patterns, prevention, and potential. *Lancet, 369,* 1220–1231.

Bearman, P., & Brückner, H. (1999). *Power in numbers: Peer effects on adolescent girls' sexual debut and pregnancy.* Washington, DC: National Campaign to Prevent Teen Pregnancy.

Boonstra, H. (2002). Teen pregnancy: Trends and lessons learned. *The Guttmacher Report on Public Policy, 5,* 7–12.

Boonstra, H. (2007). The case for a new approach to sex education mounts: Will policymakers heed the message? *The Guttmacher Report on Public Policy, 10,* 2–7.

Brückner, H., & Bearman, P. S. (2005). After the promise: The STI consequences of adolescent virginity pledges. *Journal of Adolescent Health, 36,* 271–278.

Buekens, P., Curtis, S., & Alayón, S. (2003). Demographic and health surveys: Caesarean section rates in sub-Saharan Africa. *British Medical Journal, 326,* 136–137.

Campa, M. I., & Eckenrode, J. J. (2006). Pathways to intergenerational adolescent childbearing in a high-risk sample. *Journal of Marriage and Family, 68,* 558–572.

Cates, W., Jr., Rolfs, R. T., & Aral, S. O. (2001). Sexually transmitted diseases, pelvic inflammatory disease, and infertility: An epidemiologic update. *Epidemiologic Reviews, 12,* 199–220.

Cavanagh, S. E. (2004). The sexual debut of girls in early adolescence: The intersection of race, pubertal timing, and friendship group characteristics. *Journal of Research on Adolescence, 14,* 285–312.

Centers for Disease Control and Prevention. (2005). *HIV prevention in the third decade.* Atlanta, GA: U.S. Department of Health and Human Services. Retrieved February 1, 2008, from www.cdc.gov/hiv/resources/reports/hiv3rddecade/index.htm

Centers for Disease Control and Prevention. (2007a). *HIV/AIDS surveillance report, 2005* (Vol. 17, Rev. ed.). Atlanta, GA: U.S. Department of Health and Human Services.

Centers for Disease Control and Prevention. (2007b). *Trends in reportable sexually transmitted diseases in the United States, 2006.* Retrieved December 14, 2007, from www.cdc.gov/std/stats/trends2006.htm

Cleland, J., Bernstein, S, Ezeh, A., Faundes, A. A., Glasier, A., & Innis, J. (2006). Family planning: The unfinished agenda. *Lancet, 368,* 1810–1827.

Cook, R. J., & Dickens, B. M. (2002). The injustice of unsafe motherhood. *Developing World Bioethics, 2,* 62–81.

Crowder, K., & Teachman, J. (2004). Do residential conditions explain the relationship between living arrangements and adolescent behavior? *Journal of Marriage and Family, 66,* 721–738.

Cubbin, C., Santelli, J., Brindis, C. D., & Braveman, P. (2005). Neighborhood context and sexual behaviors among adolescents: Findings from the National Longitudinal Study of Adolescent Health. *Perspectives on Sexual and Reproductive Health, 37,* 125–134.

Culwell, K. R., & Feinglass, J. (2007). The association of health insurance with use of prescription contraceptives. *Perspectives on Sexual and Reproductive Health, 39,* 226–230.

Dailard, C., & Richardson, C. T. (2005). Teenagers' access to confidential reproductive health services. *The Guttmacher Report on Public Policy, 8,* 6–11.

Dehne, K. L., & Riedner, G. (2001). Sexually transmitted infections among adolescents: The need for adequate health services. *Reproductive Health Matters, 9,* 170–183.

DiClemente, R., Salazar, L. F., Crosby, R. A., & Rosenthal, S. L. (2005). Prevention and control of sexually transmitted infections among adolescents: The importance of a socioecological perspective—a commentary. *Public Health, 119,* 1–12.

Dunne, E. F., Unger, E. R., Sternberg, M., McQuillan, G., Swan, D. C., Patel, S. S., et al. (2007). Prevalence of HPV infection among females in the United States. *Journal of the American Medical Association, 297,* 813–819.

Fathalla, M. F., Sinding, S. W., Rosenfield, A., & Fathalla, M. F. (2006). Sexual and reproductive health for all: A call to action. *Lancet, 368,* 2095–2100.

Filippi, V., Ronsmans, C., Campbell, O. M. R., Graham, W. J., Mills, A., Borghi, J., et al. (2006). Maternal health in poor countries: The broader context and a call for action. *Lancet, 368,* 1535–1541.

Finer, L. B., & Henshaw, S. K. (2006). Disparities in rates of unintended pregnancy in the United States, 1994 and 2001. *Perspectives in Sexual and Reproductive Health, 38,* 90–96.

Gallagher, K. M., Stanley, A., Shearer, D., & Mosca, C. (2005). Implementation of youth development programs: Promise and challenges. *Journal of Adolescent Health, 37*(3, Suppl.), S61–S68.

Geronimus, A. T. (2003). Damned if you do: Culture, identity, privilege, and teenage childbearing in the United States. *Social Science & Medicine, 57,* 881–893.

Gillespie, D., Ahmed, S., Tsui, A., & Radloff, S. (2007). Unwanted fertility among the poor: An inequity? *Bulletin of the World Health Organization, 85,* 100–107.

Glei, D. A. (1999). Measuring contraceptive use patterns among teenage and adult women. *Family Planning Perspectives, 31,* 73–80.

Gluckman, P. D., Hanson, M. A., Morton, S. M. B., & Pinal, C. S. (2005). Life-long echoes: A critical analysis of the developmental origins of adult disease model. *Biology of the Neonate, 87,* 127–139.

Grimes, D. A., Benson, J., Singh, S., Romero, M., Ganatra, B., Okonofua, F. E., et al. (2006). Unsafe abortion: The preventable pandemic. *Lancet, 368,* 1908–1919.

Guttmacher Institute. (2005). *Sexual and reproductive health information and services for men dangerously lacking.* Retrieved February 10, 2008, from http://guttmacher.org/media/presskits/2005/03/15/index.html

Hayes, C. D. (1987). *Risking the future: Adolescent sexuality, pregnancy, and childbearing.* Washington, DC: National Academy Press.

Henshaw, S. K. (1998). Unintended pregnancy in the United States. *Family Planning Perspectives, 30,* 24–29.

Hillis, S. D., Anda, R. F., Dube, S. R., Felitti, V. J., Marchbanks, P. A., & Marks, J. S. (2004). The association between adverse childhood experiences and adolescent pregnancy, long-term psychosocial consequences, and fetal death. *Pediatrics, 113,* 320–327.

Holden, C. A., McLachlan, R. I., Pitts, M., Cumming, R., Wittert, G., Agius, P. A., et al. (2005). Men in Australia Telephone Survey (MATeS): A national survey of the reproductive health and concerns of middle-aged and older Australian men. *Lancet, 366,* 218–224.

Institute of Medicine. (2002). *The future of the public's health in the 21st century.* Washington, DC: National Academy Press.

Jewkes, R. (2007). Comprehensive response to rape needed in conflict settings. *Lancet, 369,* 2187–2195.

Jones, R. K., Zolna, M. R. S., Henshaw, S. K., & Finer, L. B. (2008). Abortion in the United States: Incidence and access to services, 2005. *Perspectives on Sexual and Reproductive Health, 40,* 6–16.

Katz, J., West, K. P., Jr., Khatry, S. K., Christian, P., LeClerq, S. C., Pradhan, E. K., et al. (2003). Risk factors for early infant mortality in Sarlahi district, Nepal. *Bulletin of the World Health Organization, 81,* 717–725.

Kirby, D. (2002). Effective approaches to reducing adolescent unprotected sex, pregnancy, and childbearing. *Journal of Sex Research, 39,* 51–57.

Kirby, D., & Lepore, G. (2007). *Sexual risk and protective factors: Factors affecting teen sexual behavior, pregnancy, childbearing, and sexually transmitted disease.* Scotts Valley, CA: ETR Associates.

Kissinger, P., Schmidt, N., Sanders, C., & Liddon, N. (2007). The effect of the Hurricane Katrina disaster on sexual behavior and access to reproductive care for young women in New Orleans. *Sexually Transmitted Diseases, 34,* 883–886.

Klein, J. D., & Committee on Adolescence. (2005). Adolescent pregnancy: Current trends and issues. *Pediatrics, 116,* 281–286.

Kowaleski-Jones, L., & Mott, F. L. (1998). Sex, contraception and childbearing among high-risk youth: Do different factors influence males and females? *Family Planning Perspectives, 30,* 163–169.

Lindberg, L. D., Santelli, J. S., & Singh, S. (2006). Changes in formal sex education: 1995–2002. *Perspectives on Sexual and Reproductive Health, 38,* 182–189.

Lisle, L. (1996). *Without child: Challenging the stigma of childlessness.* New York: Ballantine Books.

Mandara, J., Murray, C. B., & Bangi, A. K. (2003). Predictors of African American adolescent sexual activity: An ecological framework. *Journal of Black Psychology, 29,* 337–356.

Marrazzo, J. M., Stine, K., & Koutsky, L. A. (2000). Genital human papillomavirus infection in women who have sex with women: A review. *American Journal of Obstetrics & Gynecology, 183,* 770–774.

Marston, C., & Cleland, J. (2003). Relationships between contraception and abortion: A review of the evidence. *International Family Planning Perspectives, 29,* 6–13.

Meade, C. S., & Ickovics, J. R. (2005). Systematic review of sexual risk among pregnant and mothering teens in the USA: Pregnancy as an opportunity for integrated prevention of STD and repeat pregnancy. *Social Science & Medicine, 60,* 661–678.

Medley, A., Garcia-Moreno, C., McGill, S., & Maman, S. (2004). Rates, barriers and outcomes of HIV serostatus disclosure among women in developing countries: Implications for prevention of mother-to-child transmission programmes. *Bulletin of the World Health Organization, 82,* 299–307.

Menacker, F. (2005). *Trends in cesarean rates for first births and repeat cesarean rates for low-risk women: United States 1990–2003* (National Vital Statistics Reports, Vol. 54, No. 4). Hyattsville, MD: National Center for Health Statistics.

Mercer, C. H., Bailey, J. V., Johnson, A. M., Erens, B., Wellings, K., Fenton, K. A., et al. (2007). Women who report having sex with women: British national probability data on prevalence, sexual behaviors, and health outcomes. *American Journal of Public Health, 97,* 1126–1133.

Miller, K. S., Levin, M. L., Whitaker, D. J., & Xu, X. (1998). Patterns of condom use among adolescents: The impact of mother-adolescent communication. *American Journal of Public Health, 88,* 1542–1544.

Miller, K. S., & Whitaker, D. J. (2001). Predictors of mother-adolescent discussions about condoms: Implications for providers who serve youth. *Pediatrics, 108,* E28.

Minkoff, H., & Chervenak, F. A. (2003). Elective primary cesarean delivery. *New England Journal of Medicine, 348,* 946–950.

Mitchell, J. C. W. (2004). Procreative mothers (sexual difference) and child-free sisters (gender). *European Journal of Women's Studies, 11,* 415–426.

Murphy, J. J., & Boggess, S. (1998). Increased condom use among teenage males, 1988–1995: The role of attitudes. *Family Planning Perspectives, 30,* 276–280, 303.

Murray, C. J. L., & Lopez, A. D. (1998). *Health dimensions of sex and reproduction. Global burden of disease and injury series* (Vol. 3). Boston: Harvard University Press.

Naz, R. K. (2004). *Endocrine disruptors: Effects on male and female reproductive systems* (2nd ed.). New York: CRC Press.

Nene, U. A., Coyaji, K., & Apte, H. (2005). Infertility: A label of choice among sexually dysfunctional couples. *Patient Education & Counseling, 59,* 234–238.

Newbold, R. R., & Jefferson, W. (2004). Developmental and reproductive abnormalities associated with environmental estrogens: Diethystilbesterol (DES) as an example. In R. K. Naz (Ed.), *Endocrine disruptors: Effects on male and female reproductive systems* (2nd ed., pp. 47–66). New York: CRC Press.

Population Reference Bureau. (n.d.). *World population clock, 2006.* Retrieved February 12, 2008, from www.prb.org/Articles/2006/WorldPopulationClock2006.aspx

Runganga, A. O., Sundby, J., & Aggleton, P. (2001). Culture, identity and reproductive failure in Zimbabwe. *Sexualities, 4,* 315–332.

Santelli, J. S., Lindberg, L. D., Finer, L. B., & Singh, S. (2007). Explaining recent declines in adolescent pregnancy in the United States: The contribution of abstinence and improved contraceptive use. *American Journal of Public Health, 97,* 150–156.

Say, L., Pattinson, R. C., & Gulmezoglu, M. (2004). WHO systematic review of maternal morbidity and mortality: The prevalence of severe acute maternal morbidity (near miss). *Reproductive Health, 1,* 3. Retrieved February 5, 2008, from www.reproductive-health-journal .com/content/1/1/3

Schwarcz, S., Scheer, S., McFarland, W., Katz, M., Valleroy, L., Chen, S., et al. (2007). Prevalence of HIV infection and predictors of high-transmission sexual risk behaviors among men who have sex with men. *American Journal of Public Health, 97,* 1067–1075.

Sedgh, G., Henshaw, S., Singh, S., Ahman, E., & Shah, I. H. (2007). Induced abortion: Estimated rates and trends worldwide. *Lancet, 370,* 1338–1345.

Sedgh, G., Henshaw, S. K., Singh, S., Bankole, A., & Drescher, J. (2007). Legal abortion worldwide: Incidence and recent trends. *Perspectives on Sexual and Reproductive Health, 39,* 216–225.

Singh, S., & Darroch, J. E. (2000). Adolescent pregnancy and childbearing: Levels and trends in developed countries. *Family Planning Perspectives, 32,* 14–23.

Small, S. A., & Luster, T. (1994). Adolescent sexual activity: An ecological, risk-factor approach. *Journal of Marriage and Family, 56,* 181–192.

Streatfield, P. K. (2001). Role of abortion in fertility control. *Journal of Health, Population and Nutrition, 19,* 265–267.

Teti, D. M., Lamb, M. E., & Elster, A. B. (1987). Long-range socioeconomic and marital consequences of adolescent marriage in three cohorts of adult males. *Journal of Marriage and Family, 49,* 499–506.

Trenholm, C., Devaney, B., Fortson, K., Quay, L., Wheeler, J., & Clark, M. (2007). *Impacts of four Title V, Section 510 abstinence education programs.* Princeton, NJ: Mathematica Policy Research. Retrieved February 1, 2008, from www.mathematica-mpr.com/publications/pdfs/ impactabstinence.pdf

Underhill, K., Montgomery, P., & Operario, D. (2007). Sexual abstinence only programmes to prevent HIV infection in high income countries: Systematic review. *British Medical Journal, 335,* 248–260.

United Nations. (2005). *World summit outcome* (General Assembly Resolution, A/RES/60/1). New York: Author.

Ventura, S. J., & Freedman, M. A. (2000). Teenage childbearing in the United States, 1960–1997. *American Journal of Preventive Medicine, 19*(1, Suppl.), 18–25.

Way, S., Finch, B. K., & Cohen, D. (2006). Hispanic concentration and the conditional influence of collective efficacy on adolescent childbearing. *Archives of Pediatric and Adolescent Medicine, 160,* 925–930.

Weinstock, J., Berman, S., & Cates, W., Jr. (2004). Sexually transmitted diseases among American youth: Incidence and prevalence estimates, 2000. *Perspectives in Sexual and Reproductive Health, 36,* 6–10.

Whitaker, D. J., Miller, K. S., May, D. C., & Levin, M. L. (1999). Teenage partners' communication about sexual risk and condom use: The importance of parent-teenager discussions. *Family Planning Perspectives, 31,* 117–121.

Widge, A. (2002). Sociocultural attitudes towards infertility and assisted reproduction in India. In E. Vayena, P. J. Rowe, & P. D. Griffin (Eds.), *Current practices and controversies in assisted reproduction* (pp. 60–74). Geneva, Switzerland: World Health Organization.

World Health Organization. (1998). *The second decade: Improving adolescent health and development.* Geneva, Switzerland: Author.

World Health Organization. (2000). *The world health report 2005: Make every mother or child count.* Geneva, Switzerland: Author. Retrieved February 1, 2008, from www.who.int/whr/2005/en/index.html

World Health Organization. (2005a). *Global prevalence and incidence of selected curable sexually transmitted infections: Overview and estimates.* Geneva, Switzerland: Author.

World Health Organization. (2005b). *The WHO definition of reproductive health.* Retrieved August 21, 2008, from www.rho.org/html/definition_.htm

World Health Organization. (2007). *Global HIV prevalence has levelled off. Improvements in surveillance increase understanding of the epidemic, resulting in substantial revisions to estimates.* Retrieved February 1, 2008, from www.who.int/mediacentre/news/releases/2007/pr61/en/print.html

World Health Organization. (n.d.). *Mother-to-child transmission of HIV.* Retrieved February 1, 2008, from www.who.int/hiv/mtct/en

WHO/UNFPA/UNICEF/World Bank. (1999). *Reduction of maternal mortality. A joint WHO/UNFPA/UNICEF/World Bank statement.* Retrieved February 2, 2008, from www.who.int/reproductivehealth/publications/reduction_of_maternal_mortality/reduction_maternal_mortality_preface.htm

Zavodny, M. (2001). The effect of partners' characteristics on teenage pregnancy and its resolution. *Family Planning Perspectives, 33,* 192–199, 205.

Zlidar, V. M., Gardner, R., Rutstein, S. O., Morris, L., Goldberg, H., & Johnson, K. (2003). *New survey findings: The reproductive revolution continues* (Population reports, Series M, No. 17). Johns Hopkins Bloomberg School of Public Health, The INFO Project, Baltimore, MD.

CHAPTER

11

Adolescent Health

Mimi Nichter

Adolescence represents a unique phase of the life span, a time marked by significant physical, emotional, and cognitive changes. It is a transitional period, when one moves away from the dependent years of childhood to the threshold of emerging adulthood. In line with the greater independence that characterizes these years, there are increased opportunities for experimentation with a range of activities and behaviors that can have long-range health implications. It has been well documented that many behaviors associated with adult morbidity and mortality, such as substance use, obesity, and physical inactivity, have their roots in adolescence.

This chapter will briefly review key developmental shifts that occur in adolescence, particularly as they relate to the adoption of positive and negative health behaviors. I discuss the concept of risk with a focus on environments of risk that influence which of the risk-taking behaviors initiated in this life stage become predominant. Focusing on tobacco use among youth, I consider what can be gained from applying a social ecological model to the study of adolescent health.

The social ecology of health model postulates that multiple levels of influence, ordered within different levels of organization, such as the individual, family, community, state, and global systems, all need to be critically examined to understand the meaning of health behaviors in context. Applied to the study of adolescent health, the social ecological perspective prompts researchers to move beyond psychosocial models that privilege individual behaviors to consider how social, cultural, and political-economic environments affect youth behavior and how youth behavior, in turn, may influence the environment (Balbach, Smith, & Malone, 2006; McLeroy, Bibeau, Steckler, & Glanz, 1988; Stokols, 1992). Moving from the micro (interpersonal) level to the macro (community/societal) level with a focus on reciprocal and bidirectional interaction, the social ecological model offers a productive frame for the discussion of behaviors and environments of risk that have an impact on adolescent health.

To date, although much research on adolescent health has focused on singular behaviors (e.g., smoking, dieting, teen pregnancy), numerous qualitative studies point to the co-occurrence and interaction of behaviors such as smoking and drinking or drinking and high-risk sex. In the public health literature, the term *syndemic* has been used to refer to two or more epidemics (i.e., notable increases in the rate of specific diseases in a population) interacting synergistically and contributing, as a result of their interaction, to the excess burden of disease in a population (Singer & Clair, 2003). Applied to adolescent health, co-occurring behaviors such as substance abuse, violence, and unprotected sex need to be recognized as closely linked and interdependent threats to health, which need to be studied in context rather than in isolation (Singer & Clair, 2003). Recognition of the existence of syndemics suggests the need for a biosocial reconception of disease and the adoption of holistic approaches that emphasize interrelationships and the influence of social and economic contexts.

THE IMPORTANCE OF A DEVELOPMENTAL PERSPECTIVE

Researchers on adolescence typically divide this period of the life span into three distinct stages: early adolescence (ages 11–14), midadolescence (ages 15–18), and emerging adulthood (ages 18–24). Adolescence begins with the significant biological change of pubertal maturation, the timing and sequence of which is extremely variable across individuals. Cognitive developmental changes that emerge during the teen years, such as the emergence of more sophisticated thinking abilities (i.e., hypothetical and abstract reasoning; the maturation of the ability to make judgments), can be thought of as both assets and liabilities in terms of experimentation with and adoption of "risky" health behaviors.

Recent research on adolescent brain development reveals that part of the vulnerability and opportunity of this life stage is a set of biologically based changes in neural systems of emotion and motivation. After the onset of puberty, changes in the brain contribute to an increase in sensation seeking and risk taking (Dahl, 2004). This may be observed in many adolescents who display a biologic proclivity toward high-intensity feelings (e.g., falling in and out of love at a rapid pace), which affects their decision-making processes. As Dahl (2004) has noted, under the influence of "hot" cognition—the process of thinking under conditions of high arousal and/or strong emotions, teens may act irrationally and engage in health-compromising behaviors. In contrast, when operating under "cool cognition"—thinking under conditions of low arousal and calm emotions, teens may be more likely to adopt health-enhancing behaviors. Like other developmental transitions, adolescence is characterized by discontinuity (Schulenberg, Maggs, & Hurrelmann, 1997) and is a period of gradual and inconsistent emergence of the skills and knowledge needed to take on adult roles and decisions (Dahl, 2004). Thus, it is not unusual for an adolescent to appear quite mature in one context (in class at school) while quite irrational in another (at a party with friends).

Relationships with others are particularly salient during adolescence. Young people are involved with identity projects and in "trying on" possible selves. Particularly during early adolescence, many teens experience heightened sensitivity about their behavior, believing that *others* are even more preoccupied with their actions and appearance than they themselves are (Elkind, 1967). This concern causes them to feel as if they are always on stage as the main actor, with peers as an "imaginary audience," looking on in judgment. Group identification is a central developmental task of early adolescence, with a more autonomous sense of identity achieved in later adolescence (Brown, Eicher, & Petrie, 1986; Eder, 1995). Notably, today's teens are more involved with peers than previous generations, with immediate and continuous access to friends and the unfolding intricacies of their lives facilitated by information technologies such as instant messaging, cell phones, and online social networking sites (e.g., Facebook and MySpace). Morbidity and mortality among teens is largely the result of "social morbidities," such as violence, motor vehicle accidents, and substance abuse, among other causes (DiClemente, Hansen, & Ponton, 1996). These preventable causes account for approximately two thirds of adolescent deaths in the United States. In part due to perceptions of youth as risk takers, there is a generalized sense of anxiety and mistrust among parents in relation to the capacities of young people to make a successful transition to adulthood (Kelly, 2003). However, research has consistently shown that most youth navigate this life stage with minimal difficulties (Arnett, 1999; Steinberg et al., 2004). The majority of teens *do not* become addicted to tobacco or other drugs, *do not* engage in violent behaviors, and *do* experience positive relationships with their peers and parents. To date, much adolescent research has focused on the pathological development of negative behaviors, and thus, it is perhaps not surprising that the teen years are considered to be inherently tumultuous.

PERCEPTIONS OF RISK

Media representations of teens as prone to risky behaviors are often supported by statistics that play up the percentage of youth that "have ever" engaged in a behavior (e.g., "75% of teens have tried smoking"), making it appear that the majority of teens are risking their health much of the time. The important distinction between experimentation and regular use of substances such as tobacco or alcohol is often obfuscated in popular discourse about youth. The downside of such representations is that they make behaviors appear more normative than they actually are and inadvertently may influence youth to believe that "everyone is doing it."

An important concept with regard to teens and risk has been termed *adolescent invulnerability.* Many teens believe that they are impervious to the consequences of their actions—they have an "it can't happen to me attitude" (Elkind, 1967). A study among smoking and nonsmoking high school students revealed that although the majority of teens recognized the harm of smoking and the habit's long-term consequences, there was a denial of short-term risks among both regular and casual smokers (Slovic, 2000).

To date, there is a paucity of studies on the meaning that risk has for young people, and their role as active agents in shaping their own health destinies has been largely ignored (Etorre & Miles, 2002; Hunt, Evans, & Kares, 2007; Nichter, 2000). While much concern has been expressed by public health practitioners about the physical risks of health-compromising behaviors, results of qualitative research reveal that what may be of greater salience to young people is "social risk," the perceived threat to existing and potential personal relationships that may be faced if one challenges or goes against the prevailing behavior or views of friends (Nichter, Quintero, Nichter, Mock, & Shakib, 2004). For example, a teen may be more concerned about the social risk of not getting into a car with a driver who has been drinking, if other friends are doing so, than about the physical risk of that behavior.

YOUTH AND CONSUMER SOCIETY

In this historical time in American society, risk is valorized, there are increased opportunities for arousal, and people express a diminishing tolerance for boredom (Stromberg, Nichter, & Nichter, 2007). A proliferation of products promises both instant gratification and an antidote to boredom (Starace, 2002). Today's youth are growing up in a high-consumption capitalist economy, where they are exposed to a constant flow of marketing messages inviting them to consume in contexts where they feel a lack, a desire to connect, or any number of other emotional deficits. In this environment, advertisers try to inculcate feelings of desire and lack in their audiences, to make it possible for their manufacturing and service-providing clients to sell and provide more and more goods and services. A panoply of high-arousal products and activities are available around the clock to youth, social connectedness is possible at almost all times, and self-medication is condoned as a way of handling negative emotional states.

In the next sections of the chapter, I turn to a discussion of tobacco as a case study to illustrate how a social ecological perspective can be applied to the examination of an adolescent health problem. I will demonstrate why it is useful to consider tobacco use among adolescents in a set of intersecting contexts including the intrapersonal, the interpersonal (including peer and family environments, school culture, media environments, and online social networking sites), and the broader contexts of public policy.

TOBACCO USE AMONG YOUTH: AN OVERVIEW

The public health impact of tobacco is many orders of magnitude greater than that of all other illegal drugs combined. Each year, smoking causes more deaths than fires, auto crashes, alcohol, cocaine, heroin, AIDS, homicides, and suicides combined (Centers for Disease Control and Prevention [CDC], 1998). Smoking causes more than 435,000 deaths each year, or one in every five deaths in the United States (Fellows, Trosclair, Adams, & Rivera, 2002). Every day, approximately 4,000 American youth aged 12 to 17 years try their first cigarette (Substance Abuse and Mental Health Administration, 2002). If current patterns of smoking behavior continue, an estimated 6.4 million of today's children can be expected to die prematurely from a smoking-related disease (CDC, 1997). In 2005, 23% of high school students reported current cigarette use.

Several surveys of college students have documented continuous high rates of smoking, with almost 30% of students reporting smoking within the past 30 days (Everett et al., 1999; O'Malley & Johnston, 2002; Rigotti, Lee, & Wechsler, 2000). Longitudinal data from multisite studies (1990–1999) document an increase in the 30-day prevalence of smoking among college students by about one third and an increase in daily smoking by about 40% (Johnston, O'Malley, & Bachman, 2001). Thus, the college years are a time of increased vulnerability to tobacco use and of a progression from occasional to regular use.

Intrapersonal Level: Tobacco Use as an Identity Project

A primary level of analysis within a social ecological framework is the intrapersonal level, which includes characteristics of the individual such as knowledge, attitudes, behavior, perceptions of risk, and self-concept (McLeroy et al., 1988). With regard to tobacco use, an important issue to consider is whether teens who smoke consider themselves smokers. In interviews with high school and college students, many students report that they "just smoke when partying." Gloss categories such as "smoker" and "nonsmoker," which are frequently used in the public health literature, do not adequately portray the smoking behavior of or identity adopted by many teens who experiment with tobacco. Ethnographic research on youth smoking has revealed that party time is considered to be "time out of time," where normal rules for appropriate behavior no longer apply (Stromberg et al., 2007).

Young people who smoke (or use recreational drugs) but do not define themselves as smokers defy ready categorization by those in the public health field who are more concerned with frequency and amount of use than smoker self-identity (Nichter, Nichter, Vuckovic, Quintero, & Ritenbaugh, 1997). Yet it is often user self-identity that determines whether youth think that particular tobacco control messages pertain to them. For example, tobacco control messages that depict adult smokers as passive and dependent may not be seen as relevant to youth, who see young smokers as exercising agency and being social (Rugkasa et al., 2001).

Smoking cigarettes can play an important role in one's self-concept, the process of self-exploration, and the presentation of self. Consumption of products has a symbolic significance in the process of defining one's identity (Pavis, Cunningham-Burley, & Amos, 1998). At parties, cigarettes may function as props, which signal to others that the user is not afraid to engage in risk taking and is open to whatever is happening.

In interviews with college students, one benefit of smoking articulated was that it enabled a person to change his or her image. In the first few months of college, when students are trying on "new selves," changing one's image may be particularly salient. Smoking at a party, students reported, not only helped define who you were but also *who you were not*. One young woman explained that not smoking could make you look uptight, whereas having a cigarette "helped you project a more fun and outgoing image." Smoking was fun because "it's good to be a little bad"—that is, smoking called attention to you as a person who was not afraid to do something others might look at with disapproval. Particularly given the proliferation of antismoking messages, many college students expressed pleasure at being able to show that they were "able to throw caution to the wind" (Nichter et al., 2006).

Interpersonal Level: Peers and Parents

A second level of analysis that is particularly relevant in relation to multiple health behaviors among adolescents is interpersonal relationships with peers and with parents and family members. Adolescent peer culture plays a key role in the development and mainte-nance of health-risk behaviors. In relation to tobacco initiation, adolescents report the pres-ence of friends or siblings in 80% of the occasions when they first experimented with cigarettes and report the presence of parents in only 3% of such occasions (Friedman, Lichtenstein, & Biglan, 1985; La Greca, Prinstein, & Fetter, 2001). Among regular smokers, lines of friendship are often characterized by smoking, in that smokers befriend smokers and nonsmokers befriend other nonsmokers (Kobus, 2003). Transitions to higher levels of smok-ing have also been traced to friends' encouragement and support of the behavior (Flay, Hu, & Richardson, 1998).

The Influence of Peers

Although the influence of peers on smoking initiation and continuation is well recognized in the literature, far less is known about how peer influence is experienced by teens themselves. The term *peer pressure* is often reified—that is, discussed as if it were a social fact exerting a constant force in the life of teens. Use of the term in the literature and in prevention programs that coach teens to "resist peer pressure" suggests that youth experience direct peer pressure to smoke. Yet social influences are often subtle and may be experienced in a variety of ways, depend-ing on context and the individuals involved. Rather than experiencing direct peer pressure, many teens report, they experience an internal self-pressure to smoke if others around them are smok-ing (Nichter et al., 1997). The decision to try cigarettes may be linked to youths' attempts to avoid potential exclusion by friends (social risk), to gain social approval from others, and to facilitate social interactions. The manner in which social influences work represents an impor-tant topic that has direct implications for smoking prevention programs developed to teach refusal skills to adolescents. It is not hard to imagine how youth can be "turned off" by the mes-sage that they should resist negative influences and peer pressure to smoke, when that belies their actual experience of being in social situations where friends do not pressure them to smoke but rather they chose to do so themselves.

To understand the patterns and trajectories of tobacco use, it is important to note that some factors may influence one to smoke in some contexts and protect against escalation of smoking in other contexts. In addition to negative social influences, it is important to consider social inter-actions that involve boundary setting. Feedback provided by friends about what constitutes nor-mative tobacco use in particular contexts may serve to control one's behavior (Kobus, 2003). For example, a young woman's friends may monitor her drinking and smoking behavior at a party and provide verbal or nonverbal communication about behavior deemed dangerous or sluttish (Nichter et al., 2006). The reason why boundary setting is important to study is that it provides insights into how the very same people who place one at risk of initiating tobacco use or drug use may serve a protective role in limiting one's frequency and amount of use. This is one of many areas in which sensitivity to gendered patterns of tobacco use is important.

Young women who smoke occasionally at parties are at risk of transitioning to higher lev-els of smoking, although the patterning and timing of this escalation may be different from those for males. While the college years do provide some monitoring and surveillance of drink-ing and smoking among girlfriends, there also exists a powerful "group think"; that is, a need to engage in behaviors similar to those of one's friends, which appears to be more salient among women (Nichter et al., 2006). As noted above, the same friend who may put one at risk of smoking by offering a cigarette in a group setting may also play a protective role by encouraging a friend not to smoke too much or to avoid smoking outside a party context. One might hypothesize that when women transition out of college and move into situations with less monitoring, social surveillance may be less and they might increase their smoking to higher levels.

Male college students may be at higher risk of escalating into regular or more patterned tobacco use, as this is believed to be a normative behavior among males and smoking is infrequently monitored by other male friends (Nichter et al., 2006). Indeed, recent longitudinal studies among college students show male gender predicting the transition from experimentation to regular cigarette use (Mayhew, Flay, & Mott, 2000; Wetter et al., 2004).

The Role of Parents

The role of parents is also important to consider in relation to youth tobacco trajectories. To date, the literature is inconsistent, with the majority of studies pointing to the greater role of peers in influencing the uptake of tobacco use (Avenevoli & Merikangas, 2003; Rose, Chassin, Presson, Edwards, & Sherman, 1999), with others reporting that parental influence is equal to or greater than that of peers (Bauman, Carver, & Gleiter, 2001; Chassin, Presson, & Sherman, 1995). Most studies of parental influence on youth smoking have used survey research that typically assesses parental smoking behavior and youth experimentation with tobacco. Some scholars suggest that parental smoking may be more strongly related to regular use and nicotine dependence than to experimentation, although this has not been investigated in the literature (Avenevoli & Merikangas, 2003). In addition, while most studies have examined parental smoking in relation to adolescent smoking, parental influence may be conceived of as not simply what parents do but also what is considered normative and acceptable behavior within the household context. Parental messages to their teens about behaviors such as drinking and smoking have not been adequately studied, nor have household rules that may determine what teens and their siblings can do in the home. In addition, it is not just whether the parent smokes that may influence child smoking behavior but also the quality of the relationship with the parent. Some research has found that adolescents are more likely to model their parent's smoking behavior if their relationship with them is close.

Parental and familial characteristics can also serve as protective factors to decrease youths' vulnerability to smoking uptake. Teens are less likely to smoke when parents monitor their behavior (Biglan, Duncon, Ary, & Smolkowski, 1995), use positive/authoritative parenting styles (Simons-Morton et al., 1999), and are supportive (Chassin, Presson, Sherman, Montello, & McGrew, 1986). Parental smoking can also serve as a deterrent to child smoking; many youth who grow up in a household of smokers develop negative feelings about the behavior, particularly if they suffer from asthma or other respiratory ailments.

Another important issue is whether there are people in whose presence teens do not smoke out of fear of censure or out of respect. This is important for several reasons. Not only does this behavior provide information on parental influence and control, but it may also have a protective influence with regard to daily consumption and age of onset. Not being able to smoke at home will make it far more difficult for a teen to progress from "party" smoking to regular smoking. This effect may vary with ethnicity. For example, smoking was found to be common among Filipino and Mexican American males in a California study, in spite of the fact that smoking in front of adults was considered disrespectful at home—even if their parents knew they smoked (Nichter, Nichter, Thompson, Shiffman, & Moscicki, 2002). Researchers studying smoking trajectories need to examine what factors determine at what age a teen no longer hides smoking from his or her parents—for example, whether this is dependent on biological age or on social status (arising out of things such as securing an independent income).

Community Level: School Culture and Beyond

Moving beyond the proximal factors affecting smoking behavior, it is important to consider wider environmental contexts including the community in which the adolescent is embedded. School environment can be a key variable affecting smoking uptake; for example, the prevalence of tobacco and drug use at a school can affect the levels of individual students' tobacco and drug use. In a qualitative study of multiethnic teens in California, adolescent informants found it easy to characterize high schools in their area as "heavy" versus "low" smoking schools (Nichter et al., 2002). Similarly, other studies have found that cigarette use is highly related to school culture, with smoking more prevalent in schools in which more students express attitudes in favor of drug and tobacco use, there is higher cigarette availability, and students express lower overall school attachment (Ennett, Flewelling, Lindrooth, & Norton, 1997). However, school culture can also provide a protective effect, deterring students from tobacco and other substance use through monitoring and surveillance of student activities (Wilcox, 2003). Enforcement of school antismoking policies by students, teachers, and others working in the school serves as support and reinforcement for classroom prevention programs.

Importantly, few school-based prevention programs have reduced smoking behavior unless combined with other environmentally based interventions that include community efforts to reduce teen smoking. For example, community mobilization in the form of local media campaigns, merchant education, and positive reinforcement for store clerks refusing to sell tobacco to minors has been shown to contribute to a decrease in the intention to smoke among adolescents (Biglan et al., 1996).

Social ecological models of health acknowledge the need to focus not just on individual-level decisions to smoke or abstain but also on involving the broader community in antitobacco awareness and smoking prevention activities. Applying the model to prevention efforts helps educators recognize the critical need to change community perceptions and mobilize communities toward structural change. To this end, local ordinances, restrictions on smoking in public places, tax increases, and media advocacy all become part of a mix of activities that facilitate reductions in smoking.

Population Level: Media Environment

Adolescents are intense consumers of the media, including television, music videos, and movies. The highest percentages of moviegoers are those in the 12 to 24 age range, with over

35% reporting attending movies regularly. Researchers have concluded that alcohol and tobacco use are ubiquitous in these media (Durant et al., 1997). The use of particular cigarette brands by actors in movies has increased 11-fold since the Master Settlement Agreement (MSA), in 1998, specifically restricted advertising and promotion of tobacco to youth (see below) (Office of the Attorney General, 2007). In addition, since 1998, smoking in PG-13 movies has increased by 50% (Glanz, n.d.).

The media traffic in scripts for how young people (segmented by age, gender, class) should behave in different contexts. (The term *script,* in social research, refers not to the text of a play or movie but to a cognitive structure that organizes comprehension of event-based situations; Schank & Abelson, 1977.) Those involved in marketing place products in scenes depicting consumption events to position and naturalize their use (Condry, 1989; Russell, 1999). TV/movie producers also enhance the realism of their shows by using products familiar in popular culture (a practice labeled "reality engineering"; Solomon & Englis, 1994). In the case of tobacco, young people learn about appropriate places to smoke from the popular media—environments both directly and indirectly manipulated by the tobacco industry (Bonnie & Lynch, 1994; Wakefield, Flay, Nichter, & Giovino, 2003). Movies and TV programs do not just lead youth to emulate the behavior of attractive main characters who may look tough or sexy when they light up. Smoking featured in the foreground of movies gives youth ideas about where, when, and how to smoke. In a social environment increasingly tolerant of smoking restrictions, giving youth ideas about where and when it is acceptable to smoke is an important agenda for the industry (Nichter, 2003).

Population Level: Advertising Environment

The 1998 MSA, a legal settlement between the states and the tobacco companies, prohibited the industry from "any action, directly or indirectly, to target youth . . . in the advertising, promotion, or marketing of tobacco products." Since that time, despite its persistent denials, the tobacco industry has continued to actively promote tobacco products and has actually increased its cigarette marketing expenditures significantly. In 2001, expenditures for domestic cigarette advertising and promotion were $11.2 billion, an increase of 17% over 2000 (Federal Trade Commission, 2003; Krugman, Quinn, Sung, & Morrison, 2005). In recent years, there has been a 66% increase in overall dollars spent, with a particular focus on advertising in youth-oriented magazines, promotional offers in bars, product placement in films, and in-store signage and displays. It seems likely that the result of decades of pervasive tobacco marketing and particularly the large increase in expenditures since 1998 have helped the industry maintain a constant rate of smoking initiation for the past 20 years. As long as industry activities continue, this pattern may be difficult to reverse (Bonnie, 2001).

From a social ecological model standpoint, it is important to recognize that the teen market represents new potential users for an industry that would otherwise be shrinking. Cigarette companies continue to reach a large number of youth with images that normalize smoking behavior. Adolescents aged 12 to 17 (the age range in which people are most likely to begin smoking) are twice as likely as adults to be exposed to tobacco advertisements and are three times more sensitive and responsive to cigarette ads than other age groups (Pollay et al., 1996). Cigarette brands that are popular among adolescents (e.g., Marlboro, Newport, and Camel) are more likely to be advertised in magazines that have a youthful readership than are brands popular among adults (King, Siegel, & Celebucki, 1998).

New products lines are continually being developed that boast new and fun flavors, such as such as Camel's "Kauai Kolada" cigarettes (pineapple and coconut flavored) and a citrus-flavored cigarette called "Twista Lime." Flavored Kool cigarettes have also emerged on the market, bearing names such as "Caribbean Chill" and "Mocha Taboo." Added to this marketing mix are products promoted as "healthy" alternatives, such as American Spirits and an array of "light" and "mild" cigarettes. Young adults—those who are legally able to purchase cigarettes—are the group most heavily targeted by the tobacco industry (Ling & Glantz, 2002). Public health practitioners need to be aware of the powerful force of the industry, which continually attempts to subvert prevention and intervention efforts.

Policy Environment

Over the past 15 years, many tobacco control initiatives have been undertaken in the states and local communities. Through increased tobacco tax, states have been able to generate large revenues, a portion of which has been directed toward school-based prevention activities and tobacco cessation programs. At the local level, communities have established innovative mass-media programs about the danger of tobacco use and have enforced legislation to limit youth access to tobacco.

National and local antismoking activities coexist with the powerful counterforce of the tobacco industry. As a result of the MSA, the industry has had to implement youth smoking prevention educational programs, and approximately $100 million per year has been spent on these efforts. The industry programs have focused largely on peer pressure and social influences, although previous research has shown that such programs are largely ineffective in reducing teen smoking unless combined with other, environmentally based interventions (Levy, Chaloupka, & Gitchell, 2004; Wakefield, McLeod, & Perry, 2006). This has allowed the industry to obfuscate other critical factors such as tobacco marketing, inaccurate risk appraisal, and the price of tobacco in smoking uptake (Wakefield et al., 2006). Critics have charged that the industry's prevention programs have until recently been highly (and purposefully) ineffective and have not been measured by behavioral outcomes. By appearing to be committed to youth smoking prevention, the tobacco industry has attempted to create a public image of youth smoking that redirects attention from the negative health effects of the behavior. Furthermore, the industry has been supportive of the health belief model and the theory of reasoned action, both of which focus attention on individual behavior and responsibility, thus diverting attention away from the activities and environments that promote and sustain smoking (Balbach et al., 2006). Tobacco researchers have been vociferous about the need for continued vigilance and monitoring of the industry.

The Online Social Networking Environment

Social ecological assessments also need to pay attention to online social networking sites, arenas of interaction that are increasingly central to communication among youth. Technologies such as instant messaging, text messaging, and cell phones and online social networking sites such as Facebook, MySpace, and Friendster are pervasive in youth culture, occupying uncalculated amounts of daily time. These technologies facilitate ready contact with peers, encouraging the sharing of information about self and others instantaneously.

Recent reports indicate that over one half of online teens have created a personal profile online and that they visit these Web sites at least daily, if not multiple times throughout the day. Facebook and MySpace pages are continually updated and often include up-to-the-minute exposés about one's social scene, including drinking, smoking, recreational drug use, and sexual exploits at parties. Taking risks is expressed visually through photos that, once posted, become the object of commentary by "friends" who, from the far reaches of the planet, can post a response evaluating the recent activities. Quick-response features such as "winking" and "poking," which provide seemingly casual forms of communication, also serve to enhance the monitoring and surveillance of others. Social networking sites allow young people to manage their identities strategically.

These networking sites have the potential to affect youth health behavior. For example, in the area of body image, dieting, and eating disorders, "pro-ana" (anorexia) Web sites have emerged (Hammersley & Treseder, 2007). While some of these sites provide encouragement for those recovering or suffering from anorexia, other—often teen-based sites—provide information on dieting and exercise. On the extreme end of the continuum are those Web sites that actively promote and encourage anorexia and bulimia nervosa, providing details and tips for starving, binging, and purging. With regard to smoking, recent YouTube videos provide visual demonstrations to neophytes on how to smoke cigarettes and not appear to choke like a novice. While it is not known to what extent information in these sites is used, social networking sites might represent an important environment of risk and possibly prevention to consider.

From a public health perspective, the digital environment may provide new avenues for conveying health messages to youth—a population that already uses the Internet frequently and values it as an all-important source of information. Developing Web-based health messages targeted for particular youth populations may be less confrontational and more user-friendly than traditional health education approaches. A challenge for health educators and social scientists working in this area will be to identify youth response to Internet education sites, as careful evaluation of what works and does not work will be critical to its ongoing success and utility.

CONCLUSION

Adolescence is an important period for the development of lifelong behaviors. Of particular concern to health educators and adolescent researchers are behaviors that have potential long-term negative effects on youth. Casual smoking during adolescence—a behavior that may appear innocuous, if not appropriate, when drinking with friends at parties—may lead to a lifelong addiction. Similarly, food and physical activity choices, such as preferences for high-calorie soft drinks and fast food and failure to exercise during adolescence, may result in obesity and a sedentary lifestyle in adulthood. Prevention and intervention programs that target youth will need to be cognizant of the significant developmental changes of this period of the life span and take into account the multiple interacting factors that influence everyday youth practices.

The social ecological model applied to adolescent health allows us to move beyond individual-level behaviors to acknowledge the interaction of multiple contexts including social, cultural, and political-economic contexts, as well as the role of the media, consumer culture, and public policy in shaping behavioral choices. Health promotion efforts for adolescents will need to consider both risk and protective factors that may exist in each of these environments as well as how public health messages are interpreted by youth.

REFERENCES

Arnett, J. (1999). Adolescent storm and stress, reconsidered. *American Psychologist, 54,* 317–326.

Avenevoli, S., & Merikangas, K. R. (2003). Familial influences on adolescent smoking. *Addiction, 98,* 1–20.

Balbach, E. D., Smith, E. A., & Malone, R. (2006). How the health belief model helps the tobacco industry. *Tobacco Control, 15*(Suppl. IV), 37–43.

Bauman, K. E., Carver, K., & Gleiter, K. (2001). Trends in parent and friend influence during adolescence: The case of adolescent cigarette smoking. *Addictive Behaviors, 26,* 349–361.

Biglan, A., Ary, D., Koehn, V., Levings, D., Smith, S., Wright, Z., et al. (1996). Mobilizing positive reinforcement in communities to reduce youth access to tobacco. *American Journal of Community Psychology, 24,* 625–639.

Biglan, A., Duncon, T. E., Ary, D. V., & Smolkowski, K. (1995). Peer and parental influences on adolescent tobacco use. *Journal of Behavioral Medicine, 18,* 315–330.

Bonnie, R. (2001). Tobacco and public health policy: A youth-centered approach. In P. Slovic (Ed.), *Smoking: Risk, perception and policy* (pp. 277–301). Thousand Oaks, CA: Sage.

Bonnie, W., & Lynch, B. (Eds.). (1994). *Growing up tobacco free in America* (National Institute of Medicine Committee on Preventing Nicotine Dependency in Children and Youths). Washington, DC: National Academy Press.

Brown, B., Eicher, S. A., & Petrie, S. (1986). The importance of peer group ("crowd") affiliation in adolescence. *Journal of Adolescence, 9,* 73–96.

Centers for Disease Control and Prevention. (1997). Smoking attributable mortality and years of potential life loss—United States, 1984. *Morbidity and Mortality Weekly Report, 46,* 444–451.

Centers for Disease Control and Prevention. (1998). Incidence of initiation of cigarette smoking: United States, 1965–1996. *Morbidity and Mortality Weekly Report, 47,* 837–840.

Chassin, L., Presson, C. C., & Sherman, S. J. (1995). Social psychological antecedents and consequences of adolescent tobacco use. In J. L. Wallander & I. J. Siegel (Eds.), *Adolescent health problems: Behavioral perspectives (Advances in pediatric psychology)* (pp. 141–159). New York: Guilford Press.

Chassin, L., Presson, C., Sherman, S., Montello, D., & McGrew, J. (1986). Changes in peer and parent influence during adolescence: Longitudinal versus cross-sectional perspectives on smoking initiation. *Developmental Psychology, 22*(3), 327–334.

Condry, J. (1989). *The psychology of television.* Hillsdale, NJ: Lawrence Erlbaum.

Dahl, R. (2004). Adolescent brain development: A period of vulnerabilities and opportunities. In R. E. Dahl and L. P. Spear (Eds.), *Adolescent brain development: Vulnerabilities and opportunities* (pp. 1–23). New York: Annals of the New York Academy of Sciences.

DiClemente, R. J., Hansen, W. B., & Ponton, L. (1996). Adolescents at risk: A generation in jeopardy. In R. J. DiClemente, W. B. Hansen, & L. E. Ponton (Eds.), *Handbook of adolescent health risk behavior* (pp. 1–4). New York: Plenum Press.

Durant, R. H., Rome, E. S., Rich, M., Allred, E., Emans, S. J., & Woods, E. (1997). Tobacco and alcohol use behaviors portrayed in music videos: A content analysis. *American Journal of Public Health, 87,* 1131–1135.

Eder, D. (1995). *School talk: Gender and adolescent culture.* New Brunswick, NJ: Rutgers University Press.

Elkind, D. (1967). Egocentrism in adolescence. *Child Development, 38,* 1025–1038.

Ennett, S. T., Flewelling, R. I., Lindrooth, R. C., & Norton, E. C. (1997). School and neighborhood characteristics associated with school rates of alcohol, cigarette, and marijuana use. *Journal of Health and Social Behavior, 38,* 55–71.

Etorre, E., & Miles, S. (2002). Young people, drug use, and the consumption of health. In S. Hendersen & A. Petersen (Eds.), *Consuming health: The commodification of health care* (pp. 173–186). London: Routledge.

Everett, S. A., Husten, C. G., Kann, L., Warren, C. W., Sharp, D., & Crosset, L. (1999). Smoking initiation and smoking patterns among U.S. college students. *Journal of American College Health, 48,* 55–60.

Federal Trade Commission. (2003, October). *Cigarette report for 2001.* Washington, DC: Author.

Fellows, J. L., Trosclair, A., Adams, E. K., & Rivera, C. C. (2002). Annual smoking attributable mortality, years of potential life lost and economic costs: United States 1995–1999. *Morbidity and Mortality Weekly Report, 51,* 300–303.

Flay, B. R., Hu, F. B., & Richardson, J. (1998). Psychosocial predictors of different stages of cigarette smoking among high school students. *Preventive Medicine, 27,* 9–18.

Friedman, L., Lichtenstein, E., & Biglan, A. (1985). Smoking onset among teens: An empirical analysis of initial situations. *Addictive Behaviors, 10,* 1–13.

Glanz, S. (n.d.). *Smoke-free movies.* Retrieved March 8, 2007, from www.SmokeFreeMovies.ucsf.edu

Hammersley, M., & Treseder, P. (2007). Identity as an analytic problem: Who's who in "pro-ana" Websites? *Qualitative Research, 7,* 283–300.

Hunt, G. P., Evans, K., & Kares, F. (2007). Drug use and meanings of risk and pleasure. *Journal of Youth Studies, 10,* 73–96.

Johnston, L., O'Malley, P., & Bachman, J. (2001). *Monitoring the future: National survey results on drug use: Vol. 2. College students and adults ages 19–40* (NIH Publication No. 01–4925). Bethesda, MD: National Institute on Drug Abuse.

Kelly, P. (2003). Growing up as risky business? Risks, surveillance, and the institutionalized mistrust of youth. *Journal of Youth Studies, 6,* 165–180.

King, C., Siegel, M., & Celebucki, C. (1998). Adolescent exposure to cigarette advertising in magazines: An evaluation of brand-specific advertising in relation to youth readership. *Journal of the American Medical Association, 179,* 516–520.

Kobus, K. (2003). Peers and adolescent smoking. *Addiction, 98*(Suppl. 1), 37–55.

Krugman, D., Quinn, W. H., Sung, Y., & Morrison, M. (2005). Understanding the role of cigarette promotion and youth smoking in a changing marketing environment. *Journal of Health Communication, 10,* 261–278.

La Greca, A., Prinstein, M., & Fetter, M. (2001). Adolescent peer crowd affiliation: Linkages with health-risk behaviors and close friendships. *Journal of Pediatric Psychology, 26,* 131–143.

Levy, D., Chaloupka, F., & Gitchell, J. (2004). The effects of tobacco control policies on smoking rates: A tobacco control scorecard. *Journal of Public Health Management and Practice, 10,* 338–353.

Ling, P. M., & Glantz, S. A. (2002). Why and how the tobacco industry sells cigarettes to young adults: Evidence from tobacco industry documents. *American Journal of Public Health, 92,* 2983–2989.

Mayhew, K., Flay, B., & Mott, J. (2000). Stages in the development of adolescent smoking. *Drug and Alcohol Dependence, 59*(Suppl. 1), 61–81.

McLeroy, K. R., Bibeau, D., Steckler, A., & Glanz, K. (1988). An ecological perspective on health promotion programs. *Health Education Quarterly, 15,* 351–377.

Nichter, M. (2000). *Fat talk: What girls and their parents say about dieting.* Cambridge, MA: Harvard University Press.

Nichter, M. (2003). Smoking: What does culture have to do with it? *Addiction, 98*(Suppl. 1), 139–145.

Nichter, M., Nichter, M., Lloyd-Richardson, E., Flaherty, B., Carkoglu, A., & Taylor, N. (2006). Gendered dimensions of smoking among college students. *Journal of Adolescent Research, 21,* 215–243.

Nichter, M., Nichter, M., Thompson, P., Shiffman, S., & Moscicki, A. (2002). Using qualitative research to inform survey development on nicotine dependence among adolescents. *Drug and Alcohol Dependence, 68*(Suppl. 1), 41–56.

Nichter, M., Nichter, M., Vuckovic, N., Quintero, G., & Ritenbaugh, C. (1997). Smoking experimentation and initiation among adolescent girls: Qualitative and quantitative findings. *Tobacco Control, 6,* 285–295.

Nichter, M., Quintero, G., Nichter, M., Mock, J., & Shakib, S. (2004). Qualitative research: Contributions to the study of drug use, drug abuse, and drug use(r)-related interventions. *Substance Use & Misuse, 39,* 1907–1969.

Office of the Attorney General. (2007). *Master settlement agreement.* Retrieved August 15, 2008, from http://ag.ca.gov/tobacco/msa.php

O'Malley, P., & Johnston, L. (2002). Epidemiology of alcohol and other drug use among American college students. *Journal of Studies on Alcohol, 14,* 23–39.

Pavis, S., Cunningham-Burley, S., & Amos, A. (1998). Health related behavioural change in context: Young people in transition. *Social Science and Medicine, 47,* 1407–1418.

Pollay, R., Siddarth, S., Siegel, M., Haddix, A., Mettritt, R., Giovino, G., et al. (1996). The last straw? Cigarette advertising and realized market share among youths and adults, 1979–1993. *Journal of Marketing, 60,* 1–16.

Rigotti, N., Lee, J., & Wechsler, H. (2000). U.S. college students' use of tobacco products: Results of a national survey. *Journal of the American Medical Association, 284,* 699–705.

Rose, J. S., Chassin, L., Presson, C. C., Edwards, D., & Sherman, S. J. (1999). Peer influences on adolescent cigarette smoking: A prospective sibling analysis. *Merrill Palmer Quarterly, 45,* 62–84.

Rugkasa, J., Kennedy, O., Baron, M., Abaunza, P. S., Treacy, M. P., & Knox, B. (2001). Smoking and symbolism: Children, communication and cigarettes. *Health Education Research, 16,* 131–142.

Russell, C. A. (1999). *Popular culture and persuasion: An investigation of product placements' effectiveness.* Doctoral dissertation, University of Arizona School of Management, Tucson, Arizona.

Schank, R. C., & Abelson, R. P. (1977). *Scripts. Plans, goals, and understanding: An inquiry into human knowledge structures.* Hillsdale, NJ: Lawrence Erlbaum.

Schulenberg, J., Maggs, J., & Hurrelmann, K. (1997). Negotiating developmental transitions during adolescence and young adulthood: Health risks and opportunities. In J. Schulenberg, J. Maggs, & K. Hurrelmann (Eds.), *Health risks and developmental transitions during adolescence* (pp. 1–23). Cambridge, UK: Cambridge University Press.

Simons-Morton, B., Crump, A. D., Haynie, D. L., Saylor, K. E., Eitel, P., & Yu, K. (1999). Psychosocial, school, and parent factors associated with recent smoking among early-adolescent boys and girls. *Preventive Medicine, 28,* 138–148.

Singer, M., & Clair, S. (2003). Syndemics and public health: Reconceptualizing disease in bio-social context. *Medical Anthropology Quarterly, 17,* 423–441.

Slovic, P. (2000). What does it mean to know a cumulative risk? Adolescents' perceptions of short-term and long-term consequences of smoking. *Journal of Behavioral Decision Making, 13,* 259–266.

Solomon, M. R., & Englis, B. G. (1994). The big picture: Product complementarity and integrated communications. *Journal of Advertising Research, 34,* 57–64.

Starace, G. (2002). New "normalities," new "madnesses." *British Journal of Psychotherapy, 19,* 21–32.

Steinberg, L., Dahl, R., Keating, D., Kupfer, D. J., Masten, A. S., & Pine, D. S. (2004). The study of developmental psychopathology in adolescence: Integrating affective neuroscience with the study of context. In D. Cicchetti (Ed.), *Handbook of developmental psychopathology* (pp. 710–741). New York: Wiley.

Stokols, D. (1992). Establishing and maintaining health environments: Toward a social ecology of health promotions. *American Psychologist, 47,* 6–22.

Stromberg, P., Nichter, M., & Nichter, M. (2007). Taking play seriously: Low level smoking among college students. *Culture, Medicine, and Psychiatry, 31,* 1–24.

Substance Abuse and Mental Health Services Administration. (2002). *Summary of findings from the 2001 National Household Survey on Drug Abuse: Vol. II. Technical appendices and selected data tables.* Rockville, MD: U.S. Department of Health and Human Services.

Wakefield, M., Flay, B., Nichter, M., & Giovino, G. (2003). Role of the media in influencing trajectories of youth smoking. *Addiction, 98,* 79–103.

Wakefield, M., McLeod, K., & Perry, C. L. (2006). "Stay away from them until you're old enough to make a decision": Tobacco company testimony about youth smoking initiation. *Tobacco Control, 15*(Suppl. IV), 44–53.

Wetter, D., Kenford, S., Welsch, S., Smith, S., Fouladi, R., Fiore, M., et al. (2004). Prevalence and predictors of transitions in smoking behavior among college students. *Health Psychology, 23,* 168–177.

Wilcox, P. (2003). An ecological approach to understanding youth smoking trajectories: Problems and prospects. *Addiction, 98,* 57–77.

12

Public Health and Aging

J. Neil Henderson and L. Carson Henderson

The success of public health in keeping the population alive has, paradoxically, caused unintended health problems for which there are no precedents. The problems are caused by the population living longer than ever before so that many years of life are experienced at the highest lifetime risk for chronic, incurable, dependency-causing diseases. For example, with longevity, people live into the ages of greatest risk for Alzheimer's disease, arthritis, cerebral stroke, diabetes, cardiovascular disease, cancer, and other conditions. The consequences for many are numerous expensive medications, financial resource depletion, and long-term care due to lowered functional status requiring at-home or institutional assistance. The interconnections of early-life health behavior, resultant later-life chronic disease, retirement, and the cost of long-term care collectively constitute a perfect example of the social ecology model in action.

Thirty years ago, the first head of the National Institute on Aging (NIA), Robert Butler, MD, titled a treatise on the American way of aging *Why Survive?* (1975). The title reflected the problems of increased longevity in the absence of quality of life due to chronic, incapacitating disease. Ten years ago, a former president of the American Public Health Association communicated the problem another way, "We live too short and die too long" (Bortz, 1991). Even in the present, a cursory examination of research shows that the social, behavioral, and medical impacts of aging remain to be solved.

The good news is that the troublesome side of aging can be offset by the fact that a long life gives the opportunity for families to have more time for elders and their younger family members to grow together and enrich the life experience by sharing intergenerational perspectives and histories. For a lucky few, late life is a highly functional continuation of earlier life with only some moderate changes. Longevity also allows individuals to gain even more mastery over occupational and common life experience. For these reasons, the elderly retiree may be the most relevant consultant for industrial, social, and political problem solving that exists. Yet, the positive side of a long life is dependent upon maintaining the physical, mental, and financial viability of the elder. Of all the health sciences, it is public health that is most appropriate for the critical task of preventing late-life elder limitations by promoting lifelong healthy living that will result in more high-quality years as people age.

Public health can vastly improve the late-life experience to the benefit of all generations by responding to rising numbers of elders in two ways: (1) address the health needs of elders living today, and (2) prepare the younger generations for a healthier late life. However, this is slow in developing. Part of the problem is found in a mismatch at the interface of current health care technology and chronic, incurable disease. People benefit from protection from early death afforded by medicine and public health only to be confronted with an extreme gap in the ability of medicine and public health to significantly reduce the impacts of chronic disease. The result is a growing elder population foundering in its own victory over early death.

DEMOGRAPHICS OF AN AGING SOCIETY

The total number of Americans over age 65 is 35 million (Administration on Aging [AoA], 2007). This number will more than double to over 70 million in only 40 years. Even more staggering is the fact that the age group 85 and older will triple in the same time period. Life expectancy for whites is 77.1 years at birth compared with 71.1 for African Americans. However, for those who survive to age 85, white life expectancy is 6.2 years whereas African American life expectancy is 6.4 years. This "demographic crossover" effect is presumed to be due to a more robust "survivability" for the minority person who has experienced the many negative effects of racism and still lived 85 years. Those long-term minority survivors may be generally better able to withstand the traumas of life. This "extra" ability becomes observable in late life. However, perhaps more importantly, the life expectancy at age 85 demonstrates that most of the whites and African Americans of this cohort will live into their ninth decade.

Along with the epidemiologic transition from infectious disease to chronic disease has been a concomitant improvement in life expectancy, and this improvement has been realized by people in every age group (Omran, 1971). The transition from high fertility and high mortality to low fertility and low mortality has resulted in a worldwide population increase in the numbers of persons ages 65 and older. Older people make up 14% of the population in Europe and 2.9% of the population of sub-Saharan Africa, a large difference being noted between developed and developing countries (Satariano, 2006).

While the focus here is on public health and aging in the United States, the issue of human longevity is a global one. In virtually all populations, the 85-years-and-older population is the fastest growing age cohort of all. This is due to reduced mortality rates compared with past generations so that survivorship beyond prior generations is more common than at any other time in world history. The health, political, and economic histories of all people are being rewritten by the phenomenon of unprecedented human longevity.

According to the U.S. government's Administration on Aging (AoA) (2007), minority elders represent 16.1% of the 65-and-over population. However, by 2030, the total minority numbers will jump by 217%, compared with an 81% increase among whites. By demographic group, African Americans will increase by 128%, Asian Americans by 301%, and Hispanics by 322%. The smallest minority elder group, American Indians and Alaska Natives, will increase by 193%. The fact that minorities are often more vulnerable to health and well-being deficits than the majority population means that public health faces a disparity crisis regarding health, aging, and minority status.

SOCIETAL SEARCH FOR ANTI-AGING MEDICINE

Longevity, defined as the length or duration of life, is determined at the species level. The maximum human life span is currently 110 to 120 years, with increased risk for disease occurring as a function of years accrued. There are multiple theories regarding the aging process. There are the "biological clock" theories that regard the aging process as one that is intrinsic to the individual, genetically determined, and thus programmed, in which the maturation of the human being is considered an extension of the normal developmental process. The "wear and tear" or "stochastic" theories regard the aging process as linked to tissue damage and abuse over time, leading to the deterioration of organ systems and subsequent failure to sustain life. These processes are considered to be random and probabilistic, and proponents of the "wear and tear" theories of aging cite lifestyle choices as contributing to the longevity of the human organism. It is within this theory base that the proponents of "anti-aging" strategies find their theoretical base.

Unfortunately, many commercial ventures seek to make a profit from the desperation caused by suffering or proximity to death. The myth of "anti-aging medicine" is one profit ploy that markets itself as a means (or set of products) to reverse aging. Such nonsense should be addressed by the communication and political channels of public health, and has indeed been addressed by biogerontologists. In their article "Position Statement on Human Aging," Olshansky, Hayflick, and Carnes (2002) addressed the issue of anti-aging entrepreneurs who make extravagant claims regarding manipulation of the aging process. The authors were concerned that fellow scientists were contributing to the proliferation of pseudoscientific anti-aging products by their failure to make definitive public statements concerning the extravagant claims. The consensus statement emphasized that the following have no effect on human aging: antioxidant intake, telomere manipulation, and hormone replacement. Caloric restriction with adequate nutrition might have some potential. No genes have yet been identified as directly responsible for aging. Replacement of body parts is interesting, especially in regard to stem cell research, but is inconclusive. While lifestyle modification may delay or prevent age-related disease, it does not modify the aging processes. In summary, "There are no lifestyle changes, surgical procedures, vitamins, antioxidants, hormones, or techniques of genetic engineering available today that have been demonstrated to influence the processes of aging" (Olshansky et al., 2002, pp. B295).

More positively, the feasible productive potential of public health is in the approach recently tagged "preventive gerontology." Gerontologists view aging as a lifelong event, not one that "begins" at age 65. More research is showing that intrauterine, childhood, and adult health, disease, and injury events are connected to late-life functional status and morbidity. Public health and preventive gerontology should go hand in hand.

While it is true that there is no scientific evidence that primary prevention and optimization of health behaviors can actually modify the process of aging, healthy lifestyles may contribute to increases in life expectancy by delaying the onset of disease and disability, thus compressing morbidity into the last remaining years of life. Public health must aggressively join the fight for optimization of functional status and quality of life for older persons.

HEALTH DISPARITIES IN AGING POPULATIONS

Despite an increase in life expectancy in the United States, disparities exist across groups in terms of healthy life expectancy. Many minority elders experience *multiple jeopardy* (Cummings & Galambos, 2004). Multiple jeopardy refers to risk and vulnerability of being not only old in an ageist society, but minority as well. Female gender has also been included as an additional layer of vulnerability because single, older, minority women are the most impoverished across populations. This is important because of the "gender gap," in which older women outnumber older men by 21.6 million to 15.7 million (AoA, 2007). Minority-aged individuals may experience inadequate access to health care, malnutrition, and substandard living conditions. Additionally, they experience more morbidity, disability, and barriers to social services than their counterparts in the majority population (Sokolovsky, 1997).

In tandem with this concept, there is the idea of "ethnicity as compensation" (Sokolovsky, 1997). That is, being a member of a close-knit ethnic group may serve to mitigate the exigencies of old age. While this premise may hold true in some instances, many times it does not. Adult children of minority-aged individuals may not conform to traditional cultural expectations, having been more assimilated into the mainstream culture. Employment opportunities separate families, and filial piety may be substantially decreased. The promotion of ethnicity as compensation in the political arena may lead to underfunding of programs designed to aid those who are experiencing multiple jeopardy, and thus an exacerbation of the problem (Sokolovsky, 1997).

Health disparities among elder minorities have been noted by government health agencies. For example, the AoA has developed a special focus on minority issues, such as a "Diversity Toolkit" for the National Association of Area Agencies on Aging, special grants for minority aging issues, and specific statistical compilations on minority elder populations. Also, the NIA has made special grants for elder health issues and developed and disseminates a national newsletter, *Minority Research and Training*. Another example is from the Office of Minority Health, which advises the Secretary of Health and Human Services and publishes *Closing the Gap*, a periodical for health professionals that includes topics on aging issues and health disparities.

COMMUNITY FACTORS

Services

Many social and health service activities can benefit the public's health without being titled "public health" or emanating from official public health agencies. Such is the case with many services for elders. Many national and local service agencies for elders contribute to their health and well-being via community-based resources, like "Meals on Wheels" and "aging and adult services," and respite care programs for caregiver relief. All of these assist elders to have a healthy physical (e.g., nutritional support, housing repair) and psychosocial (e.g., companion services, senior adult day programs) late-life experience. These collective efforts are referred to generically as the "aging network."

Besides the 1924 Social Security Act, the big push for elder well-being started with the 1965 Older Americans Act (OAA). The OAA provided for the development of Medicare and a new federal branch for aging services, the Administration on Aging. The AoA is directed by the assistant secretary of aging of the Department of Health and Human Services. As such, the director is a presidential appointee and causes the AoA to operate sensitively to changing political party enthusiasms. The primary mission of AoA is to keep elders in their homes as they age by coordinating services needed to prevent or forestall more costly institutional care.

AoA conducts its mission by organizing efforts of 56 State Units on Aging (this includes American territories), 655 Area Agencies on Aging (several per state based on population density), 233 tribal and Native entities, and two Native Hawaiian organizations. The main services funded by OAA via the AoA and its Area Agencies on Aging (AAAs) are (1) "supportive services," such as transportation to services, home chores, personal care, and adult day care; (2) "nutrition services," which include home-delivered meals, but also nutrition education and health screenings at senior citizen program sites; (3) "preventive health services," which include health education, smoking cessation, social engagement opportunities, and physical activities; (4) the National Family Caregiver Support Program, whose mission it is to provide those giving supportive care to any elder community resource information to facilitate their efforts; (5) "protection of the Rights of Vulnerable Older Persons," which specifically addresses risks and protections related to elder abuse; (6) "services to Native Americans," which include limited nutrition assistance to tribal elders; and (7) "eldercare locator," a national toll-free information service to find community resources and age-related information to assist with coping needs in late life.

While AoA and its AAAs are probably the most comprehensive "public health" outreach organization for elders, states and counties also provide specifically targeted elder services. Many states have departments of "Aging and Adult Services" or similarly named community resources. The same is true for counties. Because the names are different from one locale to another, phone books have governmental pages that have categorical headings by which to find the myriad aging services. However, consumers typically are heartened to find numerous entries for aging services only to be bitterly disappointed at the lack of capacity of these services. Most consumers report that they have to be placed on a waiting list due to agency financial limitations. The desperation of many caregivers who need immediate services (e.g., a parent has had a stroke, hip fracture, or dementia, or the caregiving group has had some failure) is extreme in the face of appearances that elder community resources are high when actually they are barely sufficient.

PRIMARY PREVENTION, PUBLIC HEALTH, AND AGING

When does "aging" begin? At 60? At 65? The Social Security eligibility age has been increased. According to the Social Security Administration, the government will decide when retirement may commence, based upon the person's year of birth. But retirement is only a milestone along life's trajectory. In essence, individuals begin to age when they are conceived, and continue until they die. From this broad view, we may now examine aging from a life span perspective. Therefore, public health interventions can truly be said to begin in utero, primary prevention during the first 50 years serving to postpone morbidity and disability in the second 50 years. Interventions in public health serve this way to effectively "compress" morbidity and disability into the last few years (or, preferably months) of life. From this life span perspective, one can examine many of the chronic conditions of the second 50 years of life in terms of primary and secondary prevention strategies during the first 50 years.

Cardiovascular Disease (CVD)

Collectively, the term *cardiovascular disease* (CVD) encompasses both coronary heart disease, the leading cause of death in the United States, and cerebrovascular disease (Satariano, 2006). These conditions fortunately have potentially modifiable risk factors: hypertension, obesity, lack of physical activity, poor nutrition, and tobacco use.

Another notable risk factor for CVD is diabetes, also potentially preventable, and which at this point in time has reached epidemic proportions worldwide. Diabetes is a risk factor for coronary heart disease, cerebrovascular disease, and cancers of the colon and rectum (Satariano, 2006). Type 2, or adult-onset diabetes, becomes more common with age, with a prevalence rate of 13% among those aged 65 and older. Risk factors for diabetes include family history, obesity, and low levels of physical activity.

In terms of primary prevention of CVD, adequate physical activity, good nutrition, and non-use of tobacco are the simplistic answers to avoidance of hypertension, diabetes, coronary heart disease, and cerebrovascular disease. Optimal primary prevention begins before birth, with research indicating that the fetal and neonatal period may play a role in the subsequent risk of adult-onset coronary heart disease (Schocken, 2000). In childhood, primary prevention may continue, in terms of laying the groundwork for future cardiovascular health. For the most part, this ideal is not achieved, and individuals will need to make substantial changes during adulthood in order to avoid the morbidity that CVD will bring to later years. For many individuals, achieving goals such as regular physical activity and optimal nutrition involve huge lifestyle changes, which are themselves a compilation of many culturally ingrained habits and choices.

Fortunately, these goals are achievable. Nutritional changes include avoidance of (a) animal and trans fats, foods high in cholesterol, and simple carbohydrates, such as sugars and high-fructose corn syrup; (b) excessive intake of alcohol; and (c) excessive intake of sodium. Emphasizing a diet high in omega-3 fatty acids, such as salmon, other cold-water fish, flax seed, and walnuts, and an increased intake of folate, whole grains, and vegetables would optimize the diet, and would be beneficial even after a lifetime of nutritional abuse.

Physical activity should optimally be at a level of 1 hour per day, 5 days a week. For most, walking can be recommended as being easy to accomplish, not requiring equipment or transportation.

Tobacco avoidance is mandatory for cardiovascular and pulmonary health. Use of tobacco is responsible for 90% of the lung disease in the United States and accounts for nearly 440,000 deaths each year, of which more than 135,000 are caused by smoking-related cardiovascular diseases (American Heart Association, 2008). Many tobacco cessation programs exist, and there are many tools that may be used.

Cancer

Cancer is the second leading cause of death in this country, and the risk of death increases with age (Satariano, 2006). The incidence of cancer among those 65 and older is 10 times that of younger individuals (National Cancer Institute, 2007). The National Cancer Institute recommends screenings for breast, colon, prostate, uterine, and skin cancers in order to begin secondary prevention strategies as early as possible.

Cancer is a collective designation for a general class of disease characterized by unrestrained cell growth. Cancers may be classified according to the primary site of origin. These diverse sites also relate to the designation of various modifiable risk factors. Lung cancer causes the most deaths among persons with cancer. This is followed by prostate disease in men and breast cancer in women. The primary risk factor for lung cancer is, of course, tobacco use, addressed above. For breast and colon cancers, nutritional strategies are paramount and consist of increasing fiber intake and decreasing fat intake. Women who are obese may put themselves at risk for breast and uterine cancers. Ingesting a high-fat diet may also put men at risk for colon and prostate cancers. Sun avoidance is key to the primary prevention of skin cancer.

Osteoarthritis

Osteoarthritis is the most common form of arthritis and is the most prevalent chronic health condition for both men and women (Albert, 2003). The site of the involvement predicts the extent of functional limitations and disability. Previous injury and age-associated stress and wearing of the joints, sometimes due to obesity, may predispose individuals to developing arthritis. There is also a genetic component to the development of the condition. Potentially modifiable risk factors include obesity, inadequate calcium and antioxidant intake, low levels of physical activity, and last, tobacco exposure.

Immunizations

The need for immunization continues throughout the life span. This concept comes as a surprise for many adults, who assume that childhood immunizations continue to convey protection. Additionally, some adults either were never vaccinated as children or received older versions of newer vaccines. Immunity may also fade over time. The Centers for Disease Control and Prevention (CDC) recommends that adults receive both diphtheria and tetanus immunizations if it has been 10 or more years since the last immunization. Also recommended is the herpes zoster, or shingles, vaccine (CDC, 2007).

Mortality from influenza is highest among those 65 years of age and older because many have medical conditions that place them at increased risk for complications. The CDC recommends that people 50 and older and their caregivers or other family members get a flu shot each year (CDC, 2006). Research indicates that adequate immunization reduces hospitalization by about 70% and death by about 85% among community-dwelling older people. Among nursing home residents, immunization may reduce the risk of hospitalization by about 50%, the risk of pneumonia by about 60%, and the risk of death by 75% to 80% (CDC, 2007).

Long-Term Care and Dementia

There is one condition of late life to which more emotional suffering and need is attributed than any other: Alzheimer's disease (AD). Consequently, it is the quintessential condition of aging in terms of triggering need for all the financial and personal resources available, from family to physician to community resources to nursing home. For these reasons, AD will receive a more in-depth overview than the other common diseases of aging noted above.

AD strikes at the core of individuality by taking away people's ability to think for themselves. Memory loss is one key symptom of AD, but judgment, planning, calculation, and decision making are also impaired and constantly worsen over 2 to 20 years. The person with AD becomes totally dependent on someone else. With this age-related disease, there is one commonly recognized patient with disease, but there are from one to several others who are also affected by providing round-the-clock supervision and care. Moreover, since most of the course of the disease and dependency occurs at home, the huge community impact remains hidden. With this disease, there are few outward physical signs of the disease, only the slowly increasing inability to recall events, recognize others, get dressed, prepare food, work, move about, and even properly manage ordinary hygiene. Eventually, the person is bedfast, requires feeding, is unable to speak, and typically dies from cardiac arrest or pneumonia, although the brain deterioration of AD is the ultimate cause.

Prevalence of AD is currently 4.5 million known cases, but will rise to 13.2 million cases by 2050, assuming that current demographic trends of aging continue and that no prevention is possible (Hebert, Scherr, Bienias, Bennett, & Evans, 2003). Monetary costs are staggering. The total Medicare spending on treating beneficiaries with AD will increase from $62 billion in 2000 to $189 billion in 2015. By 2050, Medicare will be spending more than $1 trillion on AD-related costs, which converts to 4 out of every 10 Medicare dollars. State and federal

Medicaid spending also will increase from $19 billion in 2000 to $118 billion in 2050 (Lewin Group, 2004).

Developing an appropriate public health response to AD requires a somewhat more detailed understanding of the disease. First, AD is one of several dementia types. "Dementia" simply refers to brain disorders with cognitive symptoms that can be due to many causes, such as being intoxicated, overmedicated, or having a traumatic brain injury. However, "dementia" also refers to specific pathological processes that permanently and progressively impair cognitive functions of the brain. AD is one such dementia, and another common one among elders is vascular dementia (VaD). These are the two most common causes of cognitive dysfunction in older people. AD and VaD have in common the symptoms of cognitive dysfunction manifested as memory loss, impaired thinking, and, as a result, need for constant supervision. However, the cause of each is different. While the pathophysiology is very complex and not completely understood, AD is ultimately caused by long-term chemical destruction of brain cells, whereas VaD symptoms are caused by huge numbers of very small strokes that kill brain cells. Recent autopsy studies show that most cases have both AD and VaD pathology simultaneously (Nandigam, Schneider, Arvanitakis, Bang, & Bennet, 2008).

The epidemiologic dynamics of AD include the following, based on a national survey (Plassman et al., 2007): (1) increasing risk with age, (2) increased risk with a certain gene variation (apolipoprotein E4), (3) increased risk with a family history, and (4) increased risk with low education. According to Plassman et al. (2007), the population aged 71 and over has a 13.9% prevalence rate for dementia. Of that population, 9.7% of cases are AD, and 2.4% are VaD. Consequently, AD accounted for about 70% of all dementia cases among people 71 and older. However, per age cohort, increased risk due to age is seen in prevalence rates (PR): For those aged 71 to 70, the PR is 5%; for those aged 80 to 89, the PR is 24.2%; for those aged 90 and over, the PR is 37.4%. It is worth recalling that it is the 85-and-over age cohort that is the fastest-growing of all.

The epidemiology of dementia across population groups is not well characterized or understood. However, data show that age-specific prevalence of dementia is significantly higher in non-Hispanic whites compared with other population groups. African Americans have higher PR than non-Hispanic whites for hypertension (65% vs. 51% for whites), high cholesterol, strokes, and type 2 diabetes (14.7% vs. 9.8%) (American Diabetes Association, 2008). All of these conditions are considered risk factors for AD and particularly VaD. The corresponding outcome is more VaD among African Americans than whites due to the vascular pathology associated with the disorders specified above. Combined with a significant increase in the 85-and-over cohort, African Americans will be entering the ages of greatest risk for AD in record numbers. For Hispanics, the PR of diabetes (10.4%) is close to that of non-Hispanic whites (American Diabetes Association, 2008). However, in a study of Mexican Americans, type 2 diabetes combined with hypertension was more often associated with dementia than when compared with whites. Specifically, 43% of subjects in this study with dementia also had diabetes, stroke, or both (Haan et al., 2003).

Interestingly, American Indians are the only population group that may be somewhat protected from AD specifically. This is possibly due to their very low frequency of the apolipoprotein E4 allele (Henderson et al., 2002). However, the high prevalence of diabetes causes a higher risk for VaD than in other populations, resulting in continued risk for cognitive impairment for elders, but not from AD pathology.

Current treatments for dementia include medications that work with the remaining normal neurons to chemically improve their ability to function. However, these drugs are modest in their effects. There is no dramatic recovery to predementia function. Also, the primary potency of these drugs is limited mainly to the early parts of the disease course. The result is that there currently are no drugs or other interventions that serve as a means to cure AD, VaD, or the many other forms of late-life dementia.

Public health is appropriate to address many aspects of dementia (e.g., policy, health economics, environmental issues, health administration of long-term care, epidemiology, etc.). Perhaps the main theme that relates best to dementia is prevention. Until recently, discussing the preventability of dementia was unthinkable. However, now that the disease process is better understood, prevention is seen as having great potential. In 2006, the National Institute on Aging distributed a booklet, *Can Alzheimer's Disease Be Prevented?* (NIA, 2006). The answer was "most likely," although the ultimate proof from scientific studies is not yet available. The next year, the CDC and the Alzheimer's Association convened a national task force to review current research to identify data supporting the concept of preventability of dementia, including AD and VaD. The task force created an action plan for developing the necessary research to prove the preventability of AD, titled *The Healthy Brain Initiative: A National Public Health Road Map to Maintaining Cognitive Health* (CDC and the Alzheimer's Association, 2007). One of the authors (JNH) was on the task force, which concluded that the basic principles of health promotion are not only good for cardiovascular health and overall health, but are specifically brain protective (Podewils et al., 2005). That is, physical activity (Larson et al., 2006; Weuve et al., 2004), mental activity, and proper nutrition (Kang, Ascherio, & Grodstein, 2005) over the life span will likely prevent or delay the symptoms of dementia.

These types of preventive gerontology do not actually stop the AD pathology from occurring, but health promotion can minimize the effects of AD as well as cause the symptoms to become noticeable later than otherwise. Minimizing the symptoms of AD occurs through the process of maintaining good cardiovascular health through optimal control of hypertension, diabetes, cholesterol levels, sufficient physical activity, and diet (Launer, 2005). Cardiovascular health is protective of cerebrovascular accidents (strokes). Also, continuing to use the brain in challenging ways keeps its functioning at nearly midlife levels. The presence of optimal early-life nutrition and lifelong education or learning is also associated with preservation of brain health.

Preventive gerontology action aimed at better control over dementia prevalence demands consideration of cross-cultural variance in health beliefs about its cause, course, and treatment. Anthropological research shows great variance in health beliefs across African American, Hispanic, Asian, and American Indian populations (Henderson, 1992, 1996, 1998; Henderson & Henderson, 2002; Henderson & Traphagan, 2005).

In summary, the research on dementia shows that there is no immediate cure on the horizon and that current treatments have limited value. Since the prevalence of AD alone will almost triple in the next few decades, it is urgent that public health develop messages to all age groups for primary prevention as well as secondary prevention of dementia. Such public health actions suffer from being long-term projects in the presence of immediate need. However, the demographic statistics combined with the epidemiology of dementia make it imperative that all efforts be fully applied now.

PUBLIC HEALTH: ORGANIZING FOR AN AGING SOCIETY

Economics of Aging

Who "funds" aging? The mix is varied. Through Medicare, the government funds around two thirds of health care needs for elders. Medicare is the largest source of payment for health care costs, assuming 45% of the debt. Medicaid, a source for low-income elders or those who are not eligible for Social Security, funds around 12%. The Veteran's Administration funds 6%, with other organizations assuming the remaining portions. Medicare covers hospital care through Part A, physician visits through Part B, and prescription benefits through Part D. Parts B and D have premiums that must be paid for by the individual, however. Long-term care benefits may be marginal. Therefore, those who are impoverished, have never worked in a system that withdraws salary funds for Social Security, or are homemakers are ineligible and must have health care expenses covered by other programs, one of which is Medicaid. Medicaid criteria vary from state to state, but may cover some long-term care services, costs for the disabled, prescriptions, eye care, dental care, and rehabilitative services.

With some living to advanced ages, there are concerns regarding the health care needs of the "oldest old," that is, those over the age of 75 years. However, the oldest old actually contribute little to increased health care costs overall, when compared with the increase in costs generated by the increase in health care sector inflation (prescription drugs and medical supplies) and the overall inflation of the economy. Those living to advanced old age are robust individuals. Economically, Medicare payments decrease as the age at death increases and so does the intensity of medical care required to maintain survival.

The financing of long-term care is another concern. Losers include single women, especially minority women, the chronically disabled, the impoverished, and the oldest old. There has been a changing family structure in the United States, and this change means fewer caregivers to older adults and lack of financial support for those who are in the home. Changing cultural expectations also impact the availability of long-term care. Medicare does not cover long-term care. Costs for nursing home care exceed $36,000 per year. Impoverishment may occur due to these long-term care costs.

Medicaid covers 52% of nursing home costs in this country but may be limited by state mandates. Eligibility criteria are stringent, and the individual may be required to "spend down" assets to ensure eligibility. The U.S. Department of Veterans Affairs (VA) may cover expenses for eligible persons. At this juncture, 80% of long-term care is provided by informal caregivers, the majority being family members. Political advocates for older adults continue to lobby for payment for informal caregivers so they may remain in the home, as well as increases in home health services for home-bound elders.

There are concerns surrounding the funding of Medicare and Medicaid, due to the large numbers of aged individuals expected to be utilizing the system in the near future. Medical care, social services, and economic policy reflect the outcomes of power struggles between dominant groups. Insurance companies have increased co-pays for older adults, and HMOs have rewarded physicians for undertreatment of patients. These strategies have also been relatively unsuccessful in decreasing health care costs. Political-economic actions designed to legislate Medicare benefits and do away with Social Security have thus far been unsuccessful, and the moral and cultural expectations of the population have prevailed.

Political Advocacy

The ageist nature of American society long ago provoked the development of political advocacy groups for elders. One of the best-known advocacy groups is the 37-million-member American Association of Retired Persons (AARP), which began in 1958. Today, AARP has established a set of priorities that reflects many of the problematic issues facing elders now and in the near future (AARP, 2008): (1) economic security; (2) Social Security; (3) pensions and savings; (4) the option of working; (5) security from financial harm; (6) affordable, reliable utilities; (7) health care and supportive services; (8) health care coverage; (9) improving Medicare; (10) affordable prescription drugs; (11) long-term support and services; (12) livable communities; (13) housing options; and (14) transportation. These priorities reflect the fact that longevity is currently plagued by insufficient money in the presence of lifetime high health costs and concerns for long-term care.

The Gray Panthers, started in the 1970s by Maggie Kuhn, is an organization whose name (given by a talk show host) recalls the militancy of the Black Panthers (Gray Panthers, 2008). However, the aggressive approach is for demanding quality of life for elders in the context of an ageist society. The current Gray Panthers describe themselves as "an intergenerational, multi-issue organization working to create a society that puts the needs of people over profit, responsibility over power and democracy over institutions." The Gray Panthers' priorities are to (1) create and fund a single-payer, nonprofit, and universal health care system; (2) regulate health maintenance organizations (HMOs) comprehensively, for the protection of patients and health care providers; (3) legislate a Patients' Bill of Rights; (4) provide funding for scientifically based sex education and reproductive health care; (5) legalize medical marijuana; (6) remove barriers to stem cell research; (7) give health care consumers a seat at the table in setting federal health research priorities; (8) return to the public a proper share of pharmaceutical profits, reflecting public investment in basic medical and health research; (9) repeal any privatization of Medicare and the Part D prescription drug program, replacing it with gap-free coverage under Medicare at fair and affordable prices; and (10) end constraints on government negotiation for lower prescription drug prices and on importation of foreign-made pharmaceuticals.

The Gray Panthers organization, like the AARP, reflects great concerns about the costs of aging in America, precisely about elders' lifetime high risk for multiple, chronic health problems and hospitalizations. Their political position shows that elders do not necessarily become passive in old age. This is similar to the movement known as the "Silver Haired Legislature"

(SHL). The SHL began in Texas in the 1970s and spread to Florida and then to about 30 other states. Members of the SHL are those 60 and older and who are interested in volunteering to be advocates to state legislators on laws impacting elders. The SHL is a loosely organized group that has, however, garnered much respect from elected officials in the states where members work. The demographics of aging shown earlier should give politicians pause since the elder population of the future will be better educated, have more at stake while aging, and continue to exert political influence. It is worth noting that the issues of universal health care, concerns over cost of age-related health maintenance, and valuing of human dignity have been major political issues for the American Public Health Association as well.

Research

The health sciences research branches are also very active in efforts to improve the health and well-being of elders. For example, in 1975, the National Institutes of Health created the National Institute on Aging (NIA). NIA conducts research on diseases of old age, but also on the social issues of aging, such as assessment of the most effective caregiving techniques. More specifically, NIA seeks to improve the health and quality of life of elders by (1) preventing or reducing diseases, disorders, and disabilities associated with aging; (2) discovering ways to keep physical health and high functional status; and (3) improving elders' abilities to continue active social roles and prevent social isolation. Also, NIA conducts basic research into the process of aging and its relationship to health and longevity. This effort includes (1) finding the biological and environmental wellsprings that are associated with optimal cognitive, sensory, and physical functioning; (2) conducting genetic research related to aging, longevity, age-related diseases, and behavior; (3) finding psychosocial and lifestyle factors that promote successful aging, and (4) understanding the differences between normal aging processes and those of pathology.

Additional aging research is done within the VA system. The VA system operates a 30-year-old Geriatric Research, Education, and Clinical Center (GRECC) initiative. The 18 current GRECCs conduct research on a wide range of age-related diseases and provide continuing education sessions for clinicians both within and outside the VA system. For example, areas of GRECC research include the biological mechanisms of diabetes as altered by age; falls and mobility issues, to reduce fractures with surgical repairs; and best clinical approaches to palliative care in end-of-life issues.

Geriatric Education

The Bureau of Health Professions has funded the Geriatric Education Center (GEC) program since the early 1980s. GECs are designed to get current age-related health information to providers in the communities. GECs are university based, but community oriented. While there are numerous age-related professional organizations (e.g., American Geriatrics Society, Gerontological Nursing Association, Association of Gerontological Social Workers, etc.), the GECs target not only aging experts, but also providers who work with a general patient population and need geriatric updates from experts, since the aging of America means that all providers to adults will have elders in the patient populations.

COMPRESSION OF
MORBIDITY AND QUALITY OF LIFE

Minimizing the length of time in a dependent state due to disease or disability is the basis of the concept "compression of morbidity," or "rectangularization of the morbidity curve" (Fries, 2005). Assuming that longevity extends to age 100, at about age 70, increasing dependency begins. In this scenario, the person who lives to age 100 experiences 30 years of increasing dependency prior to death. On the other hand, if increasing dependency begins at about 85 years of age, then the person living to age 100 will experience 15 years of dependency prior to death. The continued increase of the age at which dependency begins would result in fewer years of dependency prior to death. This is the compression-of-morbidity effect. If one can live with health and high functioning most of one's life, then most dependency due to chronic sickness will be compressed into a smaller period of time. The outcome would be not only a higher quality of life for most, but also a more economically feasible late-life experience.

Functional dependencies interrupt the ability of people to enjoy life, and they may require help from others just to do simple tasks like dressing, grooming, toileting, and other activities of daily life. The concept of "long-term care" reflects the lengthy delivery of services and assistance that can take place at home or in institutions. In-home care is done by a mix of helpers, some family and friends, and some direct services provided by agencies. Service delivery agencies can be public, like the Area Agencies on Aging (AAAs) and other governmental entities; but increasingly, private agencies are filling the market niche that an aging population creates. For example, the battery-powered personal chairs that allow for individual mobility are funded by the federal government. However, other devices for assistance are not. For example, increased lighting to safely walk in one's home; physical removal or modification of home interiors for safety, such as bathroom handgrips; and extra support for stair banisters, when elders' leg strength is weak and they use their upper body strength to pull themselves up, are all out-of-pocket expenditures—if one has the money to use.

The goal of the public health and aging paradigm is to minimize disease and disability in the last 50 years of life and to maximize functioning. The achievement of these goals may be assessed in some part by an examination of *perceived* quality of life (QOL). QOL has two domains: health-related QOL and non-health-related QOL. But for both of these domains, one essential concept must be acknowledged: QOL measures rely on self-report of the individual, not on objective observation of medical personnel or researchers (Albert, 2003).

Health-related QOL is a health status assessment that measures disease impact on the individual. It consists of patient reports of functional status, mental health, affective status, emotional well-being, social engagement, and symptom states, which include items such as shortness of breath, visual problems, hearing problems, and fatigue. It is most valuable for public health interventions. Interestingly, people with disease appear to rate their health-related QOL more highly than do nonpatients. Indeed, some with very low health-related QOL measures find life satisfying and meaningful. Thus, *perceived* QOL is the marker for success in this domain.

The task for gaining some assurance that a long life will be worth living is to minimize the amount of time experienced with health-related dependencies. Fortunately, most elders 65 years of age and older self-report that they have "good to excellent" health (AoA, 2007). For example, "good to excellent" health was reported by 74% of whites, 58% of African Americans, and 65% of Hispanics. These numbers reflect the existence of health disparities across elder groups. However, the self-report of "good to excellent" health dramatically drops with age. For example, for the 85-and-over age cohort (recall that this is the fastest-growing age group), "good to excellent" health was reported by 66% of whites, 50% of African Americans, and 53% of Hispanics. These numbers suggest that older elders will experience a significant number of years in suboptimal health characterized by disabilities and resultant dependencies and possible need for in-home or institutional assistance.

Non-health-related QOL assesses community-level indicators of well-being as well as social indicators. It incorporates the social equality model. Non-health-related QOL may also of course be affected by health, and it is difficult to separate the two types of indicators. This domain consists of patient reports of states such as the capacity to form friendships, appreciation of nature, and finding satisfaction in spiritual/religious activities. Also considered in this domain are features of the natural and built environment, housing, air and water quality, community stability, access to the arts and entertainment, and personal and economic resources.

With aging, QOL declines as morbidity and disability increase. With age, persons report fewer "good" physical and mental health days. The focus, therefore, with aging must be on maintenance of functional status, minimizing the effects of disease and disability, and working with the strengths retained.

PERSONAL FACTORS

Public health is generally concerned with community-level and population-level health. However, it is always true that the aggregate is made up of individuals. It is helpful to understand the unique attributes of older adults in terms of health so that clear conceptual distinctions in function can be made across the life span. Also, large-scale programs for older adults can profit from understanding the changes in health functioning of individuals.

Physiological changes in functioning in old age have been cataloged by Wachtel and Fretwell (2007) to show that, collectively, the older person is increasingly vulnerable to the ordinary insults of life and is due specific medical consideration. Wachtel and Fretwell (2007) note that pathogenesis of some diseases is altered with age. Compromised immune system function often found in old age can cause greater chance of disease onset in later life compared with early life. Also, disease risk and severity may be altered due to environmental exposures. For example, hypothermia is a greater risk for older adults than for younger adults because homeostatic regulation is suboptimal in older adults. Compounding this risk is the reduced sensitivity to awareness of warning signs in older persons. Reduced sensory sensitivity, for example, causes awareness of simple heat and cold to take longer to be "triggered" than in younger persons. Tissue damage can occur before the person takes protective action.

Older adults as patients have several characteristics that collectively produce the need for a unique knowledge base and set of skills to provide optimal care for them. First, the older adult is more likely than those in other age groups to express symptoms atypically (Ham, Sloane, Warsaw, Bernard, & Flaherty, 2006). The "atypical presentation" of symptoms occurs at all ages; however, in old age, it is more common. A propensity for atypical presentation of symptoms introduces the risk that clinicians will miss important symptoms or misinterpret them (Ham et al., 2006). For example, older adults may not have high temperatures in the presence of significant infectious disease. Also, myocardial infarction (MI) may be "silent." Medical texts usually describe the patient's complaint as a "crushing substernal chest pain with possible radiation into the left arm" and often cue the clinician to watch for the patient to place a fist over the chest in the vicinity of the heart in reaction to the severe pain typical of the classic "MI." Yet, older adults may show none of the classic signs. They often present with very vague reports of general malaise, no particular pain, and some nausea, and may walk into the hospital and not seem to be in a medical crisis.

Mental health conditions such as depression also can be expressed atypically. The "masked depression" is more common among older adults, posing a challenge for clinicians to detect the altered signs (Spar & La Rue, 2006). For example, typical signs of significant depression can include sadness of affect, expression of despair, changes in appetite, changes in sleep, and a general slowing of motion, reflexes, and movement. Among older adults, the depressed person may not clearly show any of these signs. Masked depression may present with a cheerful person who is involved in various social activities without signs of obvious distress. However, this same person may have loss of appetite; sleep disturbance; a cognitive awareness of sadness, loss, or despair; and inadequate energy to feel comfortable in conducting ordinary activities of daily living (ADLs). The problem is that some of these signs of masked depression are considered to be a normal part of the aging process. The older adult may not eat as much as in the past, may have sleep pattern change, may move generally slower, and may have less energy than in earlier life. Still, the clinician alerted to the increased probabilities of masked depression in older adults must distinguish between normal age-related changes and those associated with underlying depression.

The older adult population also has increased instances of "multiple pathologies" (Ham et al., 2006). This means that older adults often have several diseases at any one time. Many of these are chronic diseases for which there is no cure, only symptom management. However, it is very important to recognize that the older person with multiple pathologies may be quite able to perform his or her ordinary daily activities, because having several diagnosed diseases does not necessarily produce a net effect of noxious disability.

Related to the phenomenon of multiple pathologies, the older adult population is more at risk of "polypharmacy" than their younger counterparts (Ham et al., 2006). Clinicians treating multiple diseases and conditions prescribe medications to ameliorate the older adult's symptoms or improve function. However, some of the prescribing may occur among several clinicians who may not be aware of each other's actions. Even when one clinician treats one older adult patient, there is increased risk of noxious interactive effects and several predictable side effects. The collective experience of this by the older adult patients is that although their disease lab values may be improved, their overall sense of good health, well-being, and daily excitement about life may be reduced as a result of health care intervention.

"Impaired homeostasis" is another characteristic of older adult life that affects health care interventions (Ham et al., 2006). The ability of the older adult to maintain and/or recover from alterations to normal functioning is reduced in both speed and absolute terms. For example, tests of sway that measure the sensitivity of imbalance and recovery show that normal older adults will tilt out of balance a slightly farther distance before sensing the tilt and recovering from it compared with younger adults. Although the older adult may not fall and the sensory sensitivity of the antigravity centers of the brain still functions, the speed of reestablishing homeostasis is slower. Also, bed rest can produce loss of muscle tone very rapidly compared with younger adults. Some have suggested that 1 day of bed rest for older adults is equivalent to 3 days of bed rest for younger adults in terms of muscle tone and possible atrophy. Even the occurrence of acute disease such as the flu can take the older adult much longer than younger adults to recover to baseline function and subjective sense of wellness.

Iatrogenic disease is a type of malfunctioning due to the application of medical care. The term *iatros* derives from the Greek root word for "physician." The current use of *iatrogenic disease* does not always, however, mean specifically the physician, but, rather, exposure to the health care system as a whole or to individual practitioners, resulting in compromised health. All people are at some unavoidable risk, such as from postsurgical or other nosocomial infections acquired during hospital care. However, older adults are at heightened risk for several reasons. First, they experience more disease, physician visits, and hospital days than younger adults, which increases their exposure to such risks. Second, they experience increased vulnerability to medication problems due to polypharmacy. Third, ageism in health care can lead to undertreatment or unrecognized problems due to atypical presentation.

Collectively, these characteristics of older adults as patients constitute a clear statement of the need for a specific set of conceptual and practice skills to provide optimal treatment for older adults. Public health and aging must account for these unique factors in all types of population-based interventions, ranging from primary to tertiary prevention. To ignore the unique attributes of older adult health commits the "one size fits all" fallacy and, worse, heightens the vulnerability index already applicable to older adults and particularly to very old adults.

FUTURE PUBLIC HEALTH AND AGING NEEDS

The Harvard School of Public Health Center for Health Communication has launched the Harvard-MetLife Foundation Initiative on Retirement and Civic Engagement to identify and promote strategies to expand the contributions of older people to civic life ("Reinventing Aging," Center for Health Communication, 2004). The basis for the initiative is that the growing aging population of "baby boomers" could be induced to strengthen communities with their postretirement time by virtue of communications stemming from research on cultural factors in aging. For example, the well-known concept of a "designated driver" was created by these organizations and shows the possibilities of the purposeful start of a new social concept. Applying that experience to aging and community well-being was done by the idea of "Rethinking Aging."

"Rethinking Aging" is a tall order. One theme is the need to have individual planning for productive aging become an integrated certainty as a natural part of one's life. Erik Erikson's (1997) view of life included the notion that postretirement life should become a time during which the lessons of life are applied toward the good of the community. Another main issue is that the way that aging is discussed does not comprehensively convey the complexity that is there. For example, terms like "a senior moment" or "senior discount" are derived from negative contexts (e.g., memory failure, economic straits) that collapse a multitude of issues into a stereotypic word or phrase. More positive terms need to be found through the use of social surveys or strategies like social marketing. In addition, one of the best placements of these communications is thought to be the mass entertainment media: movies and television. The initiative is working with the entertainment industry to incorporate more positive images of older adults involved with communities. Next, the value of intergenerational programs should be improved. There is a benefit to social capital when generations interact in useful ways. Social capital in communities can be further enhanced by encouragement from community organizations to foster interactions with elders. Overall, the "Rethinking Aging" initiative stems from a culture of ageist bias that permeates all aspects of life. In order to bring correction to this prejudice, concepts common to public health and the promotion of health status are being mobilized. This should be just the beginning.

The MetLife Foundation also teamed with the National Area Agencies on Aging to conduct research that produced the following "best practices" for communities to consider in order to address the needs of an aging population (Maturing of America Report, 2006):

1. Preventive health care, such as health and "lifestyle" education, immunizations and screenings, to reduce injuries and the onset of chronic diseases, as well as a range of in-home health assistance to help people stay in their homes longer.

2. Nutrition education to promote healthy eating throughout a person's life span, as well as nutritional community-sponsored programs such as home-delivered meals for those who have difficulty or are unable to prepare their own meals.

3. Age-appropriate fitness programs and recreational facilities that offer walking trails, benches, and fitness equipment.

4. Larger, easier-to-read road signage, grooved lane dividers, reflective road markings, and dedicated left-turn lanes. Driver assessments and training to promote safe driving for all ages, especially after strokes or other health incidents. Transportation options for people who cannot or do not want to drive.

5. Special planning and training to help public safety personnel and other first responders locate and assist older adults during emergencies and disasters.

6. Home modification programs that make necessary adjustments for people with special needs. Zoning and subdivision plans that promote a variety of affordable, accessible housing located near medical, commercial, and other desired services, as well as shared housing options for older adults and their caregivers.

7. Tax assistance and property tax relief for those in financial need and programs to protect older adults against fraud and abuse.

8. Job training, retraining, and lifelong learning opportunities, as well as flexible employment options to attract and retain older workers.

9. Opportunities to engage older adults in community boards and commissions, as well as purposeful volunteer activities in local government and nonprofit organizations.

10. Single point of entry for information and access to all aging information and services in the community, and the strategic expansion of necessary services to support older adults in aging with dignity and independence in their homes and community.

Both the Harvard School of Public Health and the National Area Agencies on Aging work in conjunction with the MetLife Foundation have overall produced an action plan for improving not only the health of individual elders but also the health of communities and their members of all ages. Each initiative is filled with common principles and values of public health. These include the concepts of life span aging; prevention of disease; prevention of disability; environmental issues, such as housing and food; the crucial need for money; fair health care administration; and the need for proper health education. It is clear that there is an imperative for public health to include the many issues of aging in its lengthy list of foundational issues for maintaining the health of society.

CONCLUSION

The experience of late-adult life is significantly affected by early-life health behavior. Consequently, the public health principles of healthy living and disease prevention are extremely relevant to aging. The life span concept of aging is required to form a fully integrated model of the effects of the "first 50 years" on the "second 50 years." Moreover, the social ecology model is crucial to understanding the biological, social, political, and economic issues that collectively produce health status and quality-of-life indices in late life. Public health as an intervention system is probably the most important means in existence for achieving gerontologic health.

Public health interventions for elders include avoidance of acute disease through the use of vaccinations, antibiotics, risk exposure reduction, and being served in the health care system as needed. Also, chronic conditions must be optimally managed to keep the highest level of functioning possible for as long as possible. Managing chronic conditions often requires clinicians to be diligent in their treatments so that attention to small changes and treatment modifications can be properly done. Furthermore, brain failure demands full attention relative to prevention, moderation, and treatment. The long-term care needs inherent to brain failure can overburden health care systems as well as families.

Future elder needs echo the basic requirements of life with dignity, reward for a life lived, and a sense of gladness for living a long life. Unfortunately, for many elders today, these basic human needs and rights are missing. Public health should be a catalyst for improving the quality of life experienced during the number of years gained by modern health care advances.

Aggressive health promotion, policy, and environmental changes are the toolkit of public health and await full use in elder health.

REFERENCES

Administration on Aging. (2007). *A profile of older Americans: 2000.* Retrieved April 26, 2008, from www.aoa.gov/prof/Statistics/profile/2000/profile2000.pdf

Albert, S. M. (2003). *Public health and aging: An introduction to maximizing function and well-being.* New York: Springer.

American Association of Retired Persons. (2008). *AARP 2008 advocacy agenda.* Retrieved September 8, 2008, from http://assets.aarp.org/www.aarp.org_/articles/aboutaarp/AARP2008 AdvocacyAgenda.pdf

American Diabetes Association. (2008). *Total prevalence of diabetes & pre-diabetes.* Retrieved September, 1, 2008, from www.diabetes.org

American Heart Association. (2008). *Cigarette smoking and cardiovascular diseases.* Retrieved April 26, 2008, from http://www.americanheart.org/presenter.jhtml?identifier=4545

Bortz, W. (1991). We live too short and die too long. *Aging Today, 12,* 1–3.

Butler, R. (1975). *Why survive? Being old in America.* New York: Harper & Row.

Center for Health Communication. (2004). *Reinventing aging: Baby boomers and civic engagement.* Harvard School of Public Health–MetLife Foundation Initiative on Retirement and Civic Engagement. Retrieved September 1, 2008, from www.hsph.harvard.edu/chc/reinventingaging/ report_highlights.html

Centers for Disease Control and Prevention. (2006). *Flu vaccine effectiveness: Questions and answers for health professionals.* Retrieved August 8, 2008, from www.cdc.gov/flu/professionals/vaccination/ effectivenessqa.htm

Centers for Disease Control and Prevention. (2007). *Vaccine-preventable adult diseases.* Retrieved September 1, 2008, from http://www.cdc.gov/vaccines/vpd-vac/adult-vpd.htm

Centers for Disease Control and Prevention and the Alzheimer's Association. (2007). *The Healthy Brain Initiative: A national public health road map to maintaining cognitive health.* Chicago: Alzheimer's Association.

Cummings, S., & Galambos, C. (Eds.). (2004). *Diversity and aging in the social environment.* New York: Haworth Social Work Practice Press.

Erikson, E. H. (1997). *The life cycle completed.* New York: Norton.

Fries, J. (2005). The compression of morbidity. *Milbank Quarterly, 83*(4), 801–823.

Gray Panthers. (2008). *Health care issue statement.* Retrieved April 26, 2008, from http://graypanthers .org/index.php?option=com_content&task=blogcategory&id=7&Itemid=49

Haan, M. N., Mungas, D. M., Gonzalez, H. M., Ortiz, T. A., Acharya, A., & Jagust, W. J. (2003). Prevalence of dementia in older Latinos: The influence of type 2 diabetes mellitus, stroke and genetic factors. *Journal of the American Geriatric Society, 51,* 169–177.

Ham, R. J., Sloane, P. D., Warsaw, G. A., Bernard, M. A., & Flaherty, E. (2006). *Primary care geriatrics: A case-based approach* (5th ed.). Edinburgh, UK: Elsevier Mosby.

Hebert, L. E., Scherr, P. A., Bienias, J. L., Bennett, D. A., & Evans, D. A. (2003). Alzheimer disease in the U.S. population: Prevalence estimates using the 2000 census. *Archives of Neurology, 60*(8), 1119–1122.

Henderson, J. N. (1992). The power of support: Alzheimer's disease support groups for minority families. *Aging, 363/364,* 24–28.

Henderson, J. N. (1996). Dementia in Cuban and Puerto Rican populations. In G. Yeo & D. Gallagher-Thompson (Eds.), *Ethnicity and the dementias* (pp. 153–167). New York: Taylor & Francis.

Henderson, J. N. (1998). Dementia in cultural context: The development and decline of a support group. In J. Sokolovsky (Ed.), *The cultural context of aging* (2nd ed.). New York: Bergin and Garvey.

Henderson, J. N., Crook, R., Crook, J., Hardy, J., Onstead, L., Carson-Henderson, L., et al. (2002). Apolipoprotein E4 allele and tau allele frequencies among Choctaw Indians. *Neuroscience Letters, 324,* 77–79.

Henderson, J. N., & Henderson, L. C. (2002). Cultural construction of disease: A "supernormal" construct of dementia in an American Indian tribe. *Journal of Cross-Cultural Gerontology, 17,* 197–212.

Henderson, J. N., & Traphagan, J. (2005). Cultural factors in Alzheimer's disease: Perspectives from the anthropology of aging. *Alzheimer's Disease and Associated Disorders, 19,* 272–274.

Kang, J. H., Ascherio, A., & Grodstein, F. (2005). Fruit and vegetable consumption and cognitive decline in aging women. *Annals of Neurology, 57*(5), 713–720.

Larson, E. B., Wang, L., Bowen, J. D., McCormick, W. C., Teri, L., Crane, P. S., et al. (2006). Exercise is associated with reduced risk for incident dementia among persons 65 years of age and older. *Annals of Internal Medicine, 144*(2), 73–81.

Launer, L. (2005). Diabetes and brain aging: Epidemiologic evidence. *Current Diabetes Reports, 5*(1), 59–63.

Lewin Group. (2004). *Saving lives, saving money: Dividends for Americans investing in Alzheimer research.* A report commissioned by the Alzheimer's Association. Washington, DC: Author.

Maturing of America Report. (2006). *The maturing of America—getting communities on-track for an aging population.* Retrieved September 8, 2008, from http://www.n4a.org/pdf/The_Maturing_of_America.pdf

Nandigam, K., Schneider, J. A., Arvanitakis, Z., Bang, W., & Bennett, D. A. (2008). Mixed brain pathologies account for most dementia cases in community-dwelling older persons. *Neurology, 70,* 816–817.

National Cancer Institute. (2007). *NIH funds eight new grants focused on aging and cancer.* Retrieved September 1, 2008, from http://www.cancer.gov/newscenter/pressreleases/AgingGrants

National Institute on Aging. (2006). *Can Alzheimer's disease be prevented?* Retrieved September 8, 2008, from www.nia.nih.gov/Alzheimers/Publications/ADPrevented

Olshansky, S. J., Hayflick, L., & Carnes, B. A. (2002). Position statement on human aging. *Journal of Gerontology: Biological Sciences, 57A*(8), B292–297.

Omran, A. R. (1971). The epidemiologic transition: A theory of population change. *The Milbank Memorial Fund Quarterly, 49*(4), 509–538.

Plassman, B. L., Langa, K. M., Fisher, G. G., Heeringa, S. G., Weir, D. R., Ofstedal, M. B., et al. (2007). Prevalence of dementia in the United States: The aging, demographics, and memory study. *Neuroepidemiology, 29,* 125–132.

Podewils, L. J., Guallar, E., Kuller, K. H., Fried, L. P., Lopez, O. L., Carlson, M., et al. (2005). Physical activity, APOE genotype, and dementia risk: Findings from the Cardiovascular Health Cognition Study. *American Journal of Epidemiology, 161*(7), 639–651.

Satariano, W. A. (2006). *Epidemiology of aging: An ecological approach.* Boston: Jones & Bartlett.

Schocken, D. D. (2000). Epidemiology and risk factors for heart failure in the elderly. *Clinics in Geriatric Medicine, 16*(3), 407–418.

Sokolovsky, J. (1997). Bringing culture back home: Aging, ethnicity and family support. In J. Sokolovsky (Ed.), *The cultural context of aging* (2nd ed., pp. 262–275). Westport, CT: Bergin & Garvey.

Spar, J., & La Rue, A. (2006). *Clinical manual of geriatric psychiatry.* Arlington, VA: American Psychiatric.

Wachtel, T., & Fretwell, M. (2007). *Practical guide to the care of the geriatric patient.* New York: Mosby.

Weuve, J., Kang, J. H., Manson, J. E., Breteler, M. M., Ware, J. H., & Grodstein, F. (2004). Physical activity, including walking, and cognitive function in older women. *JAMA, 292*(12), 1454–1461.

PART V

Intervention, Methods, and Practice

Organized interventions to address health problems are the focus of Part V. Program planning is an important arena for applying the principles and methods of social and behavioral sciences. The first chapter overviews different planning frameworks, while the next two chapters discuss particular intervention strategies, community-based approaches, and social marketing programs. The fourth chapter addresses issues in policy and advocacy.

Chapter 13 overviews models for program planning and presents case studies of the major types. The importance of clearly defining objectives and involving key stakeholders through participatory planning is emphasized. Program planning takes the form of program development focused on a particular problem or planning for community-wide needs. Selected models for program development and community health planning are reviewed and case examples presented to illustrate their application. Issues in program evaluation are also addressed.

Community-based approaches have come to occupy a central role in public health intervention. Chapter 14 outlines key features of community-based approaches and overviews the main types of interventions involved. One key component is participatory research that involves members of the target community in planning and collecting data to guide program development. The PATCH model uses these features and is illustrated with a case example. Finally, the advantages and challenges of community-based interventions are assessed.

Social marketing approaches to intervention have gained increasing attention in recent years. Chapter 15 describes the principles and methods of social marketing, including the importance of product, competition, price, place, and promotion. How the approach works in practice is illustrated through case examples involving breastfeeding promotion and marketing of public health services.

Chapter 16 takes a different approach by presenting three in-depth case studies that illustrate policy and advocacy perspectives. The examples represent a range of public health issues—infectious disease, natural disaster, and health system analysis—and incorporate global health perspectives more directly than other chapters in the book. Policy-relevant research on cholera and volcanic threat in Ecuador and analysis of the Cuban public health model provide lessons that underscore the importance of putting community needs at the forefront in public health planning.

13

Planning Health Promotion and Disease Prevention Programs

Eric R. Buhi, Rita DiGioacchino DeBate, and Robert J. McDermott

One of the most common applications of social and behavioral science principles to public health occurs in the context of planning, implementing, and evaluating health promotion and disease prevention programs. For example, a local or state health department may request assistance in developing a program to decrease the prevalence of childhood obesity in its catchment area. How is this task approached? What steps are followed to develop such a program or intervention? What are the logical settings in which key initiatives should be implemented?

Fortunately, many tools and frameworks are available to assist public health professionals in the planning, implementation, and evaluation process. For instance, program planning frameworks such as PRECEDE-PROCEED (Green & Kreuter, 2005), Intervention Mapping (Bartholomew, Parcel, Kok, & Gottlieb, 2006), and Community Based Prevention Marketing (Bryant, Forthofer, McCormack Brown, & McDermott, 1999; Bryant et al., 2007), as well as community planning models such as Mobilizing for Action Through Planning and Partnerships (MAPP) (National Association of County and City Health Officials, 2004), Planned Approach to Community Health (PATCH) (Centers for Disease Control and Prevention [CDC], 1995), and Assessment Protocol for Excellence in Public Health (APEX*PH*) (National Association of County and City Health Officials, 2008) have been employed and well documented by public health practitioners. These frameworks can assist planners in the integration of behavioral and social science theories, such as those described in Part II, and in the development of interventions to prevent and control health problems.

The purpose of this chapter is threefold. First, we will describe the different types of prevention approaches and review the levels of the socio-ecological model. Second, we will provide an overview of the various settings—school, workplace, health care institution, community, and clinical general practice settings—in which prevention programs can be implemented, illustrating how these settings are leveraged with some examples from public health practice. Last, we will provide an overview of general frameworks for, and processes and methods of, planning, developing, and evaluating health promotion and disease prevention programs.

Public health programs have the overall goal of decreasing death, disease, and disability and increasing the quality of life for the population. Such programs comprise three main types: primary, secondary, and tertiary prevention. Primary prevention efforts are designed to preempt the onset of disease, illness, injury, or other health problem (McKenzie, Neiger, & Smeltzer, 2005). Some examples include increasing the number of sexually active individuals who use condoms correctly and consistently to prevent sexually transmitted infections (STIs); increasing the number of women of childbearing age who consume the recommended amount of folic aid to prevent birth defects in future pregnancies; and increasing the number of individuals who apply sunscreen appropriately to decrease their exposure to the sun's ultraviolet rays and, thus, reduce their risk of skin cancer.

Secondary prevention interventions are aimed at the early diagnosis and prompt treatment of a disease, illness, or injury to limit disability, impairment, or dependency and prevent the development of more severe problems (McKenzie et al., 2005). Examples include breast and cervical cancer screening for women (i.e., breast self-exams, mammograms, and Pap tests) and prostate screenings (the prostate-specific antigen blood test and digital rectal exam yearly) for men beginning at age 50 (Smith, Cokkinides, & Eyre, 2003).

When a disease, illness, injury, or other public health problem has already occurred, tertiary prevention measures can be employed to rehabilitate those affected, control the devastating complications, and avoid loss of life. Examples of tertiary prevention efforts include improving access to highly active antiretroviral treatment (HAART) for individuals infected with HIV (CDC, 2002), and routine foot and eye exams, and frequent A1c testing for persons with diabetes (American Diabetes Association, 2002).

Primary, secondary, and tertiary prevention initiatives can be employed at multiple levels of influence when planning and implementing public health interventions. Models addressing multiple levels of influence are generally termed *ecological models,* and a number of formulations have been developed. As noted in Chapter 1, most ecological frameworks share some common elements—interventions that target the individual; the person's social networks, such as family and friends; organizational and community-level institutions and environments; and governmental, political, and global systems. When developing and planning public health interventions, it is important to consider and plan for addressing the five hierarchical levels of influence discussed in Chapter 1—*intra*personal, *inter*personal, organizational, community, and society. Programs that address health issues at each of these levels, and across multiple levels, are more likely to be successful. In the next section, we revisit the ecological levels and provide examples of the interventions applied at each level.

LEVELS OF INFLUENCE REVISITED

Let's return to the opportunity presented at the beginning of this chapter. In developing and planning a program to reduce childhood obesity, it is important to assess and plan for interventions at the *intrapersonal level* of influence. At the intrapersonal level, interventions strive to shape individuals' behavior by focusing on characteristics such as knowledge, attitudes, beliefs, skills, and personality traits (National Cancer Institute, 2005). For example, in the case of childhood obesity, a child's dietary intake may be influenced by his or her primary caregiver's attitudes and behaviors regarding food. Although necessary for any type of prevention program, addressed alone, the intrapersonal level of influence is insufficient for creating changes in health behavior, as intrapersonal level factors are influenced by the other levels of the socio-ecological model.

At the next level in the ecological framework—the *interpersonal level*—health program planners develop interventions for individuals who are in a position to influence the behaviors of a specific population or group of people. Interpersonal influences may stem from interpersonal processes and primary groups, including family, friends, and peers who provide social identity, support, and role definition (National Cancer Institute, 2005). As indicated above, a child's primary caregiver has a substantial influence on his or her eating and physical activity behaviors, as do siblings and peers.

Addressing *organizational/institutional* and *community-level factors* is also very important for influencing health behaviors and health status. Organizational-level factors can include rules, regulations, policies, and informal structures that compromise or promote health (e.g., school district physical education policies and nonsmoking at the work site) (National Cancer Institute, 2005). At the community level, however, health program planners can focus their interventions on social networks and norms, or standards that exist formally or informally among individuals, groups, and organizations in addition to the physical or built environment (e.g., sidewalks, parks, and safe areas for physical activity) (National Cancer Institute, 2005).

Last, interventions that influence behavior through the highest level of influence in the ecological framework are aimed at shaping local, state, and federal policies and laws. *Society- or system-level* directed interventions support healthy actions and practices and discourage unhealthy behaviors through formal regulations (e.g., the PLAY Everyday Act) (National Cancer Institute, 2005). Chapter 17 provides an overview of factors associated with childhood obesity at the various levels of the socio-ecological model. Again, the most effective health promotion and disease prevention programs are those that focus efforts across *multiple levels of influence*. Multilevel interventions seek to change aspects at the individual, interpersonal, community, and system levels.

CASE STUDY   An Example From Public Health Practice

The following example illustrates a multilevel intervention to reduce cardiovascular disease (CVD) and diabetes among ethnic minorities. Charlotte REACH (Racial and Ethnic Approaches to

Community Health) 2010 is a good example of a coalition driven, multilevel prevention intervention for the Northwest Corridor in the city of Charlotte, North Carolina (DeBate, Plescia, Joyner, & Spann, 2004). The planning process was facilitated by a community coalition representing key leaders and organizations within the selected area. As shown in Table 13.1, Charlotte REACH 2010 intervention activities were aimed at all levels of the socio-ecological model.

Many residents participated in REACH community activities designed to increase awareness (an intrapersonal factor) of CVD and diabetes. However, to promote positive health behaviors among participants' families and to connect residents to local resources, a Lay Health Advisor (LHA) program also was included. LHAs are what are called "natural helpers"—trusted and respected members of community social networks to whom other network members turn for advice, support, and other types of aid (Israel, 1985). In addition to providing direct support, LHAs serve to link social network members to each other and to resources outside of the network, including screening, health education, and medical treatment services. The use of LHAs has emerged as an effective strategy in health promotion and disease prevention programs in many communities.

In the Charlotte REACH 2010 initiative, area YMCA and diabetes support groups collaborated on CVD and diabetes prevention programs implemented through various local health organizations and served as an informal network to promote health (DeBate et al., 2004). Such a collaborative maintains a unique advantage in better reaching the priority population of interest—in this case, ethnic minority and medically underserved children. As another illustration of the Charlotte REACH 2010 initiative, community advocacy efforts were aimed at legislating tobacco excise taxes to reduce cigarette purchases by new users (DeBate, et al., 2004). Yet another

TABLE 13.1 Charlotte REACH 2010 Program Strategies

Ecological Approach to Reducing CVD and Diabetes	
Level	*Charlotte REACH Strategy*
Intrapersonal	Community programming to increase awareness of CVD, diabetes, and related risk factors; educational and skill programming for increasing positive health behaviors
Interpersonal	Lay Health Advisor (LHA) Program
Organizational	YMCA collaborative programming; diabetes support group; secondary prevention activities; working relationship between LHA and program staff of various health organizations; primary-care provider prescription pad cues to action
Institutional	Primary-care disease management/quality assurance project for diabetes care patterns
Community	Winners Circle Program, neighborhood farmers market
Policy	Community advocacy for a state tobacco excise tax; community advocacy for statewide public health task force to address health disparities

SOURCE: Reproduced by permission from DeBate, R., Plescia, M., Joyner, D., and Spann, L. (2004). A Qualitative Assessment of Charlotte REACH: An Ecological Perspective for Decreasing CVD and Diabetes Among African Americans. *Ethnicity and Disease*, 14, S1-77–S71-82.

example included the promotion of policies regulating the sales and marketing of tobacco products in neighborhoods with higher proportions of ethnic minority children.

Program Planning and Intervention Development

Effective multilevel health promotion and disease prevention interventions are not born out of hasty or noncollaborative planning. Program development requires a structured, organized, systematic process with a collaborative team (McKenzie et al., 2005). Fortunately, there are a number of frameworks available to guide public health professionals in this systematic process of planning, implementing, and evaluating health promotion and disease prevention programs. Most of these intervention planning frameworks share similar elements or principles (Breckon, Harvey, & Lancaster, 1998; Kreuter, 1992).

One of the main shared principles among the planning frameworks is that the program development *process* should be well thought out and carefully planned (Breckon et al., 1998). Planners should carve out time "up front" to identify key stakeholders, both in the priority population and with potential collaborative organizations. This front-end analysis and planning time also should be devoted to identifying pertinent existing data sources and collecting new information to contribute to problem identification and, later, to tailoring the program to meet audience needs. Having clear planning goals, objectives, and timelines increases the match between intervention and audience.

Another shared principle among the planning frameworks is to *plan with people* (Breckon et al., 1998). Involving key stakeholders and representatives from all segments of the priority population throughout the planning, implementation, and evaluation process will help ensure that programming will not only meet the needs of the people being served but also will be embraced (Breckon et al., 1998; Kreuter, 1992). The principle of planning with people touches on the important concept of program ownership, which can result in greater community support for the program; also, the people centrally involved in the program will become program ambassadors because they believe in its merit (Strycker et al., 1997).

A third shared principle pertains to *planning with data* (Breckon et al., 1998). Local needs assessment data, such as information on both the actual and the perceived needs of the priority population, must drive the planning process. These data can be primary data (i.e., collected directly by program developers) or secondary data (i.e., existing information, such as census data, service utilization data). Moreover, they can be quantitative (i.e., in the form of numerical data and statistics), qualitative (i.e., data collected through interviews, observations, and written documents), or both. Social indicators; the perceived needs of the community; epidemiologic indicators; behavioral risk factors; access to health care; and the health knowledge, attitudes, beliefs, and skills necessary for behavior change and health status improvement are all rich sources of program planning information.

The fourth shared principle is that planners should *plan and develop objectives* to assess short-term and long-term program outcomes. An objective is a brief statement specifying the desired effect of a program. Well-written objectives state *how much* of *what* happens (*to whom*) *by when* (see Figure 13.1). Measurable objectives guide the program implementation process and, later, assist with program evaluation efforts.

FIGURE 13.1   Writing SMART Objectives

To be most effective, objectives should be clear and leave no room for misinterpretation.

S-M-A-R-T is a helpful acronym for developing objectives that are Specific, Measurable, Achievable, Relevant, and Timebound.

The following is an example of an S-M-A-R-T objective for decreasing childhood obesity:

By 2010, the proportion of overweight and obese children and adolescents aged 6–19 years (as measured by gender- and age-specific 95th percentile of BMI based on the revised CDC Growth Charts for the United States) who live in State X will decrease to 5%. (Baseline: 11% in 1994; Data Source: National Health and Nutrition Examination Survey [NHANES], CDC, NCHS)

The objective is *specific* because it identifies a priority population: children and adolescents between the ages of 6 and 19 who reside in State X. The objective is *measurable* because it specifies a baseline value and the quantity of change the intervention is designed to achieve: from 11% (baseline) to 5% (target objective). As in the example, it is worthwhile to note whether there is an existing data source for the objective. The objective is *achievable* because it is realistic given the greater than 15-year time frame and the fact that the reduction of obesity is a long-term issue. The objective is also *relevant* because it is pertains to reducing an epidemiological indicator, in this case childhood obesity. Finally, the objective is *timebound* because it provides a specified time frame by which the objective will be achieved (i.e., by the year 2010).

A tool to help write SMART objective:

Objective	By 2010, the proportion of overweight and obese children and adolescents aged 6–19 years (as measured by gender- and age-specific 95th percentile of BMI based on the revised CDC Growth Charts for the United States) who live in State X will decrease to 5%. (Baseline: 11% in 1994; Data Source: National Health and Nutrition Examination Survey [NHANES], CDC, NCHS). (CDC, 2007a)						
Breakdown	Verb	Metric	Population	Object	Baseline Measure	Target Measure	Time Frame
	Decrease	Percent	Children and adolescents aged 6 to 19 years who reside in State X	Overweight/ obesity	11%	5%	By 2010

SOURCE: Adapted from Writing SMART Objectives (CDC, 2007b).

Finally, apparent in most frameworks is the importance for planners to *plan for evaluation* (Breckon et al., 1998). If incorporated well, evaluation is a tool that can assist in every step of the process, from planning to implementation and beyond. For instance, process evaluation procedures can be conducted during the program planning and implementation phases and will answer questions such as "Did we do what we said we were going to do and in the manner that was planned?" On the other hand, impact and outcome evaluations assist in answering questions related to the short- and longer-term impacts, respectively, of a program. Program evaluation will be addressed in greater detail at the end of this chapter. To assist planners in reaching priority populations where they live, interact, and work, in the next section of this chapter, the various settings in which prevention programs can be implemented and evaluated are presented.

INTERVENTION SETTINGS

The nature of multilevel interventions necessitates that programs are planned for implementation in a variety of settings. Prominent settings or venues include schools, workplaces, health care institutions, community locations, and clinical general-practice settings. The particular venue or combination of venues to be accessed depends on the intervention and the priority population(s).

Since the early 1900s, when school nurses battled poor sanitation and infectious diseases, schools have been an important setting for implementing primary and secondary prevention programs (Marx, Wooley, & Northrop, 1998). Health promotion and disease prevention programs are ideal in such settings because lifelong health habits, both good *and* poor ones, develop at an early age. Additionally, children and youth are in school for most of their childhood and, thus, can serve as a "captive audience" for health programming and health screenings for 12 or more years. Moreover, a healthy child is more likely to achieve academically than an unhealthy one (Dewey, 1999; Dunkle & Nash, 1991; Ellickson, Tucker, & Klein, 2003; Mandell, Hill, Carter, & Brandon, 2002; Shephard, 1996; Swingle, 1997; Valois, MacDonald, Bretous, Fischer, & Drane, 2002). There are a number of evidence-based health promotion and disease prevention programs that are appropriate for school settings. One example is Safer Choices, a 2-year, school-based HIV/STI and teen pregnancy prevention program. Evaluations of Safer Choices in schools reveal that the program increased students' use of effective contraception and condoms (Coyle et al., 1999, 2001; Kirby et al., 2004).

Health promotion and disease prevention programs also have been widely implemented in workplace settings, and for good reason. Labor statistics reveal that employed Americans work an average of 8.0 hours on weekdays—about half of their waking hours (Partnership for Prevention, 2001; U.S. Bureau of Labor Statistics, 2007). The implementation of workplace health promotion (WHP) programs has resulted in a number of positive health and work-related outcomes. Such outcomes include increased employee productivity, reduced employee absenteeism, reduced health care costs, and, probably most important, reduced employee health risks (O'Donnell, 2001; Partnership for Prevention, 2001). One example of an effective WHP program is provided by the Du Pont Company. An evaluation of this comprehensive WHP program—which included health risk appraisals and a variety of self-directed and group health education opportunities—indicated a reduction in disability days among blue-collar employees and, subsequently, lower disability costs at intervention sites, when compared with control sites not receiving the program (Bertera, 1990).

In addition to schools and workplaces, the community has been an important venue for implementing health promotion and disease prevention programs. A community can refer to a group of people connected by a common physical/spatial arrangement (i.e., geography, such as a neighborhood or city) or a group sharing special social ties, such as ethnicity, nationality, age, or religious affiliation (Stephens, 2007). Primary and secondary prevention interventions have been implemented focusing on both conceptualizations of community. An example of an effective community-based intervention activity, limited by geography, is the implementation of sobriety checkpoints to reduce alcohol-impaired driving. The use of such checkpoints by community law enforcement agencies has decreased motor vehicle crashes related to alcohol use (Shults et al., 2001; Task Force on Community Preventive Services, 2001). An example of a community-based intervention tailored to focus on people with shared ties includes the case of the Witness Project™, a theory-based cancer education program designed to provide culturally sensitive messages to African American women. Evaluation findings from the Witness Project™ have indicated increases in the practice of breast self-examination and mammography among participating women (Erwin, Spatz, Stotts, Hollenberg, & Deloney, 1996). The next chapter further examines community-based approaches to health promotion.

Finally, health care institutions and clinical general practice settings are important for reaching certain priority populations. Secondary prevention activities (e.g., blood pressure monitoring, diabetes control, and cancer screening) have been implemented in such settings. However, health care institutions and clinical general practice settings are also important venues for conducting primary prevention activities. An example of this activity is the "brief intervention." Brief interventions can last between 5 and 60 minutes (Higgins-Biddle & Babor, 1996), and are often initiated by a primary-care physician or nurse. Brief interventions are usually followed by a referral for counseling and education with a health education specialist. Sometimes, however, there are multiple sessions involved in brief interventions. Another example of effective interventions in health care institutions and clinical general-practice settings is formalized HIV testing and counseling. For instance, face-to-face HIV prevention counseling, held in conjunction with HIV testing at public health clinics, has demonstrated a reduction of high-risk sexual behaviors (e.g., due to increased use of condoms) and new STIs among clients (Kamb et al., 1998).

APPROACHES TO PROGRAM PLANNING

Program Development

PRECEDE-PROCEED

Among the various public health prevention program planning frameworks, perhaps the most commonly used and best known is PRECEDE-PROCEED. There are more than 900 documented applications of PRECEDE-PROCEED, which address multiple health issues and concerns in a number of public health settings (Blake, Green, & Rootman, 1999). The PRECEDE-PROCEED framework consists of two basic components, each comprising multiple phases. The first component, called PRECEDE, is made up of a series of planned assessments and data collection steps. PRECEDE is an acronym for *predisposing, reinforcing,* and *enabling constructs in ecosystem diagnosis and evaluation* (Figure 13.2). The second component, called PROCEED, is an acronym for *policy, regulating* (or *resourcing*), and

FIGURE 13.2   Schematic of the PRECEDE-PROCEED Framework

Precede

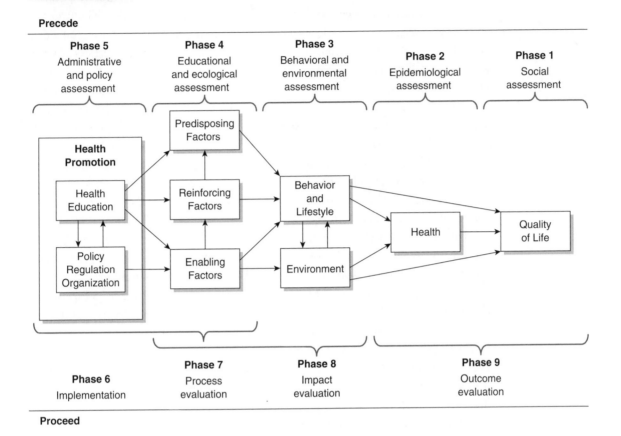

SOURCE: Green, L. W., and M. W. Kreuter. (2005). *Health Program Planning: An Educational and Ecological Approach.* (4th ed.). New York: McGraw-Hill. Reproduced by permission of McGraw-Hill.

organizing constructs for educational and environmental development and "is marked by the strategic implementation of multiple actions based on what was learned from the assessments in the initial phase" (Green & Kreuter, 2005, p. 9). Green and Kreuter (2005) identified two important assumptions about the PRECEDE-PROCEED framework. The first assumption is that the planning process to address health behavior and behavior change should be driven by more than simply knowledge, beliefs, and attitudes. That is, behavior and behavior change must be enabled (e.g., by eliminating barriers to or identifying the resources that can facilitate behavior change). Second, health behavior and behavior change usually must be sustained over long periods of time to achieve health benefits. In other words, behavior must be reinforced (e.g., rewarded) as well as enabled to be sustained.

There are five phases in the PRECEDE component (Figure 13.2). Program planners following this framework begin the planning process by considering the health outcomes, or desired ends, for a community or population of interest (i.e., the priority population); they then work backward to determine the factors influencing success in reaching those ends (Green & Kreuter, 2005).

Phase 1, a *social assessment and situational analysis,* entails an appraisal of both the real and the perceived needs of the priority population. In Phase 1, important social indicator data are collected on the priority population, from unemployment and crime statistics to data on absenteeism, alienation, achievement, and happiness. Data also should be collected regarding a community's quality of life, including the subjectively defined problems and priorities of the priority population. Finally, data should be collected regarding existing human resource assets that can help provide program support (Green & Kreuter, 2005). These assets include skills and other resources of residents; businesses, nonprofit organizations, and social services agencies; institutions of higher education; cultural and religious associations; and public institutions and schools. The identification of assets in a community is known as asset mapping (Kretzmann & McKnight, 1993) and is an essential step to prevent duplication of services and optimal investment of resources.

One of the hallmarks of the PRECEDE-PROCEED framework is that it is guided by a participatory process. It is in Phase 1 that community members play a key role in the planning process. At its core, a social assessment and situational analysis of the priority population entails an understanding, through "the eyes of the community residents themselves" (Green & Kreuter, 2005, p. 34), of what matters most, in their context, in terms of health and quality of life. Information on subjective health concerns and quality of life is collected in this phase, often through surveys, interviews, and focus groups. The products of Phase 1 are engaged community partners, prioritization of social problems important to the priority population, and an understanding of assets available in the community from which planners can draw to help address the social problems identified.

Phase 2, an *epidemiologic assessment,* involves the identification of health status indicators that contribute to the social problems identified in Phase 1. Health status indicators are identified by consulting vital statistics indicators and existing data sources, including the morbidity, mortality, disability, and fertility statistics of the priority population.

Phase 3 includes the identification of behavioral and environmental factors associated with the health issue identified in Phase 2. Behavioral indicators are those practices, both risk and protective behaviors, associated with the health problem. Environmental assessment examines genetic contributors, as well as elements of the social and built environment. Genetic indicators assess the association of genes with various illnesses and conditions (i.e., genes that predispose someone to a certain disease). Environmental indicators assess the modifiable factors that support health and quality of life and can include both the economic and the physical environment. Note that these indicators occur at multiple levels of influence (e.g., intrapersonal, organizational, and community). Up to this point in the planning process, Phases 1 and 2 are equivalent to conducting a community needs assessment (Witkin & Altschuld, 1995).

Once the health issue and associated behavioral and environmental factors have been prioritized and selected (Phases 1–3), an *educational and ecological assessment* is conducted that explores and prioritizes the predisposing, reinforcing, and enabling factors that influence the behavioral and environmental risk factors identified. Predisposing factors "include a person's or population's knowledge, attitudes, beliefs, values, and perceptions that facilitate or hinder motivation for change" (Green & Kreuter, 2005, p. 14). Reinforcing factors are the rewards received and feedback an individual gets from others following adoption of a behavior. Such feedback can promote or dissuade continuation of the behavior. Enabling factors are "skills, resources, or barriers that can help or hinder the desired behavioral changes as well as environmental changes" (Green & Kreuter, 2005, p. 15). The products of Phase 4 include improved understanding of the modifiable factors that have a direct impact on the social and health problems identified in the earlier phases. These factors represent the best variables for programmatic focus (Green & Kreuter, 2005), to be addressed in subsequent phases.

Once information is gathered and program priorities, determinants of change, and objectives for change have been identified (Phases 1–4), planners next determine the program strategies needed to influence the desired behavioral and environmental changes. In Phase 5, planners also identify the settings in which health promotion and disease prevention activities will take place—school, workplace, health care institution, community, and clinical general-practice settings. The products of Phase 5 are an intervention design, intervention objectives, and the accompanying program budget and timeline.

With the completion of PRECEDE's Phase 5, planners move on to PROCEED with program implementation and evaluation (Green & Kreuter, 2005). This second component in the PRECEDE-PROCEED framework comprises four additional phases (Figure 13.2). The first phase of PROCEED, Phase 6, entails an assessment of organizational readiness and capacity to carry out the program activities and, subsequently, implementation of the program. Phase 7, the second phase of PROCEED, involves *process evaluation*. Process evaluation, as noted previously, focuses on examining "the processes by which the actual interventions (as program components) and programs themselves take shape" (Green & Kreuter, 2005, p. 192). The third phase of PROCEED, Phase 8, entails an evaluation of *program impact,* or the immediate effects program activities have on participants' behaviors and their mediating factors (i.e., predisposing, enabling, and reinforcing antecedents to the desired behavior). The final phase of the PRECEDE-PROCEED framework, Phase 9, evaluates *program outcomes.* In this last step, longer-term program effects are assessed, such as the overall health status and quality of life of the priority population.

Intervention Mapping

Intervention mapping (IM) was developed as a planning framework, building on PRECEDE-PROCEED but also emphasizing the importance of planners' use of social and behavioral science theory and empirical data to develop health promotion and disease prevention programs (Bartholomew, Parcel, & Kok, 1998). IM comprises six cumulative steps (Bartholomew et al., 2006). IM's first step involves the planning and execution of a community needs assessment, which is similar to Phases 1 to 3 in PRECEDE-PROCEED. The second step entails the creation of a matrix of proximal program objectives—that is, what participants will learn from their involvement in the program and what environmental changes can be expected as a result of the program. Program objectives created in this second step should represent each level of influence (e.g., *intra*personal, *inter*personal) to be addressed by the program strategies. The third step in IM involves the selection of theory-based intervention methods and practical strategies. In this step—similar to other planning frameworks—program ideas should be reviewed with members of the priority population. Unique to IM, however, this step emphasizes the use of behavioral theory and existing empirical research to facilitate behavior change. Step 4, designing and organizing a program, consists of planning the scope and sequence of intervention components, considering what the program will "look like," and designing and pretesting program materials. In this step, planners should again involve members of the priority population to ensure that their opinions about, and preferences for, program design are taken into account. The fifth step involves the specification of adoption and implementation plans. Such specification includes, but is not limited to, a delineation of the exact roles and responsibilities of program personnel, such as who is in charge of program implementation or carrying out certain program activities. As with other planning frameworks, the sixth and final step in IM involves the generation of program evaluation plans.

IM has been applied in many countries to address a number of different public health issues. For instance, Tortolero and colleagues (2005) described how IM was used to adapt a theory-based, effective HIV, sexually transmitted disease, and pregnancy prevention program to a new priority population. Murray and colleagues (1998) used IM to develop a violence prevention intervention for Hispanic parents. Kraag and colleagues (2005) developed a stress management program for Dutch fifth and sixth graders using IM. Finally, Hoelscher and colleagues (2002) described how IM can be used to design effective nutrition education programs for adolescents.

Other Program Development Frameworks

Whereas the PRECEDE-PROCEED and IM frameworks lack the principle of *planning with people* as a *major* focus, Community-Based Prevention Marketing (CBPM) employs this principle as its initial step: *community mobilization.* CBPM is described as follows:

> A community directed social change process that applies marketing theories and techniques to the design, implementation, and evaluation of health promotion and disease prevention programs. CBPM integrates community capacity building principles and practices, behavioral theories, and marketing concepts and methodologies into a synergistic framework for directing positive change among selected audience segments. (Bryant et al., 1999, p. 54)

CBPM places the individual (or consumer) at the center of an exchange process involving four key concepts: (1) the *product* (the behavior being promoted and the benefits it offers adopters); (2) the *price* (social, emotional, and monetary costs exchanged for the product's benefits); (3) the *place* (where the target behavior is practiced); and (4) *promotion* (activities used to communicate about and promote the product). As a relatively new program planning framework, CBPM has been used to develop strategies to prevent smoking (Zapata et al., 2004) and drinking (Eaton et al., 2004) among middle school students, promote physical activity among "tweens" (Bryant et al., 2007), and prevent eye injuries among Florida's citrus workers (Luque et al., 2007).

CASE STUDY   An Application of Intervention Mapping

A worthy illustration of program development in action was the use of IM to adapt an existing, effective program to a different community and priority population (Tortolero et al., 2005). The existing program, Safer Choices (which was described briefly in the section Intervention Settings), was originally developed—based on elements from social learning theory, the theory of reasoned action, and the health belief model—to reduce adolescent sexual risk-taking behaviors. The program comprises a school curriculum, a parent component, a peer education module, community linkages and resources, and school organization components. Evaluations of Safer Choices have indicated reduction in the number of sexual partners and frequency of sexual intercourse without a condom and increase in the use of condoms and effective contraceptive methods at last intercourse (Coyle et al., 1999, 2001) among students attending regular high schools. However, the interest of program planners in this case was to adapt Safer Choices for use with higher-risk students attending alternative schools (i.e., youth who are at risk of dropping out of high school). Table 13.2 lists the IM steps employed to adapt Safer Choices to this new priority population.

The first step, a needs assessment of the students attending the targeted alternative schools, revealed that these students were more sexually active, less likely to use condoms, and more likely to use illicit drugs than students in regular high schools. Researchers learned through focus group discussions that many girls attending alternative schools had dated older men. The age gap presented a challenge for the younger girls to negotiate sexual relationships (including condom use). The needs assessment also revealed that alternative school students maintained negative attitudes underscoring "a level of disrespect and depersonalization associated with sexual relationships" (Tortolero et al., 2005, p. 291). For instance, students often used language to refer to sexual intercourse as "banging" and "smashing" and to members of the opposite sex as "whores" and "pimps." Finally, the needs assessment indicated that it was not uncommon for alternative-school girls to provide sexual relations in exchange for material goods (e.g., jewelry).

In IM, Step 1, Tasks 1 and 2, program planners adapted the behavioral outcomes and performance objectives for Safer Choices to the new priority population to reflect the findings of the needs assessment. For instance, one of the original expected outcomes of Safer Choices was reduction in the number of students who *began* having sexual intercourse during their high school years. Because most alternative school students were sexually active already, planners eliminated this as an outcome for the alternative school adaptation. Instead, program planners chose to focus their efforts on the second original expected outcome: increased use of condoms among students.

TABLE 13.2   Using Intervention Mapping Steps to Adapt a Program to a New Population

Step 0: Needs Assessment

What new cultural or other population issues are present?

What new environmental issues must be considered?

What is the community capacity for the new population?

Step 1, Task 1: Review Behavioral Outcomes

What behavioral outcomes need to be added for the new population?

Which behavioral outcomes need to be deleted as inappropriate?

Which behavioral outcomes need to be deleted or adapted as impractical?

Step 1, Task 2: Specify Performance Objectives

Which performance objectives should be deleted as irrelevant?

Given the new or revised behavioral outcomes:

   What performance objectives need to be added?

   What performance objectives need to be revised?

Step 1, Task 3: Specify Determinants

What determinants were used in devising the original program?

What is the supporting evidence for those determinants?

Does the evidence indicate the determinants are relevant to the new population?

Which determinants should be deleted or revised?

What determinants need to be added for the new population?

What determinants need to be added for the new performance objectives?

Step 1, Task 4: Develop Proximal Program Objectives

For each determinant of each performance objective:

   What are the learning objectives of the existing program?

Given the changes in determinants and performance objectives:

   What learning objectives should be deleted?

   What learning objectives should be revised?

   What learning objectives should be added?

Step 2, Part 1: Identifying Theoretical Foundation

What behavioral theory is associated with each determinant in the original program?

Which of these theories is relevant to the new population?

Which of these theories is appropriate for the new determinants?

What part of the theoretical foundation should be discarded?

What should be added to the theoretical foundation of the revised program?

Step 2, Part 2: Selecting Methods and Strategies

Are the methods and strategies of the original program effective for the new population?

Are they feasible given the new study design?

Are they practical given the new community context?

Given that methods and strategies are specific to learning objectives:

Which methods or strategies should be deleted?

Which methods and strategies should be revised?

Looking at the new learning objectives and the relevant theories:

Which methods can be expanded to cover new learning objectives?

What new intervention methods or strategies need to be added?

SOURCE: Reproduced by permission from *Health Promotion Practice*. Tortolero, S. R., Markham, C. M., Parcel, G. S., Peters, R. J., Jr., Escobar-Chaves, S. L., Basen-Engquist, K., et al. (2005). Using Intervention Mapping to Adapt an Effective HIV, Sexually Transmitted Disease, and Pregnancy Prevention Program for High-Risk Minority Youth. *Health Promotion Practice, 6*(3), 286–298.

The next step, IM, Step 1, Task 3, involved an analysis of the theoretical determinants for behavior and behavior change guiding the original Safer Choices program, as well as identification of any new determinants that may be particularly important for the new priority population. Three new determinants were identified based on the needs assessment results: (1) power in relationships, (2) gender role expectations, and (3) future orientation. The first two new determinants stemmed from the focus group discussions. The third was added because evidence in the sexual behavior literature supports the notion that improving students' educational investment and plans to attend college increases condom use.

In terms of selecting theory-based, practical methods and strategies for addressing these determinants of behavior (IM, Step 2), some existing strategies were retained; however, new strategies were also developed to reflect the new determinants added to the program. One new strategy, the use of a video, was designed to assist students in recognizing healthy and unhealthy relationships (in order to address gender role expectations and power in relationships). Theory-based strategies employed in the original Safer Choices program, such as role modeling sex refusal skills—a central construct of social learning theory—were retained in the revised Safer Choices program for alternative schools.

One of the last adaptations of the original Safer Choices program for the new priority population pertained to adoption and implementation (IM, Step 4). The original program was designed to be executed over a 2-year period among 9th and 10th graders. However, alternative schools have high student turnover, and alternative school students have high drop-out rates. Thus, program planners chose to adopt a more intensive Safer Choices program, implemented more frequently and over a shorter time period. Finally, because the alternative school students "seemed to have more mistrust of the educational system and authority figures such as teachers, trained facilitators with similar ethnic backgrounds to the [priority] population were used to deliver the program in a classroom setting" (Tortolero et al., 2005, p. 296).

Community Health Planning

Mobilizing for Action Through Planning and Partnerships

MAPP is a process developed in 2001 by the National Association of County and City Health Officials (NACCHO) and the CDC as a tool to assist "communities improve health and quality of life through community-wide and community-driven strategic planning" (National Association of County and City Health Officials, 2004, p. 3). The model portrayed in Figure 13.3 illustrates the MAPP process. In this model, the six essential MAPP phases are outlined in the center. The MAPP process begins with strong organizational, community, and partnership/stakeholder development. Once commitment from community partners has been solidified, a shared vision for pursuing common goals is identified.

Next, planners can use any one of the four or *all* four MAPP assessments. These assessments are illustrated in the four outer arrows of Figure 13.3. The *Community Themes and Strengths Assessment* helps planners understand issues the priority population feels are important. This assessment asks, "What is important to our community?" The *Local Public Health System Assessment,* on the other hand, evaluates the activities and capacities of the local public health system. The *Community Health Status Assessment* assists planners in identifying the overall health status of the priority population. This assessment is equivalent to

---

FIGURE 13.3   MAPP Framework Showing Assessment Processes

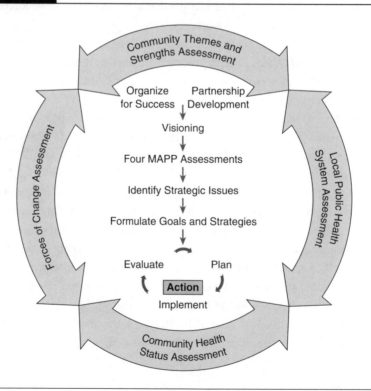

SOURCE: National Association of County and City Health Officials. (2004). *Mobilizing for Action Through Planning and Partnerships: Achieving Healthier Communities Through MAPP: A User's Handbook.* Washington, DC: Author.

Phase 2 of the PRECEDE-PROCEED framework. Last, the *Forces of Change Assessment* component identifies elements that can influence both the health and quality of life of the priority population and the work of the local public health system in carrying out its 10 essential public health services (National Association of County and City Health Officials, 2004).

The next phase involves an examination of the four assessments "to determine the most critical issues that must be addressed for the community to achieve its vision" (National Association of County and City Health Officials, 2004, p. 7). After strategic health issues have been identified, planners formulate goals and strategies to address each issue. Finally, they plan, implement, and evaluate the selected strategies and activities. A step-by-step MAPP handbook and field guide can be retrieved from the NACCHO Web site, www .naccho.org/MAPP/.

Other Community Health Planning Frameworks

MAPP is an important and useful community health planning model; however, it is not the only one. The PATCH was developed in the 1980s as another community health planning model, allowing for community variation in the process of assessing needs, setting priorities, formulating solutions, and owning programs (CDC, 1995). Developed by the CDC in collaboration with local health departments and community groups, PATCH has been used in many communities, states, and nations to address public health issues, including physical activity, CVD, tobacco use, HIV, breast cancer, unintentional injuries, child abuse, teenage pregnancy, and access to health care (CDC, 1995; Freudenberg, 2000; Valdiserri, Aultman, & Curran, 1995). PATCH is discussed in greater detail in Chapter 14.

Another community planning framework, developed in the 1990s through a partnership involving the CDC, NACCHO, the American Public Health Association, and several other organizations, is the APEX*PH* (National Association of County and City Health Officials, 2008). Like PATCH, APEX*PH* leverages community groups to prioritize health problems. The APEX*PH* framework focuses attention on the organizational and service delivery capacity of the local public health department.

CASE STUDY   An Application of Mobilizing Actions Through Planning and Partnerships (MAPP)

A useful illustration of community health planning in action is the use of MAPP by the Chicago Department of Public Health (CDPH) to support organized community-based public health improvement planning through the Turning Point initiative (Salem, Hooberman, & Ramirez, 2005). The purpose of the Turning Point initiative, coordinated by the W. K. Kellogg and Robert Wood Johnson foundations, was to make public health systems "more effective, more community-based, and more collaborative in protecting and improving the public's health and well-being" (Nicola, Berkowitz, & Lafronza, 2002, p. iv):

> The goals of CDPH's efforts were to use MAPP to (a) increase the capacity of Chicago communities to participate in public health decision making; (b) promote new partnerships, both within

individual communities and across the city; (c) provide communities with an organized voice and access to decision makers; and (d) determine an appropriate role for the public health department in supporting community-based health improvement activities. (Salem et al., 2005, p. 394)

Based on needs, available resources, history of collaboration, and other factors, five Chicago communities were selected as CDPH partners to achieve these goals. Beginning with community coalition development, the planning process followed the steps prescribed by MAPP (see Table 13.3).

TABLE 13.3 Overview of the Chicago Department of Public Health Community-Based Public Health Improvement Planning Process, Using the MAPP Model

Process Phase	How It Was Done	Who Participated
Vision development	At facilitated meeting, five questions posed about the communities' strengths and future	Full coalitions and subcommittees
Community perceptions	28 focus groups convened to discuss community assets and challenges	252 participants included youth, adults, seniors, and immigrant populations
Health status assessment	Gathered and organized data on indicators recommended by coalition members in six categories	Full coalitions and subcommittees
Forces and trends assessment	At 1–2 meetings, matrix used to identify current influences on community health system and related threats and opportunities	Coalitions
Community health system assessment	Quantitative data on local system considered; asset mapping	Coalition members Community residents
Strategic issue identification	Based on review of vision and assessment findings, key issues that could be addressed at community level were selected	Full coalitions
Strategy development	Small groups organized around strategic issues to brainstorm strategies; consolidation by coalitions as a whole	Coalition subgroups Full coalitions
Action planning, implementation, evaluation	Action area workgroups established to develop plans, lead implementation, and monitor it	Coalition subgroups

SOURCE: Reproduced by permission from the *Journal of Public Health Management and Practice*. Salem, E., Hooberman, J., and Ramirez, D. (2005). MAPP in Chicago: A Model for Public Health Systems Development and Community Building. *Journal of Public Health Management and Practice, 11*(5), 393–400, Table 2.

Outcomes achieved from this community health planning process included increased community participation in crime reduction efforts, reduced barriers to health care access, and newly forged partnerships, resulting in less duplication of services and a pooling of community resources and thus strengthening the quality of health services and programming. Another important outcome attained was increased access to healthy foods for community members. Stemming from community assessment results, as guided by the MAPP model, coalition members from one of the five Chicago communities discovered that less than one third of their area's 26 grocery and convenience stores sold fresh produce. Subsequently, the community coalition worked to increase the availability of healthy foods in these stores. The first efforts focused on three area grocery stores that did not carry produce at all. To stimulate a supply-and-demand effect, the community coalition supplied these stores with crates of a "Food of the Month," with financial assistance from the local chamber of commerce. The proportion of neighborhood stores selling fresh produce subsequently increased, from 32% to 58% (Salem et al., 2005). Additionally, three area grocery stores agreed to host monthly samplings of the community coalition's food of the month and monitor sales of these foods. Evaluation revealed that between 2003 and 2004, sales of jars of nopales (cactus), cases of cucumbers, and cases of kiwi fruit increased by 40%, 31%, and 41%, respectively (Salem et al., 2005). Finally, the community coalition was instrumental in developing a community garden that not only increases access to fresh produce for community members but also may help improve the beautification of urban areas and bolster feelings of community, thereby increasing social capital.

Summary of Intervention Frameworks

Frameworks and models such as PRECEDE-PROCEED, IM, CBPM, MAPP, PATCH, and APEX*PH* are step-by-step guides that can be used to assist public health professionals in developing multilevel prevention interventions that engage the community in the planning initiatives. Although each of these frameworks describes a different approach to program development and community health planning, they share important principles such as community input, data-driven decision making, and evaluation, which is discussed next in greater detail.

PROGRAM EVALUATION

Evaluation has been defined as "the process of determining the merit, worth, and value of things, and evaluations are the products of that process" (Scriven, 1991, p. 1). However, the following is a more encompassing definition of program evaluation:

> A collection of methods, skills, and sensitivities necessary to determine whether a human service is needed and likely to be used, whether the service is sufficiently intensive to meet the unmet needs identified, whether the service is offered as planned, and whether the service actually does help people in need at a reasonable cost without unacceptable side effects. (Posavac & Carey, 2007, p. 2)

As stated earlier, evaluation can provide valuable information for planning, implementing, and sustaining effective and efficient public health interventions. Whereas this discussion of evaluation comes at the end of this chapter on program and community health planning, it should be noted that evaluation should never be an afterthought or left until the end of the program (e.g., "We have developed and implemented the program, and now we need to figure out if it works"). Instead, planners should incorporate the four types of evaluation—(1) evaluation of a need, (2) evaluation of a process, (3) evaluation of outcomes, and (4) evaluation of efficiency (Posavac & Carey, 2007)—throughout the program planning process.

The first type of evaluation, evaluation of a need, is often referred to as a needs assessment. Keeping in mind the definition above, the aim of this evaluation type is to determine not only whether a health and human service is needed but also whether such a service is likely to be used by members of the priority population. In evaluating needs, planners determine who needs a potential program, how great the need is, and what might work to meet the need.

The second type of evaluation, evaluation of a process, examines whether the health and human service offered is sufficiently intensive to meet the unmet needs identified and whether the service is being offered as it was planned/intended (i.e., program fidelity). In evaluating program processes, planners collect important data focusing on the activities, services, materials, staffing, and administrative arrangements that make up a program and how they operate (Posavac & Carey, 2007). Data collection may also include assessments of the barriers encountered during program implementation and the extent to which the priority population has been reached, as well as the numbers of staff/volunteers trained, people participating in program activities, and program sessions held.

The third type of evaluation, evaluation of outcomes, is likely to be the type with which people are most familiar. In evaluating program outcomes, planners investigate whether the program produced demonstrable effects on specifically defined target outcomes and assess the overall or net effects of the program as a whole (Trochim, 2006). Outcome evaluations collect data to examine the immediate effects of programs on participants' knowledge, attitudes, awareness, and behaviors, and the long-term effects, such as impacts on participants' maintenance of positive behaviors and/or behavior change, morbidity and mortality rates, and the overall quality of life of the priority population. Outcome evaluations focus on answering the question "Does the program work?" However, answering this question is only part of assessing outcomes. Sometimes, programs have *unintended* effects, similar to the side effects of a medication, which are as (if not more) important to uncover as the *intended* program effects. The unintended effects of health promotion and disease prevention programs are not often studied. However, a documented example of an unintended effect has been provided by Smith (2006):

> In the Philippines, an HIV/AIDS program designed to debunk the myth that mosquitoes carry HIV had the unintended consequence of reducing empathy for HIV+ individuals. The public reasoning was that one cannot be blamed for mosquito behavior, but people can be blamed for their own sexual activity. (p. i39)

Unintended effects may hamper public health efforts to combat the spread of HIV and provide health and social services to individuals affected by HIV and AIDS.

The fourth and final type of evaluation, evaluation of efficiency, is also called a cost-effectiveness analysis. This type of evaluation examines how similar outcomes can be achieved by programs with different levels of resources. In the case study example of the Safer Choices program adaptation provided earlier, the original version of the program was designed to be implemented over a period of 2 years, whereas the adapted version was designed to be implemented over an 8- to 10-week period. If the latter version of Safer Choices yields better (or at least comparable) effects, in terms of condom use by high school students, then the latter version may be more cost-effective (cost is equal to time in this case) to implement.

CONCLUSION

This chapter reemphasized the importance of focusing health promotion and disease prevention programs ecologically, at multiple levels; provided a general overview of frameworks for planning, implementing, and evaluating public health programs; and illustrated the various settings in which prevention interventions can be implemented. Unfortunately, there is much more to planning, implementing, and evaluating prevention programs than what can be offered in this chapter. Numerous books and resources are available (Anspaugh, Dignan, & Anspaugh, 2006; Bartholomew et al., 2006; Green & Kreuter, 2005; Grembowski, 2001; McKenzie et al., 2005; Posavac & Carey, 2007; Valente, 2002), in addition to university-level courses that are devoted completely to addressing these important topics. However, the necessary foundations readers can use as a starting point for planning health promotion and disease prevention programs and for understanding their underlying social and behavioral science foundations have been provided.

Through advances in prevention science, developing, implementing, and evaluating public health programs for sustainability should no longer be a "shot in the dark." Practical frameworks to guide the delivery of evidence-based interventions exist that are grounded in sound theory and that scientists and public health practitioners working together have had opportunity to test and refine. Continued experience in developing and disseminating effective programs in multiple settings is expected to help combat the public health disparities that exist in the United States and around the world.

REFERENCES

American Diabetes Association. (2002). Clinical practice recommendations. *Diabetes Care, 25*(Suppl. 1), S1–S147.

Anspaugh, D. J., Dignan, M. B., & Anspaugh, S. L. (2006). *Developing health promotion programs* (2nd ed.). Long Grove, IL: Waveland Press.

Bartholomew, L. K., Parcel, G. S., & Kok, G. (1998). Intervention mapping: A process for developing theory- and evidence-based health education programs. *Health Education and Behavior, 25,* 545–563.

Bartholomew, L. K., Parcel, G. S., Kok, G., & Gottlieb, N. H. (2006). *Planning health promotion programs: An intervention mapping approach* (2nd ed.). San Francisco: Jossey-Bass.

Bertera, R. L. (1990). The effects of workplace health promotion on absenteeism and employment costs in a large industrial population. *American Journal of Public Health, 80*(9), 1101–1105.

Blake, D. P., Green, L. W., & Rootman, I. (Eds.). (1999). *Settings for health promotion: Linking theory and practice.* Thousand Oaks, CA: Sage.

Breckon, D., Harvey, J., & Lancaster, B. (1998). *Community health education: Setting, roles, and skills for the 21st century* (4th ed.). Gaithersburg, MD: Aspen.

Bryant, C. A., Courtney, A. H., Baldwin, J. A., McDermott, R. J., Nickelson, J., & McCormack Brown, K. R. (2007). The VERB™ Summer Scorecard. In G. Hastings (Ed.), *Social marketing: Why should the devil have all the best tunes?* (pp. 272–277). Oxford, UK: Elsevier.

Bryant, C. A., Forthofer, M. S., McCormack Brown, K., & McDermott, R. J. (1999). Community-based prevention marketing. *Social Marketing Quarterly, 5*(3), 54–59.

Bryant, C. A., McCormack Brown, K. R., McDermott, R. J., Forthofer, M. S., Bumpus, E. C., Calkins, S. A., et al. (2007). Community-based prevention marketing: Organizing a community for health behavior intervention. *Health Promotion Practice, 8*(2), 154–163.

Centers for Disease Control and Prevention. (1995). *Planned approach to community health: Guide for the local coordinator.* Atlanta, GA: U.S. Department of Health and Human Services, Public Health Service, Centers for Disease Control and Prevention, National Center for Chronic Disease Prevention and Health Promotion.

Centers for Disease Control and Prevention. (2002). Guidelines for preventing opportunistic infections among HIV-infected persons: 2002. *Morbidity and Mortality Weekly Report, 51*(RR08), 1–46.

Centers for Disease Control and Prevention. (2007a). *National Health and Nutrition Examination Survey.* Retrieved May 1, 2008, from www.cdc.gov/nchs/nhanes.htm

Centers for Disease Control and Prevention. (2007b). *A guide to developing a TB program evaluation plan, Appendix B: Writing SMART objectives.* Retrieved May 1, 2008, from www.cdc.gov/TB/Program_Evaluation/Guide/AppB_Writing_Smart_Objectives.htm

Coyle, K., Basen-Engquist, K., Kirby, D., Parcel, G., Banspach, S., Collins, J., et al. (2001). Safer Choices: Reducing teen pregnancy, HIV, and STDs. *Public Health Reports, 116*(Suppl. 1), 82–93.

Coyle, K., Basen-Engquist, K., Kirby, D., Parcel, G., Banspach, S., Harrist, R., et al. (1999). Short-term impact of Safer Choices: A multicomponent, school-based HIV, other STD, and pregnancy prevention program. *Journal of School Health, 69,* 181–188.

DeBate, R., Plescia, M., Joyner, D., & Spann, L. (2004). A qualitative assessment of Charlotte REACH: An ecological perspective for decreasing CVD and diabetes among African Americans. *Ethnicity and Disease, 14*(3, Suppl. 1), S77–S82.

Dewey, J. D. (1999). Reviewing the relationship between school factors and substance use for elementary, middle, and high school students. *Journal of Primary Prevention, 19*(3), 177–225.

Dunkle, M. C., & Nash, M. A. (1991). *Beyond the health room.* Washington, DC: Council of Chief State School Officers, Resource Center on Educational Equity.

Eaton, D. K., Forthofer, M. S., Zapata, L. B., McCormack Brown, K. R., Bryant, C. A., Reynolds, S. T., et al. (2004). Factors related to alcohol use among 6th through 10th graders: The Sarasota County demonstration project. *Journal of School Health, 74*(3), 95–104.

Ellickson, P. L., Tucker, J. S., & Klein, D. J. (2003). Ten-year prospective study of public health problems associated with early drinking. *Pediatrics, 111*(5, Pt. 1), 949–955.

INTERVENTION, METHODS, AND PRACTICE

Erwin, D. O., Spatz, T. S., Stotts, R. C., Hollenberg, J. A., & Deloney, L. A. (1996). Increasing mammography and breast self-examination in African American women using the Witness Project™ model. *Journal of Cancer Education, 11*(4), 210–215.

Freudenberg, N. (2000). Health promotion in the city: A review of current practice and future prospects in the United States. *Annual Review of Public Health, 21,* 473–503.

Green, L. W., & Kreuter, M. W. (2005). *Health program planning: An educational and ecological approach* (4th ed.). New York: McGraw-Hill.

Grembowski, D. (2001). *The practice of health program evaluation.* Thousand Oaks, CA: Sage.

Higgins-Biddle, J. C., & Babor, T. F. (1996). Reducing risky drinking via screening and brief intervention. *Alcohol and Drug Abuse Weekly, 8,* 5.

Hoelscher, D. M., Evans, A., Parcel, G. S., & Kelder, S. H. (2002). Designing effective nutrition interventions for adolescents. *Journal of the American Dietetic Association, 102* (3, Suppl. 1), S52–S63.

Israel, B. A. (1985). Social networks and social support: Implications for natural helper and community level interventions. *Health Education Quarterly, 12,* 65–80.

Kamb, M. L., Fishbein, M., Douglas, J. M., Rhodes, F., Rogers, J., Bolan, G., et al. (1998). Efficacy of risk-reduction counseling to prevent human immunodeficiency virus and sexually transmitted diseases: A randomized controlled trial. *Journal of the American Medical Association, 280*(13), 1161–1167.

Kirby, D. B., Baumler, E., Coyle, K. K., Basen-Engquist, K., Parcel, G. S., Harrist, R., et al. (2004). The "Safer Choices" intervention: Its impact on the sexual behaviors of different subgroups of high school students. *Journal of Adolescent Health, 35*(6), 442–452.

Kraag, G., Kok, G., Huijer Abu-Saad, H., Lamberts, P., & Fekkes, M. (2005). Development of a stress management programme—Learn Young, Learn Fair—for fifth and sixth formers in the Netherlands using intervention mapping. *International Journal of Mental Health Promotion, 7*(3), 37–44.

Kretzmann, J. P., & McKnight, J. L. (1993). *Building communities from the inside out: A path toward finding and mobilizing a community's assets.* Chicago: Northwestern University, Center for Urban Affairs and Policy Research, Neighborhood Innovations Network.

Kreuter, M. W. (1992). PATCH: Its origin, basic concepts, and links to contemporary public health policy. *Journal of Health Education, 23*(3), 135–139.

Luque, J. S., Monaghan, P., Contreras, R. B., August, E., Baldwin, J. A., Bryant, C. A., et al. (2007). Implementation evaluation of a culturally competent eye injury prevention program for citrus workers in a Florida migrant community. *Progress in Community Health Partnerships, 1*(4), 359–369.

Mandell, D. J., Hill, S. L., Carter, L., & Brandon, R. N. (2002). *The impact of substance use and violence/delinquency on academic achievement for groups of middle and high school students in Washington.* Seattle, WA: University of Washington, Evans School of Public Affairs, Human Services Policy Center, Washington Kids Count.

Marx, E., Wooley, S. F., & Northrop, D. (Eds.). (1998). *Health is academic: A guide to coordinated school health programs.* New York: Teachers College Press.

McKenzie, J. F., Neiger, B. L., & Smeltzer, J. L. (2005). *Planning, implementing, and evaluating health promotion programs: A primer* (4th ed.). San Francisco: Benjamin Cummings.

Murray, N. G., Kelder, S. H., Parcel, G. S., & Orpinas, P. (1998). Development of an intervention map for a parent education intervention to prevent violence among Hispanic middle school children. *Journal of School Health, 68*(2), 46–52.

National Association of County and City Health Officials. (2004). *Mobilizing for Action Through Planning and Partnerships: Achieving healthier communities through MAPP: A user's handbook.* Washington, DC: Author. Retrieved February 10, 2008, from www.naccho.org/pubs/documents/na64_ mapphandbook.pdf

National Association of County and City Health Officials. (2008). APEX*PH.* Washington, DC: Author. Retrieved March 18, 2008, from www.naccho.org/topics/infrastructure/APEXPH.cfm

National Cancer Institute. (2005). *Theory at a glance: A guide for health promotion practice.* Retrieved February 20, 2008, from www.nci.nih.gov/theory/pdf

Nicola, R. M., Berkowitz, B., & Lafronza, V. (2002). A turning point for public health. *Journal of Public Health Management and Practice, 8*(1), iv–vii.

O'Donnell, M. P. (2001). *Health promotion in the workplace* (3rd ed.). Albany, NY: Thomson Delmar Learning.

Partnership for Prevention. (2001). *Healthy workforce 2010: An essential health promotion sourcebook for employers, large and small.* Washington, DC: Author.

Posavac, E. J., & Carey, R. G. (2007). *Program evaluation: Methods and case studies* (7th ed.). Upper Saddle River, NJ: Pearson Education.

Salem, E., Hooberman, J., & Ramirez, D. (2005). MAPP in Chicago: A model for public health systems development and community building. *Journal of Public Health Management and Practice, 11*(5), 393–400.

Scriven, M. (1991). *Evaluation thesaurus* (4th ed.). Newbury Park, CA: Sage.

Shephard, R. J. (1996). Habitual physical activity and academic performance. *Nutrition Reviews, 54*(4, Pt. 2), S32–S36.

Shults, R. A., Elder, R. W., Sleet, D. A., Nichols, J. L., Alao, M. O., Carande-Kulis, V. G., et al. (2001). Reviews of evidence regarding interventions to reduce alcohol-impaired driving. *American Journal of Preventive Medicine, 21*(4, Suppl.), 66–88.

Smith, R. A., Cokkinides, V., & Eyre, H. J. (2003). American Cancer Society guidelines for the early detection of cancer, 2003. *CA: A Cancer Journal for Clinicians, 53,* 27–43.

Smith, W. A. (2006). Social marketing: An overview of approach and effects. *Injury Prevention, 12*(Suppl. 1), i38–i43.

Stephens, C. (2007). Community as practice: Social representations of community and their implications for health promotion. *Journal of Community and Applied Social Psychology, 17*(2), 103–114.

Strycker, L. A., Foster, L. S., Pettigrew, L., Donnelly-Perry, J., Jordan, S., & Glasgow, R. E. (1997). Steering committee enhancements on health promotion program delivery. *American Journal of Health Promotion, 11*(6), 437–440.

Swingle, C. A. (1997). *The relationship between the health of school-age children and learning: Implications for schools.* Lansing, MI: Michigan Department of Community Health.

Task Force on Community Preventive Services. (2001). Motor-vehicle occupant injury: Strategies for increasing use of child safety seats, increasing use of safety belts, and reducing alcohol-impaired driving. *Morbidity and Mortality Weekly Report, 50*(RR07), 1–13.

Tortolero, S. R., Markham, C. M., Parcel, G. S., Peters, R. J., Jr., Escobar-Chaves, S. L., Basen-Engquist, K., et al. (2005). Using intervention mapping to adapt an effective HIV, sexually transmitted disease, and pregnancy prevention program for high-risk minority youth. *Health Promotion Practice, 6*(3), 286–298.

Trochim, W. M. K. (2006). *Introduction to evaluation.* Retrieved April 18, 2008, from www.social researchmethods.net/kb/intreval.htm

U.S. Bureau of Labor Statistics. (2007). *American Time Use Survey: Charts by topic: Work and employment.* Retrieved March 5, 2008, from www.bls.gov/tus/charts/work.htm

Valdiserri, R. O., Aultman, T. V., & Curran, J. W. (1995). Community planning: A national strategy to improve HIV prevention programs. *Journal of Community Health, 20*(2), 87–100.

Valente, T. W. (2002). *Evaluating health promotion programs.* New York: Oxford University Press.

Valois, R. F., MacDonald, J. M., Bretous, L., Fischer, M. A., & Drane, J. W. (2002). Risk factors and behaviors associated with adolescent violence and aggression. *American Journal of Health Behavior, 26*(6), 454–464.

Witkin, B. R., & Altschuld, J. W. (1995). *Planning and conducting needs assessments: A practical guide.* Thousand Oaks, CA: Sage.

Zapata, L. B., Forthofer, M. S., Eaton, L. K., McCormack Brown, K., Bryant, C. A., Reynolds, S. T., et al. (2004). Cigarette use in 6th-10th grade youth: The Sarasota County demonstration project. *American Journal of Health Behavior, 28*(2), 151–165.

14

Community-Based
Approaches to Health Promotion

Carol A. Bryant

With the increasing popularity of the social ecological perspective, many public health professionals have turned their attention to community-level factors that influence disease and joined hands with community partners to bring about population-level changes. This chapter examines how an imaginary Director of Health Promotion would proceed if she decided to adopt a community-based approach to solve public health problems. This chapter begins with an examination of the concept of community and includes the key features and the various types of community-based frameworks. The final section discusses the benefits and challenges associated with community-based approaches to health promotion and disease prevention.

COMMUNITY

Community has been defined in numerous ways depending on the theorist's discipline and practitioner's purpose (Patrick & Wickizer, 1995); however, most definitions fall into two primary categories: community as *place* (e.g., a neighborhood) and community as *identity* (e.g., the gay community) (Campbell & Murray, 2004). Early theoretical discussions of community focused heavily on community as locality, and many public health scholars (e.g., Baker & Goodman, 2003, p. 178) still define community as "a collection of individuals who live within a geographic area that can be specified." These definitions of community work well for public health agencies because their political mandate and service boundaries typically correspond with geographically defined boundaries, that is, a state, a county, a city, or a reservation. However, most theorists would argue that not all neighborhoods, cities, or other geographic units represent communities; rather, they must share some sense of belonging or common interests to be considered a community.

Locality-based definitions of community have fallen into question as societal trends toward greater geographic mobility and increased reliance on technology for communication have weakened the ties between people living in proximity. In fact, in many neighborhoods, social ties are too weak to provide residents the support and interdependency needed to function as a community, and many people seek social support from other groups, including those they find or form on the Internet. As a result, many definitions of community now focus on social interaction and shared identity. These definitions emphasize the social ties or networks that arise from interaction among people and the goals, values, and symbols they come to share. For instance, we can talk about virtual communities of breast cancer survivors or occupational communities, such as citrus pickers, who share common goals, concerns, norms, and the use of symbols as they interact with each other.

In this chapter, we look at interventions designed in communities defined as place and shared identity; but in each circumstance, the elements required for a group to be considered a community include a shared sense of belonging; shared values and symbols; and shared constraints or conditions, such as limited access to power (Campbell & Jovchelovitch, 2000). Underlying our definition of community is the premise that a shared identity and sense of belonging develop when people come together to share problems, and the resulting social ties protect health and prevent disease. Like Christine Stephens (2007), we believe that a community is socially constructed and can serve as "a location for support and succour, a representation of need for assistance from outside, a site for competition for resources, a forum for action, a place of identity, or as a site for the integration of identified groups" (p. 106).

KEY FEATURES OF COMMUNITY-BASED INTERVENTIONS

Community-based interventions are guided by a philosophy that is characterized by three major principles: the social ecological framework, respect for community values and needs, and community participation and control (Brownson, Baker, & Novick, 1999). The multilevel social ecological framework is the central organizing structure for community-based public health and guiding principle for all community-based interventions (Baker & Goodman, 2003). Because individual, interpersonal, community, organizational, and societal factors are believed to affect individual health status, community-based programs attempt to address multiple factors, either simultaneously or sequentially (Brownson et al., 1999). For example, a community-based approach to breast-feeding promotion might address individual factors by offering classes or individual counseling to increase knowledge and build skills. At the same time, peer counselors or lay health advisors might be trained to act as local advisors and referral sources as a way to build social ties. Community members might advocate for changes in hospital policies to make lactation management and support more readily available and encourage employers to allow mothers to pump their breasts or breastfeed during their breaks.

Finally, a community coalition might lobby for changes in federal policies to guarantee women the right to breastfeed in public settings or require employers to make special provisions for mothers while they are nursing their infants.

Second, community-based interventions are designed to meet the perceived needs and wants of community members. The notion of "starting where the people are" (i.e., the issues they consider important) is a fundamental principle of health promotion dating back to the Ottawa Charter for Health Promotion (World Health Organization, Health and Welfare Canada, & Canadian Public Health Association, 1986). This principle is realized by listening to what community members want and respecting their rights to select the problems they would like to address. For this reason, community-based interventions typically begin with an assessment of local needs and assets and the development of ties with community leaders who understand the community's strengths and problems. However, if a group's "sense of community" (their shared identity and ability to work together) is poorly developed, then work must first begin toward the development of trust, mutual support, and leadership needed to work together to understand and solve common problems (Brownson et al., 1999). In working with citrus pickers in Immokalee, Florida, an agricultural community that had received little previous attention, the Florida Prevention Research Center devoted the first year of their project to mobilizing a board of community members made up of pickers, citrus industry representatives, migrant worker advocates, social service personnel, and other stakeholders. Only after the group had formed and developed guidelines for working together could research be done to assess the community's needs, assets, and preferences and the results then used to select project goals.

The third, and most distinctive, characteristic of community-based interventions is community participation. Community participation is the process by which individuals and families take an active part in discussions and activities to improve community life, services, or resources (Bracht & Tsouros, 1990). In contrast to public health interventions planned and implemented by public health professionals *for* communities where they neither work nor live, community-based approaches place public health professionals in a collaborative partnership *with* community members. These community members may include community professionals, lay leaders, activists, representatives of local businesses, members of the religious community, volunteers, and other citizens. This partnership brings together people who share common goals, resources, and problems (McWilliam, Desai, & Greig, 1997). Working together, partners define and critically analyze community problems, set goals, and design, implement, and evaluate interventions aimed at achieving these goals.

Whereas all community-based approaches involve community members in some activities, they differ in the degree to which community members actually control and direct the process. At one end of the continuum are programs in which public health professionals work in communities using a predetermined or structured planning framework. Although community input or feedback is valued, the professionals control key decisions and direct program activities. More common are programs that fall in the middle of the continuum: Professionals use a process flexible enough to allow community members to participate in all phases of the process and share decision making as equal partners. In programs that fall at the other end of the continuum, community members are given control of the change process, and outside experts provide technical assistance and training. When community members have the power to select the problems they want to address and direct efforts to achieve their goals, the process is referred to as *community organization* (Minkler & Wallerstein, 1998).

Community organizers believe that it is essential for the community to set the agenda, determine the goals, and assume control and ownership of the intervention strategies used to achieve the group's goals. Control of the direction of the change process empowers the community and increases the likelihood that local institutions will adopt and sustain these activities after outside funding ceases.

Other principles that guide community-based approaches to health promotion (Baker & Goodman, 2003; Bond & Hauf, 2007; Bracht & Kingsbury, 1990) are as follows:

- Planning is based on a historical understanding of the community.
- Prevention initiatives are based on sound theory and research.
- Program strategies build on community strengths or assets.
- Work is conducted using existing community organizations and members as a means to strengthen their capacity and promote social justice.
- All participants are respectful and act in ways to build trust.
- Coalitions or similar bodies are formed so that the intersectoral components of the community can work together to address the problem in a comprehensive manner (Butterfoss & Kegler, 2002).

When carrying out community-based interventions, especially those that give community members control of the process, it is important to assess their capacity or readiness to undertake the project. Whereas some communities have the assets or resources needed to initiate and carry out health promotion projects independently, many need technical and financial assistance from public health specialists outside the community. Assessing a community's capacity or readiness to work together provides valuable insights into the resources needed to mobilize its members and enables the selection of the best framework for planning and implementing community-based interventions.

Community Assessment and Community-Based Participatory Research

As we saw in the previous chapter, most community-based approaches include a community assessment phase. *Community-based participatory research* (CBPR) describes the active involvement of community members in community assessment and other research activities. In many community organization projects, community members work with researchers to define the research problem and set research objectives, design the methodology and data collection instruments, collect and interpret data, and use the results to guide program planning and evaluation (Schulz et al., 1999). Through their involvement in creating new knowledge and using information to address underlying social and political inequities, community members acquire valuable skills. Participatory research also empowers and democratizes program planning and evaluation by putting community members in control of the types of questions that are asked and issues that are investigated (Coombe, 1998).

Barbara Israel and her associates (Israel et al., 2003; Israel, Schulz, Parker, & Becker, 1998) have developed key principles for conducting CBPR, which are summarized in Table 14.1.

TABLE 14.1   Principles for Conducting Community-Based or Participatory Research

Key Factors	Description
Focus on the community	The concept of community as a unit of social identity is central to community-based research. Community-based research attempts to identify and work with communities and strengthen social relationships through collective engagement.
Community assets	Community-based research attempts to identify and build on community assets—skills, resources, and social relationships—as a way to address communal health concerns.
Equal participation	Community members are equal partners in all phases of the research process. Individuals from outside the community who can assist the community in improving the health and well-being of its members may also participate in research activities.
Beneficial knowledge	Community-based research generates knowledge that is mutually beneficial to all partners by informing the social change process and contributing to a broad understanding of the factors related to health and well-being.
Empowerment	Community-based research encourages colearning and empowerment. Community members acquire new skills, while academic researchers learn from community members' knowledge, experience, and unique perspectives of local problems. By acknowledging the inequalities between researchers and community members and by enabling power sharing, research helps empower the community.
Cyclical and iterative research	Community-based research is cyclical and iterative. Steps include "partnership development and maintenance, community assessment, problem definition, development of research methodology, data collection and analysis, interpretation of data, determination of action and policy implications, dissemination of results, action taking (as appropriate), specification of learnings, and establishment of mechanisms for sustainability" (Israel et al., 1998, p. 180). Ideally, as one problem is resolved, research identifies other issues requiring attention, and the process begins again.
Ecological perspective	Community-based research uses an ecological model of health and addresses the concept of health from a positive model, emphasizing physical, mental, and social well-being.
Broad dissemination	All partners have access to research findings. Results are disseminated to community members and other partners in a format and language that is easy to understand and use. Community participants all have a voice as to how the results are published, and their contributions/ownership of the information is acknowledged.

SOURCE: From Israel et al. (1998, 2003).

TYPES OF COMMUNITY-BASED APPROACHES

There is no widely accepted taxonomy of community-based intervention models; however, a popular typology (Rothman, 1970; Rothman & Tropman, 1987) categorizes these approaches into three models of practice, compared in Table 14.2: locality development, social planning, and social action.

Locality or community development emphasizes community participation and consensus building, with the goal of increasing community competence. Community development is heavily process oriented, drawing on a broad cross-section of people to determine and solve their own problems. A major goal of these projects is to enhance community capacity and empower community members and organizations to change the social and political environment (Minkler & Wallerstein, 1998). Professionals who live outside the community may help citizens learn new skills or provide important resources needed to implement change strategies; however, community members are actively involved in prioritizing health problems in their communities, selecting the health condition(s) to be addressed, and designing interventions to achieve the goals they have set. Community members also have the primary responsibility for program implementation, including community education and grassroots organizing.

During this process, indigenous leaders are developed who can stimulate critical problem-solving activities and direct sustainable change activities (Minkler & Wallerstein, 1998). As community members work together to solve their problems, they gain a stronger sense of collective efficacy and learn how to engage in effective problem solving. Participation increases community members' sense of mastery and their realization that they can improve their lives and those of others. Through participation and increased competence, citizen groups gain more power over resources—social and tangible assets—and learn to use their collective skills and power to obtain a more equitable share of resources (Israel, Checkoway, Schulz, & Zimmerman, 1994).

TABLE 14.2   Comparison of Community-Based Planning Models

Locality Development	Social Action	Social Planning
Process oriented.	Mix of process and task orientations.	Task oriented.
Community leads effort.	Outside experts help organize grassroots organizations to lead the effort.	Outside professionals lead effort.
Outcomes focused on enhanced collective efficacy and community empowerment.	Outcomes focused on enhanced power or equity and problem-solving skills.	Outcomes focused on solving problems.

SOURCE: From Rothman (1970); Rothman and Tropman (1987).

Photovoice provides an innovative example of a community development approach that is heavily participatory and process oriented, with the goal of empowering disenfranchised peoples (Wang, 2003). Photovoice gives community members cameras to document their health and work realities. The photographers select images that represent the issues of greatest importance in their community and then discuss their experiences and ideas about the factors associated with these problems. The photographs and stories serve as their "voice" as they advocate for change with policymakers and the broader society. Developed by Wang, Burris, & Ping (1996) in their work for Women's Reproductive Health and Development Program in Yunnan, China, the process has been applied in a wide variety of international and U.S. settings, empowering rural women, the homeless, economically disadvantaged youth, and other disenfranchised populations. Steps in the Photovoice process, ethical issues associated with documentary photography, and case studies featuring community members' photographs and stories can be found at www.photovoice.org.

The second model, *social action,* focuses on a disadvantaged segment of the population that needs to be organized in order to achieve equity and justice. Conflict and dissatisfaction with the status quo are often used to create pressure for change and place demands on the larger community for increased resources or just more treatment. The ultimate goal of social action is to enable communities to change institutions or community practices in order to redistribute power, resources, and decision making (Minkler & Wallerstein, 1998; Rothman & Tropman, 1987). Saul Alinsky's work in Chicago and other urban settings is a good example of how social action strategies can be used to promote social justice. For more than three decades, Alinsky taught disenfranchised citizens the nature of power and mobilized them into grassroots organizations that changed the political agenda. Alinsky's social action strategies produced a grassroots "people movement" that bolstered the civil rights struggle and farm workers movement in the United States (Cart, 1998; Minkler & Wallerstein, 1998).

Social planning is a more carefully controlled approach to solving substantive community problems such as crime, HIV/AIDS, or drug use. This approach is heavily task oriented and based on empirical problem-solving methods. Social planning is usually directed by external planners who "through the exercise of technical abilities, including the ability to manipulate large bureaucratic organizations, can skillfully guide complex change processes" (Rothman & Tropman, 1987, p. 27). Social planners often rely on research and the manipulation of formal organizations or power structures to achieve specific program goals in order to solve specific community problems. This model is often mixed with elements of community development. The Planned Approach to Community Health (PATCH) model described below is a good example of a social planning model that also includes elements of the locality or community development model.

Planned Approach to Community Health

PATCH is a planning model that provides communities with a structured process for identifying and prioritizing health problems and then implementing and evaluating programs to resolve them (U.S. Department of Health and Human Services, 1993). The

PATCH process is usually directed by a local or state health department; however, other organizations (hospitals, military institutions, universities, and voluntary groups) have used PATCH to address a variety of health concerns. Because PATCH uses data in a systematic approach to solving substantive health problems, it can be classified as a social planning model for community organizing. However, PATCH is similar to locality or community development models in its "use of broad participation of a wide spectrum of people at the local community level in goal determination and action" (Rothman & Tropman, 1987, p. 26).

Community participation is a central feature of PATCH—community members form health promotion committees/groups; collect and use data; establish health priorities; and design, implement, and evaluate activities to modify established behavioral risk factors (U.S. Department of Health and Human Services, 1993). PATCH is predicated on the belief that empowerment and community capacity are essential for improving the health of individuals and communities by increasing people's sense of control over their health (Kreuter, 1992). For this reason, a primary goal of PATCH is to increase a community's capacity to solve its own problems by teaching its members the skills necessary to critically analyze health problems; set goals; and plan, implement, and evaluate programs aimed at increasing the health of the community.

PATCH also encourages collaboration among academic-based researchers; local public health professionals; state representatives; lay leaders and activists; representatives of local business, churches, and voluntary organizations; and residents. This collaboration brings people together who share common goals, offer a variety of resources and expertise, and share a vested interest in solving the problem (McWilliam et al., 1997). The end result of a successful PATCH process is greater collaboration between state and local public health agencies and increased communication among local agencies and organizations and state and federal agencies. This collaboration also results in decreased risk of duplicated services being directed to the same health priority (Kreuter, 1992). Most important, the use of PATCH can increase community members' capacity to work together in addressing behavioral risk factors and obtaining the knowledge, funding, and other resources that can enable them to help themselves (Bogan, Omar, Knobloch, Liburd, & O'Rourke, 1992; Katz & Kreuter, 1997).

History and Theory

PATCH was created through a collaborative effort between state and local health departments and community groups in the mid-1980s (U.S. Department of Health and Human Services, 1993). It was designed to be a user-friendly, community-based process that incorporated information from health education, health promotion, community organizations, and development theories within the context of the PRECEDE model (Green & Kreuter, 1991). (PRECEDE is an acronym for predisposing, reinforcing, and enabling constructs in ecosystem diagnosis and evaluation.)

The following elements are considered critical to the success of PATCH:

- An inclusive array of *community members participate* in the processes of analyzing community data, setting priorities, planning interventions, and making decisions about the health needs of their communities. This participation should result in a greater sense of community ownership of the program.
- *Data guide the process* from planning to implementation and evaluation. Community members use many types of data in an effort to gain a comprehensive view of the health status of the community.
- *Participants develop and implement a comprehensive promotion strategy* based on community data.
- *Evaluation activities emphasize feedback and improvement,* to make timely changes if needed. Both process and impact evaluations are crucial.
- The *community's capacity* for health education and health promotion is *strengthened,* and community members are better equipped to repeat the process as they address other health priorities (U.S. Department of Health and Human Services, 1993).

Phases in the Process

The PATCH process is made up of five phases:

Phase I: Community mobilization

Phase II: Data collection and organization

Phase III: Selection of health priorities

Phase IV: Intervention plan development

Phase V: Evaluation

Mobilization begins with attempts to define the community and gain commitment from organizations and individuals to participate in the PATCH process. This phase often takes several months to a year. An important part of this phase is the creation of an organizational structure, such as a coalition, that will guide the PATCH process. This structure typically consists of a local coordinator, a steering committee, and a larger planning committee. Evaluations of PATCH in several communities reveal that some local coordinators need training in volunteer recruitment and retention to ensure involvement of a diverse assortment of community members in PATCH committees and activities (Orenstein, Nelson, Speers, Brownstein, & Ramsey, 1992).

Once the community is mobilized, *community members collect and analyze data* on mortality, morbidity, and factors related to health risk behaviors. These include information on opinions, beliefs, knowledge, and motivating, enabling, and rewarding factors (U.S. Department of Health and Human Services, 1993). Communities are encouraged to use preexisting sources of data and to collect data via focus groups, face-to-face interview, surveys, and other combinations of qualitative and quantitative methods to examine factors at all levels in the ecological framework. Data collection activities are essential to the success of PATCH programs; however, community members may grow impatient if large amounts of time and effort are spent on these activities, especially if insufficient attention is devoted to the development and implementation of interventions (Bogan et al., 1992; Orenstein et al., 1992).

The *selection of health priorities* to be addressed begins once the community data have been analyzed. In keeping with the social ecological framework, the community group reviews the individual, interpersonal, community, and societal factors that influence health behaviors. A review of existing programs and policies helps the community group assess local capacity to address the health problems under consideration. Guided by the PRECEDE model, prioritization of health problems includes an evaluation of the "importance" and "changeability" of the behavioral risk factors. Once the health problems have been prioritized, the group selects the health issues to be addressed in the next phase in the process.

In the fourth phase, *a comprehensive intervention plan is developed.* During this stage, the community group uses data from the previous phases to create a health promotion strategy, establishes objectives, and develops a plan. Guided by the social ecological framework, the multilevel intervention typically includes education, policy formulation, and environmental change strategies.

Evaluation is labeled "Phase V"; however, monitoring and assessment activities should occur throughout all phases of the PATCH process. The community establishes evaluation criteria to measure program success in achieving the shared goals and objectives. Process and impact evaluations are crucial to the PATCH process. Process evaluations allow the community to compare actual implementation with ideal implementation. Impact evaluations measure changes in both intermediate outcomes, such as behavior or behavioral intentions, as well as longer-term outcomes, such as changes in the environment, policies, and health status. Process and impact evaluation data are particularly important for planners to use for program improvement purposes.

CASE STUDY   **PATCH in Sarasota County, Florida**

In 1984, Sarasota County was the first county in Florida selected by the Centers for Disease Control and Prevention (CDC) and the State of Florida's Chronic Disease Program to become a PATCH program. Sarasota County is located in southwest Florida and is home to approximately 360,000 individuals. The U.S. Census Bureau (2007) indicates that the population of Sarasota County is predominantly white (87% white, 6% Hispanic, 4% black), older (42% of the population is 55 years of age or older), and divided almost evenly between males and females (52% female vs. 48% male). Approximately 13% of the population has less than a high school education and 8% fall below the poverty level. While Sarasota County is not representative of the state of Florida, due to its lower number of minority residents (7% vs. 29%) and lower percentage of people falling below the poverty level (7% vs. 13%), it was selected because the community's capacity (local leadership and other resources) would enable it to test this new planning model and support the process once initiated.

Sarasota County provides a good example of activities that constitute the stages in the PATCH process. Efforts to *mobilize the community* began with the initiation of a PATCH coalition in Sarasota County. Public health leaders from the Sarasota County Public Health

Department initiated the process by contacting representatives of local community organizations, including hospitals, local foundations, national foundations (e.g., American Cancer Society), schools, senior centers, fire departments, and mental-health centers. A community outreach subcommittee was responsible for generating a comprehensive list of organizations in the local area, which would serve as resources for a wide variety of community activities. The use of local representatives and health leaders also was an important component of the mobilization efforts. Word-of-mouth, meetings, newsletters, and personal letters were used to invite people to participate in a partnership comprising the community of Sarasota County, the state of Florida, and the CDC in order to address the local health problems in a unique way.

After the initial community structure was developed in Sarasota County, a workshop, "Diagnosing the Community," was held to discuss ways in which the current health status of community residents could be assessed. Workshop participants identified the existing sources of information (e.g., the Behavioral Risk Factor Surveillance System) and conducted an opinion survey of health officials, religious leaders, civic members, business leaders, and local community members. Community members were asked three questions: (1) What are the major health problems in Sarasota County? (2) What do you think are the causes? and (3) How should these problems be reduced?

A second workshop was conducted to prioritize the local health problems and set objectives to reduce the major health problems. Workshop participants selected six areas of major concern in Sarasota County: HIV/AIDS, inadequate community wellness education, lack of access to affordable health care, geriatric problems, substance abuse, and teen problems. Six corresponding committees were formed to address these areas. Ultimately, the Teen Problems committee moved from PATCH to become a committee of the Sarasota County Youth Related Services Associate, and four additional committees were formed: (1) Mental Health Issues, (2) Environmental Health Issues, (3) Perinatal Resource Network, and (4) Healthy Sarasota 2000. Each committee set objectives for their specific health priority area and developed *interventions* to achieve them. Figure 14.1 provides an early representation of PATCH in Sarasota County.

Specific evaluation activities and outcomes are beyond the scope of this discussion due to the large number of PATCH committees involved in Sarasota County; however, the overall results of the program suggest that PATCH has been successful in mobilizing the community to address the priority health concerns and in enabling the community members to develop skills that can be generalized to a variety of health issues in a variety of settings. PATCH members remain active and continue to generate new interests.

During the past 5 years, PATCH has incorporated new topics, and many committees have merged with other community groups, such as the Sarasota County Openly Plans for Excellence and the Community Health Improvement projects. These community teams have reassessed the local needs and used the same community participatory process to establish teams, review results, prioritize problems, and develop plans for addressing selected problems. For instance, community action teams have advocated for policy changes and successfully developed the following:

- A leadership development program to nurture and support promising individuals
- A low-cost medical/dental service center

Figure 14.1 Early Representation of PATCH in Sarasota County

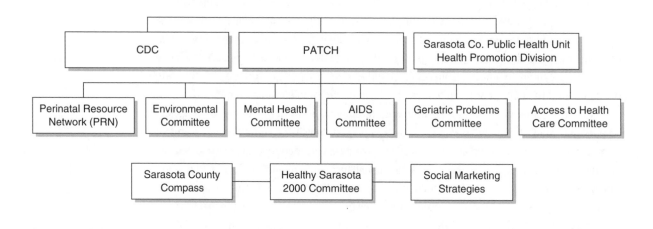

- A local health service directory that improves access to health information and preventive care
- A novel program providing integrated at-home services for patients with type 2 diabetes.

For more examples of how these community teams have intervened at multiple levels in the ecological model, you can visit their Web sites, www.scopexcel.org/ and www.chip4health.org.

ADVANTAGES OF COMMUNITY-BASED INTERVENTIONS

Community-based approaches offer many benefits to public health professionals attempting to address population-level problems. First, as already noted, community-based approaches recognize that health problems have multiple causes, and multiple interventions are required to change individual behavior and modify the interpersonal, community, organizational, social, political, and economic environment in which health conditions are based (Butterfoss, Goodman, & Wandersman, 1993). Community-based approaches focus on multiple environmental and interpersonal factors and avoid an overreliance on education, communications, and other strategies criticized for "blaming the victim" (Ling, Franklin, Lindsteadt, & Gearon, 1992; Rothschild, 1997). This approach also encourages the introduction of supportive norms, policies, and environmental changes that make it easier for individuals to adopt healthier lifestyles.

Second, community participation has an indirect effect on health by strengthening the social networks of community members as they work together to define and solve problems. Thus, community participation enhances participants' sense of social connectedness, perceived control, individual coping capacity, and health status (Minkler & Wallerstein, 1998).

Evidence for the positive health benefits of social connectedness or cohesion comes from the small town of Roseto, Pennsylvania (Patrick & Wickizer, 1995). Roseto captured researchers' interest because its residents had dramatically lower myocardial infarction mortality rates than neighboring communities with similar demographic characteristics. Studies conducted in the late 1950s and early 1960s found an important association between mortality rates and social cohesion. In addition to having lower mortality rates than neighboring communities, Roseto's citizens enjoyed closer family ties, more ethnic and social homogeneity, and more social support. Even the poorest citizens shared a sense of connectedness and benefited from social ties to other community members. Additional support for the link between social cohesiveness and health came from a longitudinal study of myocardial infarction rates in Roseto over the next 30 years. As the community's stability, family cohesion, and supportiveness declined, myocardial infarction rates climbed. Other studies have focused on the flip side of social cohesion, documenting increased rates of suicide and other health problems among socially isolated individuals. As discussed in previous chapters, people who are socially isolated have far higher rates of death from many causes than those with one or more close social ties.

A third benefit of community-based interventions comes from community participation and a shared sense of ownership that citizens develop together. In addition to the impact this sense of ownership has on participants' own health, local control also ensures the longevity of change. Members are more likely to sustain efforts that they have had a role in designing and implementing.

Fourth, the community's participation facilitates the development of interventions that are integrated into the existing community structures; programs, services, and other activities are more likely to be compatible with community norms, values, and beliefs, and the endorsement of local leaders or opinion makers fosters acceptance by other community members (Bracht, 1990).

Fifth, community-based approaches can be very cost-effective. Even small successes reap important economic benefits because of the large number of people reached. Compare the impact of a community-wide program that assists just 5% of its 50,000 members to exercise regularly with a 75% success rate among 500 participants in an exercise class or other intervention targeting small groups of individuals. Economic benefits are especially impressive when community-based interventions bring about permanent changes in community norms or provide for environmental structures that reinforce and thus facilitate long-term change (Bracht, 1990; Frankish & Green, 1994).

CHALLENGES ASSOCIATED WITH COMMUNITY-BASED INTERVENTIONS

Community-based interventions can also be challenging. Because community control of the change process is a defining theme in community-based intervention models, success requires the formation of an effective working relationship between public health professionals and community members. Many factors have been reported to affect these partnerships and the effectiveness of their work:

- Community relevance and self-determination, central tenets of community organizing, are often difficult to implement. Funding sources frequently limit issue selection to specified categories or health problems (e.g., HIV prevention). Even when funding is not categorically limited, health departments or other lead community organizations may be unable to make the transition from a strict problem-solving focus to a broader community development project (Baker & Goodman, 2003). Time constraints may also affect a program's potential for success and comprehensiveness. Many funding agencies expect observable results within 5 years or less—an unrealistic expectation for community-based projects that see their efforts as a long-term investment in building local capacity. Even very successful community-based projects that focus on specific health problems may not be able to report significant health outcomes within this time frame (Israel et al., 1994, 2003).

- Community-planning coalitions vary in terms of how well its members represent the larger community. Community leaders may not understand issues of importance beyond their individual concerns. For this reason, many community-based interventions rely on research with representative samples to understand the views of community members whose time and interest preclude more active participation in community affairs.

- CBPR also poses special challenges. As David Katz (2004) has noted,

> Diversity of perspectives and expertise is valuable, but it can also lead to diversity of opinion— as well as conflict. For CBPR to work well, all partners must commit to the project goals, remain well informed at each step of the research process, be willing to work through disagreement, and maintain mutual respect if consensus does not form easily. Project ownership and influence must also be shared equitably. (p. 3)

- Power differentials between public health professionals and community members may hinder the development of collaborative relationships. To build trust, public health professionals must be willing to be guided by the needs and desires of the community representatives and ultimately the community itself.

- Confusion over lines of authority and/or the roles individual members play in the collaborative process can seriously inhibit the achievement of program goals. Community organizations tend to be more democratic and focus on shared decision making and responsibility, while public health organizations (e.g., health departments and schools of public health) are accustomed to hierarchical leadership with a "clear chain of command" (Buchanan, 1996, p. 265). The difference between structures has the potential to paralyze the collaborative process unless an explicit delineation of roles and leadership responsibilities is made at the onset of the program (Brownson, Riley, & Bruce, 1998).

- The development of community-based interventions is a complex, time-consuming process. If the intervention is begun before the community is ready or if the evaluation is done before adequate time is allowed for the intervention to have an impact, the program may falsely appear to have been inadequate. Public health professionals must be prepared to allocate sufficient time for community members to feel comfortable participating in the program and for the actual intervention and evaluation of the program (Brownson et al., 1998).

CONCLUSION

When addressing public health problems that affect large segments of a population, many public health professionals collaborate with community members in their effort to design comprehensive, multilevel interventions. The community-based health promotion frameworks described in this chapter are guided by a social ecological perspective of health, a commitment to design or tailor programs to reflect community needs and preferences, and the active participation of community members in the planning and implementation of programs. Additionally, community organization approaches emphasize community empowerment and capacity building by helping members work together to set goals, develop strategies for achieving those goals, and gain mastery over the social and political environmental factors that influence their health and well-being.

Community-based approaches can be challenging because of the additional time and skill needed to build effective partnerships with community members. Many public health practitioners are used to controlling planning activities and find it difficult to allow the community to be in the driver's seat. When successful, however, community-based interventions can be more effective in addressing the multiple factors that influence health and in bringing about changes that are sustained longer than changes brought about by agencies outside the community.

REFERENCES

Baker, E. A., & Goodman, R. M. (2003). Community assessment and change: A framework, principles, models, methods, and skills. In F. D. Scutchfield & C. W. Keck, (Eds.), *Principles of public health practice* (pp. 177–190). Clifton Park, NY: Thomson Learning.

Bogan, G., Omar, A., Knobloch, S., Liburd, L. C., & O'Rourke, T. W. (1992). Organizing an urban African-American community for health promotion: Lessons from Chicago. *Journal of Health Education, 23*(3), 157–163.

Bond, L. A., & Hauf, A. M. C. (2007). Community-based collaboration: An overarching best practice in prevention. *The Counseling Psychologist, 35*(4), 567–575.

Bracht, N. (1990). *Health promotion at the community level.* Newbury Park, CA: Sage.

Bracht, N., & Kingsbury, L. (1990). In N. Bracht (Ed.), *Health promotion at the community level* (pp. 66–88). Newbury Park, CA: Sage.

Bracht, N., & Tsouros, N. (1990). Principles and strategies of effective community participation. *Health Promotion International, 5*(3), 199–208.

Brownson, R. C., Baker, E. A., & Novick, L. F. (1999). *Community-based prevention: Programs that work.* Gaithersburg, MD: Aspen.

Brownson, R. C., Riley, P., & Bruce, T. A. (1998). Demonstration projects in community-based prevention. *Journal of Public Health Management and Practice, 4*(2), 66–77.

Buchanan, D. R. (1996). Building academic-community linkages for health promotion: A case study in Massachusetts. *American Journal of Health Promotion, 10*(4), 262–269.

Butterfoss, F. D., Goodman, R. M., & Wandersman, A. (1993). Community coalitions for prevention and health promotion. *Health Education Research, 8,* 315–330.

Butterfoss, F. D., & Kegler, M. C. (2002). Toward a comprehensive understanding of community coalitions. In R. J. DiClemente, R. A. Crosby, & M. C. Kegler, (Eds.), *Emerging theories in health promotion practice and research: Strategies for improving public health* (pp. 157–193). San Francisco: Jossey-Bass.

Campbell, C., & Jovchelovitch, S. (2000). Health, community and development: Towards a social psychology of participation. *Journal of Community and Applied Social Psychology, 10,* 255–270.

Campbell, C., & Murray, M. (2004). Community health psychology: Promoting analysis and action for social change. *Journal of Health Psychology, 9,* 187–195.

Cart, C. U. (1998). Online computer networks: Potential challenges for community organizing and community building now and in the future. In M. Minkler & N. Wallerstein (Eds.), *Community-based participatory research for health* (pp. 325–338). San Francisco: Jossey-Bass.

Coombe, C. M. (1998). Using empowerment evaluation in community organizing and community-based health initiatives. In M. Minkler (Ed.), *Community organizing and community building for health* (pp. 291–307). New Brunswick, NJ: Rutgers University Press.

Frankish, C. J., & Green, L. W. (1994). Organizational and community change as the social scientific basis for disease prevention and health promotion policy. In G. L. Albrecht (Ed.), *Advances in medical sociology: Vol. 4. A reconsideration of health behavior change models* (pp. 209–233). Ipswitch, CT: JAI Press.

Green, L. W., & Kreuter, M. W. (Eds.). (1991). *Health promotion planning: An educational and environmental approach* (2nd ed.). Mountain View, CA: Mayfield.

Israel, B. A., Checkoway, B., Schulz, A., & Zimmerman, M. (1994). Health education and community empowerment: Conceptualizing and measuring perceptions of individual, organizational, and community control. *Health Education Quarterly, 21*(2), 149–170.

Israel, B. A., Schulz, A. J., Parker, E. A., & Becker, A. B. (1998). Key principles of community-based research. *Annual Review of Public Health, 19,* 173–202.

Israel, B. A., Schulz, A. J., Parker, E. A., Becker, A. B., Allen, A. J., & Guzman, J. R. (2003). Critical issues in developing and following community based participatory research principles. In M. Minkler & N. Wallerstein (Eds.), *Community-based participatory research for health* (pp. 53–71). San Francisco: Jossey-Bass.

Katz, D. L. (2004). Representing your community in community-based participatory research: Differences made and measured. *Preventing Chronic Disease, 1*(1), 1–3. www.cdc.gov/pcd/issues/2004/jan/toc.htm

Katz, M. F., & Kreuter, M. W. (1997). Community assessment and empowerment. In F. D. Scutchfield & C. W. Keck (Eds.), *Principles of public health practice* (pp. 147–157). Albany, NY: Delmar.

Kreuter, M. W. (1992). PATCH: Its origin, basic concepts, and links for contemporary public health policy. *Journal of Health Education, 23*(3), 135–139.

Ling, J. C., Franklin, B. A., Lindsteadt, J. F., & Gearon, S. A. N. (1992). Social marketing: Its place in public health. *Annual Review of Public Health, 13,* 341–362.

McWilliam, C. L., Desai, K., & Greig, B. (1997). Bridging town and gown: Building research partnerships between community-based professional providers and academia. *Journal of Professional Nursing, 13*(5), 307–315.

Minkler, M. (Ed.). (1998). *Community organizing and community building for health.* New Brunswick, NJ: Rutgers University Press.

Minkler, M., & Wallerstein, N. (1998). Improving health through community organization and community building: A health education perspective. In M. Minkler (Ed.), *Community organizing and community building for health* (pp. 30–52). Gaithersburg, MD: Aspen.

Minkler, M., & Wallerstein, N. (Eds.). (2003). *Community-based participatory research for health.* San Francisco: Jossey-Bass.

Orenstein, D., Nelson, C., Speers, M., Brownstein, J. N., & Ramsey, D. C. (1992). Synthesis of the four PATCH evaluations. *Journal of Health Education, 23*(3), 187–192.

Patrick, D. L., & Wickizer, T. M. (1995). Community and health. In B. Amick, S. Levine, A. R. Tarlov, & D. C. Walsh (Eds.), *Society and health* (pp. 64–92). New York: Oxford University Press.

Rothman, J. (1970). Three models of community organization practice. In F. M. Cox, J. L. Erlich, J. Rothman, & J. E. Tropman (Eds.), *Strategies of community organization* (pp. 20–36). Itasca, IL: Peacock Press.

Rothman, J., & Tropman, J. E. (1987). Models of community organizing and macro practice: Their mixing and phasing. In F. M. Cox, J. L. Erlich, J. Rothman, & J. E. Tropman (Eds.), *Strategies of community organization* (4th ed., pp. 25–45). Itasca, IL: F. E. Peacock.

Rothschild, M. (1997). A historic perspective of social marketing. *Journal of Health Communication, 2,* 308–309.

Schulz, A. J., Parker, E. A., Israel, B. A., Becker, A. B., Maciak, B. J., & Hollis, R. (1999). Conducting a participatory community-based survey. In R. C. Brownson, E. A. Baker, and L. F. Novick (Eds.), *Community-based prevention: Programs that work* (pp. 84–105). Gaithersburg, MD: Aspen.

Stephens, C. (2007). Community as practice: Social representations of community and their implications for health promotion. *Journal of Community and Applied Social Psychology, 17,* 103–114.

U.S. Census Bureau. (2007). *Sarasota County, Florida general demographic characteristics: 2005.* Retrieved November 2, 2007, from http://factfinder.census.gov/home/saff/main.html?_lang=en

U.S. Department of Health and Human Services, Centers for Disease Control and Prevention, National Center for Chronic Disease Prevention and Health Promotion. (1993). *Planned approach to community health: Guide for the local coordinator.* Atlanta, GA: Author.

Wang, C. (2003). Using Photovoice as a participatory assessment and issue selection tool: A case study with the homeless in Ann Arbor. In M. Minkler & N. Wallerstein (Eds.), *Community-based participatory research for health* (pp. 179–196). San Francisco: Jossey-Bass.

Wang, C., Burris, M. A., & Ping, X. Y. (1996). Chinese village women as visual anthropologists: A participatory approach to reaching policymakers. *Social Science and Medicine, 42*(10), 1391–1400.

World Health Organization, Health and Welfare Canada, and Canadian Public Health Association. (1986, November 21). *Ottawa charter for health promotion.* Presented in the First International Conference on Health Promotion, Ottawa, Ontario, Canada.

15

Social Marketing in Public Health

Carol A. Bryant

Social marketing is a planning framework that has gained widespread acceptance in public health during the past 25 years (Grier & Bryant, 2005). In the United States, it is used by a wide range of governmental agencies and social service organizations, including the Centers for Disease Control and Prevention, U.S. Department of Agriculture, the National Cancer Institute, and the American Association of Retired Persons. Social marketing is also commonly applied by government agencies in other European countries, Australia, New Zealand, and Canada. The United Kingdom, for instance, has created the National Social Marketing Center to develop and implement large-scale health promotion interventions and reduce health care costs (Hastings, 2007; National Social Marketing Center, 2007).

In public health, social marketing has shown great promise in addressing a wide range of problems, including the following:

- Diabetes (Jones & Hall, 2007)
- HIV/AIDS (Deshpande, 2007; Lee et al., 2006)
- Smoking (Evans et al., 2007; Hicks, 2002; Lavack, Watson, & Markwart, 2007)
- Drunk driving (Rothschild, Mastin, Karsten, & Miller, 2003)
- Adolescent substance abuse (Denniston, 2004)
- Physical inactivity (Bryant et al., 2007; Wong et al., 2004)
- Poor dietary practices (Bellows, Cole, & Anderson, 2006; John, Kerby, & Landers, 2004)
- Population control (Dholakia & Dholakia, 2001; Harvey, 1999)
- Environmental degradation (McKenzie-Mohr & Smith, 1999)

In addition to programs targeting individual behavior change, social marketing has been used to promote public health services (Bryant & Lindenberger, 2002; Carroll & VanVeen, 2002; McCormack Brown et al., 2000) and policy changes (McDermott et al., 2005; Siegel & Lotenberg, 2007).

Social marketing uses marketing principles and techniques to promote socially beneficial behaviors and to create, communicate, and deliver socially beneficial programs and other products. In this chapter, we examine the distinguishing features of the social marketing approach, the steps used to design social change interventions, and the common criticisms and challenges facing the field. A case study is used to illustrate how social marketing can be applied to improve public health program design and delivery.

DISTINGUISHING FEATURES OF THE SOCIAL MARKETING APPROACH

Social marketing is distinguished from other planning frameworks discussed in this book by four principles: (1) a commitment to create satisfying exchanges, (2) the use of marketing's conceptual framework to design interventions, (3) a data-based consumer orientation, and (4) segmentation of populations and careful selection of target audiences.

Satisfying Exchanges

In commercial marketing, consumers are expected to act largely out of self-interest by finding ways to optimize the benefits they gain and minimize the costs they pay in their exchanges with others (Bagozzi, 1979). In most commercial transactions, consumers exchange money for tangible commodities (e.g., clothing) and services (such as dry cleaning). They feel satisfied when their purchases provide them with assets (pleasure, pride, hope, prestige) at an affordable price and are delighted when they pay less than what they believe the product is worth.

This notion of exchange is not new. As discussed in Chapter 4, it is a central component of the health belief model and other behavior change theories that assert that people make comparisons between the benefits they will reap and the sacrifices they must make when deciding to adopt a new health behavior, participate in a public health program, or vote for a public health policy. Unfortunately, the exchanges involved with many public health products are less intrinsically satisfying than they are for commercial transactions. All too often, public health professionals ask their consumers to exchange immediate pleasure, discomfort, and the hassle of changing daily habits for a somewhat lowered risk of developing disease at a future time. Despite these challenges, social marketers are committed to understanding what their customers *want* and try to create products that deliver benefits that truly outweigh the costs. They may do this by promoting non–health benefits that satisfy customers' more immediate desires (e.g., looking good, fitting into favorite clothes), finding ways to make the health benefits more compelling, and/or finding creative ways to make products more affordable (e.g., recommending diet plans that are tasty and easy to follow, reducing the waiting time to be served in a health clinic).

Conceptual Framework

In addition to the notion of exchange, social marketing is distinguished by its reliance on additional concepts known as the marketing mix: *product, price, place,* and *promotion.*

Product is conceptualized on three levels: the actual product, the core product, and the augmented product (Kotler & Lee, 2007). In public health, the actual product refers to a protective behavior (e.g., start a regular exercise regimen), a health program or service (with the behavioral objective of getting people to use it), or a protective health policy. Social marketers search for ways to design the actual product so that it is compatible with consumers' realities and preferences and also meets their health needs. For example, if consumer research reveals that a sedentary segment of the population is clearly unable and unwilling to exercise for 60 minutes a day, the marketing intervention may recommend an amount they would embrace, such as three 10-minute exercise sessions most days each week.

The second level—the core product—refers to the benefits consumers gain when adopting the actual product. Social marketers search for ways to give their products a sustainable competitive advantage; that is, they make their products more attractive than competing products (Hastings, 2007). Research known as competitive analysis is conducted to understand how consumers view the competition: the products they currently use and the needs and wants these products satisfy. Competitive analysis reminds us that people always have a choice: They can continue to smoke and eat too much, dismiss our appeals to be immunized, or vote against smoking bans. As Gerard Hastings (2007) explains, "[Competitive analysis] . . . compels us to think about what we are offering and the extent to which it meets people's real needs" (pp. 160–161). In some instances, these needs and the most attractive product benefits may not be health related, such as when weight loss is promoted as a way to look and feel more attractive instead of as a preventive health measure.

Breast-feeding is a product that clearly illustrates the importance of finding the right benefits needed to create a sustainable competitive advantage. For over a decade, public health professionals in federal, state, and local public health agencies promoted breast-feeding as the superior infant feeding choice for infants and their mothers. They touted its nutritional composition, immunological protection for acute and chronic diseases, cost savings, and convenience. However, as breast-feeding rates continued to slump throughout the 1980s, some public health professionals turned to social marketing for a new perspective on the problem (Bryant, Coreil, D'Angelo, Bailey, & Lazarov, 1992). Their marketing research revealed that while mothers clearly want their babies to be healthy, the medical risks associated with bottle-feeding are not visible enough in the United States to convince many women that breast milk is truly superior to formula. Moreover, pregnant women's aspirations as mothers focus on the love they expect to give and receive and the special bonds they want to establish with their babies, not health concerns. In marketing terms, breast-feeding's emotional benefits give it a more competitive edge over bottle-feeding than the health benefits public health professionals had been emphasizing. Building on these findings, a marketing intervention called *Loving Support Makes Breastfeeding Work* was designed to emphasize the close, loving bond and special joy that breast-feeding mothers share with their babies (Bryant et al., 1992; Lindenberger &

Bryant, 2000). Health and other benefits were discussed in promotional materials, but breast-feeding's emotional advantages were used to give it a sustainable competitive edge over infant formula.

In some cases, products have a third level, the augmented product, which has additional features that add value and enhance its attractiveness to consumers. In a project to prevent eye injuries among citrus pickers, researchers at the Florida Prevention Research Center at the University of South Florida found that safety eyewear use (the actual product) increased when workers were offered a brand of safety glasses with special features that improved their comfort and antifogging capabilities (Monaghan et al., in press.). Other examples of augmented products are colors and textures added to condoms and slender, suspender-like straps used to make life vests more comfortable (Kotler & Lee, 2007).

The second P in the marketing mix, *price,* refers to monetary outlays (fees, lost wages) and nonmonetary costs (time, effort, embarrassment, loss of pride and dignity, and the psychological discomfort associated with behavior change). With respect to breast-feeding promotion, research among pregnant women revealed that many women are attracted to the products' benefits but are deterred by the costs. They worry that breast-feeding in front of others will be embarrassing and expose them to criticism from friends or relatives. Some women are unwilling to invest the additional time it takes to nurse a baby and worry about how breast-feeding will affect their ability to return to work, school, or an active social life. Other "costs" associated with breast-feeding are the pain associated with nursing, the changes women think they must make in dietary and health practices, and anxiety about their ability to produce the quality and quantity of breast milk needed to meet their child's nutritional needs. Also, some women are afraid that they will alienate spouses, boyfriends, or their own mothers, who might feel left out of the special relationship breast-feeding creates between a mother and her child.

To make the exchange more affordable for pregnant women, the *Loving Support* program teaches health providers to use a three-step counseling strategy to quickly identify a woman's perception of the costs of breast-feeding and help her develop acceptable ways to overcome them. Public information and consumer education materials are used to change family members' attitudes about breast-feeding in public and counter misperceptions about the time required to breast-feed. These materials also inform people of how they can breast-feed after returning to work. Even the overall theme of the program—"Loving Support Makes Breastfeeding Work"—and television and radio advertising is designed to encourage family, friends, and the public at large to support breast-feeding (Lindenberger & Bryant, 2000).

Place, the third P, also has several levels depending on the type of product being marketed. When promoting healthy behaviors or services, place refers to where the exchange takes place (e.g., where people can be physically active or the time and location clinic services are offered). When promoting tangible products, such as condoms, place refers to distribution channels and retail outlets where products can be purchased. Place also refers to intermediaries or partners: people who can facilitate change (e.g., bartenders who can encourage intoxicated customers to take a taxi home). In promoting breast-feeding, the *Loving Support* campaign developed motivational, training, and support materials to equip WIC staff and prenatal care providers to encourage their participants to breast-feed. As trusted medical spokespersons, these intermediaries play an essential role in endorsing breast-feeding and providing help if and when women encountered problems (Coreil, Bryant, Westover, Bailey, & d'Angelo, 1995; Lindenberger & Bryant, 2000).

The fourth P refers to *promotion*—communication and other activities used to facilitate change. Many public health professionals equate social marketing with social advertising, so it may be surprising that marketing interventions do not necessarily use mass media to bring about change. In fact, social marketing programs vary widely in how they structure their promotional strategy: Some, such as *VERB™: It's What You Do,* use large-scale advertising campaigns to build awareness and promote product benefits to large populations; others use a more limited range of communication activities, including consumer education materials, direct mail, and interpersonal communications, to reach narrower target audiences. In the project to prevent eye injuries among citrus workers, peers are trained to promote safety glass use through role modeling, informal interpersonal communication, and distribution of safety wear. Television, radio, and print materials would be inappropriate for reaching this special audience.

In many public health projects, the promotional strategy also includes other activities, such as service delivery improvements, community-based activities, the use of incentives, and many other means for satisfying consumers' desires and needs. We have just seen the mix of health communication, policy changes, personal counseling strategies, consumer education, and other activities used in the *Loving Support* program. The Texas WIC case described below gives another example of a multifaceted marketing plan.

Finally, to be effective, all aspects of the marketing mix are integrated to reinforce each other. The promotional strategy is carefully crafted to ensure that consumers know and value the benefits being offered, believe that the product is "affordable," and are inspired to act (Kotler, Roberto, & Lee, 2002). When designing and disseminating communication materials, the promotional strategy guides the development of persuasive messages; the selection of credible, trustworthy spokespersons to achieve these goals; and the selection of cost-effective information channels.

In promoting breast-feeding, the *Loving Support* television ads would be foolish to feature the Surgeon General or tout breast milk's amazing nutritional value because the product strategy emphasizes the emotional benefits women value so highly. Far more effective is the program's use of a warm, emotional appeal from other women who have experienced the joys of breast-feeding and can offer advice about overcoming embarrassment and other costs. To develop a well-integrated marketing plan, social marketers rely on consumer research— the next distinguishing feature of the social marketing approach.

Product

- The actual product: behavior, good, service, or policy being promoted
- The core product: benefits that consumers find attractive and that distinguish the actual product from its competition
- The augmented product: features that add value to the actual product

Competition

  – Products (services, behaviors, or commodities) that compete with the product

Price

  – The costs consumers exchange for product benefits, including monetary and other costs

Place

  – The locations where services are provided and consumers practice new behaviors, channels for distributing tangible products, and people who can facilitate adoption

Promotions

  – Communications and other activities designed to bring about behavior change

Data-Based Consumer Orientation

An inherent feature of the marketing mind-set is a steadfast commitment to understand the consumer. Social marketers want to know everything they can about the people who will adopt their products—their dreams, fears, beliefs, attitudes, and current behavioral patterns. Formative research is used to analyze the public health problem; identify appropriate audiences and the actions they can take to prevent or resolve the problem; and develop preliminary strategies for helping them adopt the desired behaviors, services, or policies. Of special importance is identifying the benefits consumers value most, the costs they are willing to pay, other factors that influence their behavioral decisions, the spokespersons they find the most credible, ways to frame messages, and channels to distribute tangible products—all key elements of an integrated marketing plan. Pretesting research is then used to assess consumers' responses to marketing materials and tactics and revise them as necessary (Siegel & Lotenberg, 2007).

Marketing research is guided by a variety of theoretical frameworks or models. Especially powerful is the social ecology model, which directs social marketers' attention to the multiple levels of intrapersonal, interpersonal, organizational, community, and broader societal factors that influence social change. This framework reminds marketers to address environmental factors that make adoption of new behaviors easier, services more accessible, and support from friends and relatives more readily available (Bryant & Dunlevy, 2007; Donovan & Henley, 2003). Behavioral theories are also important in pointing to the interpersonal and intrapersonal factors that affect individual behavior change, for example, perceived susceptibility and severity, self-efficacy, social norms, beliefs and values, previous behavior, and intentions to change (Lefebvre, 2001). However, because social marketing typically intervenes at multiple levels, no single theory or framework dominates the field.

To save time and money, social marketers rely on existing or secondary data to make key marketing decisions whenever possible. For example, routine information collected by most public health programs provides valuable clues about the characteristics of people who continue or stop using services. Publications and technical reports conducted for similar projects, products, or audiences (e.g., those available on CDC's Audience Communication Research

Database at www.health.gov/communication/default.asp) also offer valuable marketing insights.

When existing information is unavailable or inadequate, a mix of qualitative and quantitative research is conducted with consumers and those that have the greatest influence on their behavior. The most common data collection techniques used in the field are described in Table 15.1 (Kotler & Lee, 2007).

Audience Segmentation

Marketers know that one size does not fit all. People differ in terms of the benefits they find most attractive, the price they are willing to pay, the places they are most comfortable purchasing products or using services, and their differential responsiveness to promotional tactics. Just think of the variety of cereals produced to meet the varying wants and needs of American consumers. Cereal makers know that some people are limited in what they are willing to pay for a box of cereal and offer large, economy sizes and generic brands. They also know that the public can be divided into segments based on the features or benefits they value most. Cereals designed for children are usually sweet and feature well-known animated characters, such as those in the movie *Shrek*. Those produced for adults are more likely to promote their fiber and vitamin content or promise weight loss and a sexier image.

Marketers use a process called audience segmentation to divide large heterogeneous populations into more homogeneous subgroups based on the characteristics that influence their responsiveness to marketing interventions. This process gives public health program planners several advantages. First, segmentation allows public health professionals to optimize resource allocation by deciding to which subgroups to give the greatest priority when funds and/or time are limited. In designing a program to promote low-cost mammograms, for instance, program planners might segment the population based on stages of change (Prochaska, DiClementi, & Norcross, 1992) and discover that 20% of women are in precontemplation, 60% are in contemplation, 5% are in preparation, 15% are in action, and the rest are screened annually as recommended. Based on these findings, it would be wise to focus the efforts of the program on contemplators because they comprise such a large proportion of women and because they are already thinking about being screened. Without taking the time to segment the population, program planners would not have known which groups provide the best "return on investment" and may have designed a program with little relevance for those who could benefit most readily.

Another function of segmentation is to determine the most effective strategies for reaching high-priority segments. In the mammogram example, after selecting contemplators as a high-priority group, program planners would most likely rely on the processes of change shown to be effective in moving women from contemplation to preparation, such as self-reevaluation, social support, modeling, focusing on positive outcomes, and providing them an easy, low-cost way to try out the behavior (Prochaska et al., 1992). If they had sufficient funds, the program planners might also design activities appropriate for precontemplators.

TABLE 15.1   A Marketing Research Primer

Marketing Research is the systematic design, collection, analysis, and reporting of data and findings relevant to a specific marketing situation facing the organization.[a]

Characterized by Research Objective:

- *Exploratory* research helps define problems and suggest hypotheses.
- *Descriptive* research helps understand marketing problems, situations, or markets.
- *Causal* research tests hypotheses about cause-and-effect relationships.

Characterized by Stage in Planning Process:

- *Formative* research is used to help select and understand target markets and develop the draft marketing strategy.
- *Pretest* research is used to evaluate draft marketing mix strategies and then make changes prior to finalizing the marketing plan and communication elements.
- *Monitoring* research provides ongoing measurement of program outcomes through periodic surveys.
- *Evaluation* research most often refers to research conducted at the conclusion of a campaign effort.

Characterized by Source of Information

- *Secondary* data are collected for another purpose and already exist somewhere.
- *Primary* data are freshly gathered for a specific purpose or for a specific research project.

Characterized by Approach to Collecting Primary Data

- *Key informant* interviews are conducted with colleagues, decision makers, opinion leaders, technical experts, and others who may provide valuable insight regarding target markets, competitors, and strategies.
- *Focus groups* usually involve 8 to 10 people gathered for a couple of hours with a trained moderator who uses a discussion guide to focus discussion.
- *Surveys* use a variety of contact methods, including mail, telephone, online/Internet, intercept, and self-administered surveys, asking people questions about their knowledge, attitudes, preferences, and behaviors.
- *Experimental* research is used to capture cause-and-effect relationships, gathering primary data by selecting matched groups of subjects, giving them different treatments, controlling related factors, and checking for differences in group responses.[b]
- *Observation* is the gathering of primary data by observing target audiences in action, in relevant situations.
- *Ethnographic* research is considered a holistic research method, founded in the idea that to truly understand target markets, the researcher will need an extensive immersion in their natural environment.
- *Mystery shoppers* pose as customers and report on strong or weak points experienced in the buying process.

Characterized by Technique:

- *Qualitative* research is exploratory in nature, seeking to identify and clarify issues. Sample sizes are usually small, and findings are not usually appropriate for projections to larger populations.
- *Quantitative* research refers to research that is conducted in order to reliably profile markets, predict cause and effect, and project findings. Sample sizes are usually large, and surveys are conducted in a controlled and organized environment.

SOURCE: Kotler and Lee (2007, p. 74).

a. Kotler and Armstrong (2001, p. 140).
b. Kotler and Armstrong (2001, p. 146).

Some public health professionals object to social marketing's use of segmentation, claiming that public health programs must attempt to reach everyone rather than focus on specific subgroups. They do not recognize that, in fact, segmentation always occurs—some respond and some do not. Without strategically assessing and selecting one or more groups to give the greatest priority to, public health programs are less likely to reach those who would benefit most and more likely to miss a large portion of the population. As Craig Lefevbre, a pioneer in the field, concludes, "*The only issue is whether the targeting is done based on research and strategic analysis or by happenstance and default* [italics added]" (Lefebvre et al., 1995, p. 222).

STEPS IN THE SOCIAL MARKETING PROCESS

The social marketing process is a continuous, iterative process that can be conceived as consisting of five major phases or tasks:

1. Audience analysis

   Problem description

   Formative research

2. Strategy development

3. Program development

4. Implementation

5. Tracking and evaluation

Audience Analysis

The overall goal of the first stage is to determine program goals and identify preliminary behavioral objectives, target markets, factors believed to influence the desired change, and potential strategies (e.g., evidence-based practices) for achieving program goals. During the problem description phase, program planners determine the program focus, conduct a SWOT (Strengths, Weaknesses, Opportunities, and Threats) assessment, and review past and similar programs and relevant research and other existing data (Kotler & Lee, 2007).

Because prior research and available data often fail to provide the insights needed to plan the product, pricing, placement, and program strategies, additional formative research is typically needed. Situational factors affecting the project are also considered at this time, and special attention is paid to consumers' perceptions of product benefits, costs, placement, and potential promotional strategies.

Strategy Development

During the strategy development phase, a realistic marketing plan is developed that specifies measurable objectives and a step-by-step work plan to guide the development, implementation, and tracking of the demonstration project. The marketing plan contains a clear statement of the overall goals or mission of the project, a vivid description of the audience segments to be given the highest priority, the actual and core products to promote with each audience segment, and strategies for addressing the critical factors associated with the health behaviors being promoted.

The marketing plan is organized around marketing's conceptual framework of the four Ps. The product strategy delineates the benefits that target audience members find most attractive about the recommended product and determines how the product should be distinguished from its competition (e.g., exercise can be something fun and easy to do). Depending on the nature of the actual product, branding, packaging, and other value-added features may be considered at this time.

The pricing strategy proposes ways to lower costs or make them more acceptable. Other barriers that impede adoption and recommendations for overcoming them are also delineated. In setting the monetary price for tangible commodities, social marketers consider what consumers are willing and able to pay, if they view products given away or priced too low as inferior to those with a higher cost, and whether they prefer to pay more to obtain certain "value-added" benefits.

The placement strategy specifies distribution channels for tangible products and the location and hours of clinic-based services. It may include decision prompts or reminder systems to cue people to action or a plan for recruiting, training, and motivating the people who will work directly with consumers, for example, health providers or business personnel involved in promotional activities. The placement strategy's goal is to make behaviors easy to practice, products easy and convenient to acquire, and services accessible and comfortable to use.

The promotional strategy specifies the communication guidelines that will guide message design, media and other informational channels that will be used to reach priority segments, and the activities proposed to facilitate change, for example, professional training, peer counselor programs, media advocacy, and grassroots advocacy.

The product, price, place, and promotional strategies are accompanied by a step-by-step implementation plan, a timetable, and a budget for each campaign component. Health and behavioral outcome measures are identified, and methods for monitoring these are specified. An evaluation and monitoring plan is also developed at this time, so that baseline measures can be assessed and program tracking can begin as soon as the program is launched.

Program Development

This phase involves the development of program materials and tactics. Often, an advertising agency or other creative team is hired to design messages and prepare communication materials. Instructional designers, professional trainers, and public relations firms develop new products, curricula, campaign messages and materials, and public relations activities. Program strategies, campaign messages and materials, and other products are pretested and revised.

Program Implementation

Many social marketing projects do not reach the implementation phase until after months of planning. Although coordination is important for any program, social marketing projects typically require managers to balance an unusually large number of staff, consultants, or subcontractors and manage multiple activities, each of which requires careful timing. Proper sequencing of legislative advocacy, organizational policy and procedural changes, professional training, distribution of materials, public relations, and public policy formation is essential to the success of a project.

Tracking and Evaluation

As social marketing interventions are implemented, each component is monitored to identify activities that (1) are effective and worthy of being sustained and (2) require midcourse revision. Social marketers are constantly checking with target audiences to gauge their responses to all aspects of an intervention, from the broad marketing strategy to specific messages and materials.

After the program has been implemented for sufficient time to bring about the desired changes, assessment of program outcomes can be conducted. Evaluation of overall program performance (media exposure, product/service usage patterns, number of staff trained, adoption rates) allows managers to decide what to continue to do, what to refine, and what to abandon.

CASE STUDY   Public Health Services Marketing

Although social marketing is most often used to promote healthy behaviors, it has tremendous potential to help public health professionals design and improve public health services. Social marketing has proven effective in increasing program utilization, improving consumer satisfaction, increasing employees' job satisfaction and productivity, and making service delivery more consumer-friendly (Grier & Bryant, 2005; Kotler & Lee, 2007). One example of how public health administrators have applied social marketing to increase program utilization comes from the Texas Special Supplemental Nutrition Program for Women, Infants, and Children (WIC).

The Texas WIC program provides target populations of women, infants, and young children with nutrition education, supplementary nutritious foods, and referrals to appropriate health and social services. Numerous studies have documented WIC's positive impact on birth weight and other birth-related outcomes and its ability to lower birth-related Medicaid costs (Fox, Hamilton, & Lin, 2004); however, many families who could benefit from WIC do not participate in the program. To meet the challenge of offering the Texas WIC program to more families in need of its services, public health administrators contracted with a social marketing firm, Best Start Social Marketing, to develop marketing strategies to increase enrollment among the state's diverse, rapidly growing population (Bryant et al., 1998, 2001; Lindenberger & Bryant, 2000).

Steps in the Texas WIC Marketing Project

During the initial planning phase, Texas public health administrators and Best Start staff identified pregnant women who had never enrolled in the WIC program as a high-priority audience for the project. A large proportion of women who were receiving Medicaid benefits, and thus automatically income eligible for the WIC program, were not enrolled. A comparison of census data and WIC program participant data (pregnant women enrolled in the program) suggested that program participation was higher among women whose incomes fell below 150% of the poverty guidelines than those whose incomes fell between 150% and 185%—the upper limit for eligibility in WIC. The behavioral objective set for this target audience was to motivate the latter group to enroll in the program.

Relatively little was known about this particular segment's reluctance to use the program, so extensive formative research was needed to identify the program benefits women in this group desired and the perceived costs and other factors that influenced their decision to participate in WIC. A computer match of pregnant women enrolled in the Texas Medicaid and Texas WIC programs generated a list of 36,743 Medicaid recipients who were eligible but not currently participating in WIC. A 28-item mail survey was sent to a random sample of 15,000 of these women. Of these, 20% returned the survey on time to be included in the study. Five focus groups and 81 telephone interviews were also conducted with women who indicated on the survey that they would be willing to talk further with researchers.

Research results revealed important attitudes and perceptions that influenced their decision to use the WIC program. Overall, women had a positive impression of the program but did not know its full service offerings. Focus group discussions, for example, revealed that most women were familiar with the infant formula and dairy products provided by WIC but few knew that WIC also offered many other nutritious foods and services they valued, such as individualized nutritional risk assessment and counseling, education classes, and immunizations.

Research also indicated several costs or barriers to program participation. One of the most formidable barriers was the embarrassment some women said they would feel if identified as a recipient of free food. For many, enrollment in WIC, which they viewed as a government welfare program, would "rob" them of their sense of self-sufficiency. Another reason women were reluctant to accept WIC benefits was the misperception that WIC program services were in short supply and should be limited to those with the greatest need. Some eligible women feared that their enrollment would displace other women and children whose needs were far greater than their own. This was especially true for those who believed that the program should be available only to those who cannot provide for themselves. While they did not think that it was shameful for people to accept help when it was truly justified, they felt that it would be wrong from them to enroll, because they were not destitute.

Other major barriers were created by confusion about WIC's eligibility criteria. Almost half of the survey respondents who were not enrolled in WIC did not recognize that they were automatically income eligible for WIC. Focus group discussions provided insight into the source of confusion. The most common misconceptions were that the family income had to be lower than theirs; they were not qualified if they or their husbands worked; and they were ineligible because they lived with relatives whose incomes were too high. Many believed that they were ineligible because they had been denied Food Stamps despite the fact that the Supplemental Nutrition Assistance Program has much stricter income guidelines than WIC.

Finally, some women did not enroll because of problems that friends and relatives had encountered as WIC recipients. Long waits at WIC clinics to obtain food cards and to listen to educational videotapes, rude treatment by WIC staff, lack of Spanish-speaking staff members, and rude treatment while redeeming WIC food vouchers at the grocery store were mentioned repeatedly. Together, these inconveniences and insensitive treatment represented an unacceptable "price" or barrier to participation. Nonenrollees did not want to encounter the shame that their friends and relatives felt because of being forced to wait what seemed like unnecessarily long periods of time and/or being spoken to discourteously. Instead, they chose to forego the benefits of the program in order to avoid being treated poorly.

Audience segmentation research made it possible to identify subgroups of women who had never enrolled and provided insights into the most effective ways to recruit them. For example, women who were employed, who had completed high school, and whose incomes were 135% to 185% of the federal poverty level were the least likely to be enrolled and the least likely to know that they were income eligible for WIC. Women in this segment also were the least likely to know that they were qualified. This segment was selected as an important target for outreach efforts designed to clarify eligibility requirements.

In the next phase, strategy development, research findings were used to develop a comprehensive social marketing plan. The portion of the plan targeting women who had never enrolled focused on countering misperceptions of the program's benefits. Outreach materials were designed to emphasize the nutrition education, health checkups, immunizations, and referrals that WIC provided. These materials featured the variety of nutritious foods WIC offers in an attempt to reframe WIC as a program that parents can be proud to use because it helps them raise healthy children.

The plan also included recommendations for lowering the price of participating in WIC. To make participation less embarrassing, the program's image was redefined from a "free food" or government assistance program to a health and nutrition program. In light of women's concerns about self-sufficiency, WIC's image was also reframed as a nutrition and health education program, "Helping Families Help Themselves," in which families can maintain their pride and self-esteem as they earn their WIC benefits and learn about nutrition and other ways to help their families.

Because many women did not know that they were eligible for the program, the marketing plan also emphasized ways to help families understand eligibility guidelines, streamline the certification process, and make it easier for health and social service professionals to refer eligible women. One television advertisement addressed the most common misperceptions about WIC eligibility, featuring a working father and his two daughters, a pregnant teen who lives with relatives, and a married woman as participants who are qualified for program benefits. During the ad, the narrator informs people that many families do not realize that they qualify for this valuable program and encourages people who do not qualify for Food Stamps, working families, and those living with relatives to call a toll-free line to find out if they are eligible.

Placement and promotional strategies were also designed for the Texas WIC program. Message design guidelines were developed to guide the creative team in preparing television, radio, and print messages consistent with the plan's overall goals. Audience segmentation results were used to determine the regions within the state, and specific stations, to air radio and television spots and purchase billboards. Audience segmentation results showing that whites or

Anglos were the most likely to believe that it is embarrassing to accept government assistance guided the decision to cast a family with these characteristics in a second television spot. This advertisement was designed to reposition or redefine the WIC program as a health and nutrition program that "brings lots to the table."

Finally, service delivery improvements were planned to make the program more consumer-friendly, making it possible to retain women who enrolled and to minimize the number of complaints participants made to other eligible families. A training program was designed to teach grocery store cashiers how to handle difficult WIC transactions while treating WIC participants respectfully. In addition, a permanent data collection procedure was designed for tracking program enrollment and program satisfaction. A summary of the Texas WIC Marketing Plan is displayed in Table 15.2.

Using the social marketing plan as a guide, Best Start social marketers, health department personnel, and an advertising agency then developed the messages, outreach materials, training programs, data collection instruments, and other resources needed to implement and evaluate the program. A key element in this phase was ensuring that each component was consistent with the overall marketing strategy. Marketing messages and mass media materials were rigorously pretested and redesigned until they proved to be effective. Communication materials included a new WIC logo, two television spots, three radio spots (each of which were in English and Spanish), billboards, a set of outreach brochures and posters, a community organizer's kit to facilitate coalition building at the local-agency level, several training modules, and data collection instruments for tracking and evaluating the program.

The Texas WIC program was launched in the fall of 1995. Approximately $250,000 was used to purchase television and radio air time and billboard space. Mass media and consumer education was augmented with other outreach efforts, service improvements, and other activities. To increase referrals from other social service programs and prenatal care providers, materials clarifying WIC services and eligibility guidelines and offering helpful suggestions were distributed to health providers and social service workers who service people eligible for WIC. User-friendly certification procedures were designed to help each new enrollee feel like a very important person in order to create a positive introduction to WIC, and the program was made more consumer-friendly by offering child-safe play areas, a peer-buddy system, decreased waiting times, new educational materials, and customer relations training for clinic staff and grocery store cashiers.

Finally, a permanent data collection system was designed to collect baseline data from new participants, regular participants, and program employees. These satisfaction surveys were designed to identify problems that affect satisfaction among these three groups and make midcourse revisions. Unfortunately, the Texas WIC Program has not continued to collect these data, and funds were not released for a formal evaluation of the program's impact. Program data, however, point to significant increases in the number of families who called the toll-free number for more information after the program was launched and, most important, the number of people participating in Texas WIC. The program's caseload grew from 542,000 in 1993 to almost 700,000 in 1998, and in 2007, the program served almost 1 million Texas families.

TABLE 15.2 The Texas WIC Social Marketing Plan

Major Components	Examples of Specific Strategies
Policy recommendations	1. Recognition for staff performance, including customer service awards. 2. Career growth opportunities for staff, with a clear career ladder structure. 3. Use of computers to communicate policy changes more effectively between state and local staff. 4. Revised appointment scheduling policies to improve clinic efficiency and create more "user-friendly" certification and food card issuance procedures (e.g., online, computerized policy manuals for staff).
Service delivery	1. Increased accessibility by offering WIC services at daycare centers, employers, grocery stores, and migrant camps and more flexible clinic hours (night, lunch time, and one Saturday per month). 2. Child-friendly clinics, where children can play, eat nutritious snacks, and learn about nutrition in child-proofed areas supervised by staff, paraprofessionals, and volunteers. 3. Peer-buddy system—paraprofessionals act as advocates/guides for participants waiting for clinic services, ensure that participants have required documentation, answer questions about certification and food cards, and give "smart shopping" tips. 4. Improvements in grocery store experiences with a new food card redemption system (fewer cards to be signed in the register) and a "products brochure" to depict allowable WIC foods for participants and serve as a reference for cashiers.
Training	1. Staff training and continuing education. 2. Grocery store cashier training program, videotape about customer service and the WIC transaction.
Nutrition education	1. Nutrition education facilitator training in interactive teaching skills to discuss nutrition and new, nontraditional WIC subjects (e.g., parenting, child development) issues with participants. 2. *Food and Family*, educational magazine for WIC participants.
Tracking system	1. Monitoring system to track participant satisfaction with the food package, nutrition education, food redemption, clinic service, and clinic environment and staff satisfaction with supervision, clinic environment, ability to provide WIC services, and participant contact. 2. Training for local agency directors in interpreting results and identifying and overcoming service delivery problems.
Health communication plan	1. Messages to reposition WIC's image to a comprehensive health and education program offering nutritious foods, screening, social support, and referral to other services, for example, through 30-second "Nutrition Tips" radio spots. 2. Messages to increase awareness of income eligibility criteria.
Community outreach	1. Community organizers' kit to assist local agency directors in working with program partners in increasing referrals of eligible families to WIC. 2. Kit includes outreach materials targeted to health professionals and eligible families.

SOURCE: From Bryant et al. (2001).

NOTE: This chart includes examples of the many strategies that have been developed for each component of the social marketing plan.

The first five components are designed to increase participant and staff satisfaction; the last two are intended to increase participant enrollment.

CRITICISMS AND CHALLENGES

While its use has increased dramatically over the past 20 years, social marketing faces many challenges before it can realize its full potential (Grier & Bryant, 2005). The most common include the following:

- *An overemphasis on interventions that "blame the victim"* (Wallack, 2002): In the past, many social marketing interventions were guilty of overrelying on communications to address knowledge, attitudes, and other intrapersonal factors. More recently, the field has responded to this criticism by placing more importance on community-level and broader societal-level factors that underlie health problems and by designing multilevel interventions to make the social environment more conducive to individual healthy behavior (Donovan & Henley, 2003).

- *Confusion between social marketing and social advertising or health communication:* Many public health professionals still apply the label social marketing to campaigns that rely exclusively on mass media messages to bring about change. Even when the promotional strategies are well designed, these programs do not qualify as social marketing because they have not segmented the audience or used consumer research to create a carefully integrated marketing plan based on the full marketing mix of product, price, and place, as well as promotion.

- *Failure to invest time and money on formative research needed to understand consumers' wants and needs:* While marketing research does not have to be expensive or complex, it is essential to understand how consumers view the product benefits, costs, placement, and promotion. Ideally, data already exist that provide the insights needed to create an integrated marketing plan, but all too often additional data must be collected.

- *Overuse of focus groups:* Focus groups can provide valuable insights into consumers' aspirations, fears, and perceptions of the product; but far too many social marketing programs have relied on them exclusively, failed to conduct them rigorously, and/or interpreted results inappropriately. Like all qualitative data collection methods, focus group results cannot be verified statistically or used to estimate the prevalence of views within a target population. A far better approach is to use a mix of qualitative and quantitative methods for audience segmentation and analyses.

- *Failure to segment populations and carefully select priority audiences:* Many public health professionals still hope to reach everyone with the same intervention. If they segment at all, they do so exclusively with demographic variables instead of more powerful behavioral and attitudinal characteristics.

- *Failure to rigorously evaluate social marketing interventions* (McDermott, 2003): As noted in the WIC case study, many public health agencies are reluctant to allocate funds for program evaluation.

CONCLUSION

Social marketing offers public health professionals an effective approach for developing programs to promote healthy behaviors. It is distinguished from other program-planning models by its use of the marketing conceptual framework (exchange theory and the 4 Ps), consumer orientation, reliance on formative research to understand consumers' desires and needs, and audience segmentation. Although social marketing often uses mass media to communicate with its target audiences, it should not be confused with health communication, social advertising, or educational approaches that simply create awareness of a behavior's health benefits or attempt to persuade people to change through motivational messages. Social marketers use data to identify the product benefits that are most attractive to target audiences, determine which costs will be acceptable and those that must be lowered, identify the best places to offer products, and design the best mix of promotional tactics to communicate with consumers and elicit behavior change.

Social marketing also offers public health a new institutional mind-set, one in which solutions to problems are solicited from consumers. An organization that adopts the social marketing mind-set continually evaluates and remakes itself so as to increase the likelihood that it will meet the needs of its ever-changing constituency. This mind-set makes social marketing an effective tool for increasing enrollment in public health programs and enables them to ensure continued satisfaction and program participation.

REFERENCES

Bagozzi, R. P. (1979). Toward a formal theory of marketing exchanges. In O. C. Ferrell, S. W. Brown, & C. W. Lamb Jr. (Eds.), *Conceptual and theoretical developments in marketing* (pp. 431–447). Chicago: American Marketing Association.

Bellows, L., Cole, K., & Anderson, J. (2006). Assessing characteristics, needs, and preferences of a secondary audience for the development of a bilingual parent component to the food friends social marketing campaign. *Social Marketing Quarterly, 12*(2), 43–57.

Bryant, C. A., Coreil, J., D'Angelo, S., Bailey, D., & Lazarov, M. (1992). A new strategy for promoting breastfeeding among economically disadvantaged women and adolescents. *NAACOG's Clinical Issues in Perinatal and Women's Health Issues: Breastfeeding, 3*(4), 723–730.

Bryant, C. A., Courtney, A. H., Baldwin, J. A., McDermott, R. J., Nickelson, J., & McCormack Brown, K. R. (2007). The VERB™ Summer Scorecard. In G. Hastings (Ed.), *The potential of social marketing: Why should the devil have all the best tunes?* (pp. 272–275). Oxford, UK: Elsevier.

Bryant, C. A., & Dunlevy, K. (2007). Social marketing: Why should the devil have all the best tunes? [Book review]. *Social Marketing Quarterly, 12*(2), 72–77.

Bryant, C. A., Kent, E., Brown, C., Bustillo, M., Blair, C., Lindenberger, J., et al. (1998). A social marketing approach to increase customer satisfaction with the Texas WIC Program. *Marketing Health Care Services, Winter,* 5–17.

Bryant, C. A., & Lindenberger, J. H. (2002). Increasing utilization in the Texas WIC Program. In P. Kotler, N. Robert, & N. Lee (Eds.), *Social marketing: Improving the quality of life* (pp. 190–194). Thousand Oaks, CA: Sage.

Bryant, C. A., Lindenberger, J. H., Brown, C., Kent, E., Schreiber, J. M., Bustillo, M., et al. (2001). A social marketing approach to increasing enrollment in a public health program: Case study of the Texas WIC Program. *Human Organization, 60*(3), 234–246.

Carroll, T. E., & Van Veen, L. (2002). Public health social marketing: The Immunise Australia program. *Social Marketing Quarterly, 8*(1), 55–61.

Coreil, J., Bryant, C. A., Westover, B., Bailey, D., & d'Angelo, S. (1995). Breastfeeding counseling by health care professionals: Client and provider views. *Journal of Human Lactation, 11,* 265–271.

Denniston, R. (2004). Planning, implementing, and managing an unprecedented, government-funded prevention communications initiative. *Social Marketing Quarterly, 10*(2), 7–27.

Deshpande, S. (2007). The challenges of using social marketing in India: The case of HIV/AIDS prevention. In G. Hastings (Ed.), *The potential of social marketing: Why should the devil have all the best tunes?* (pp. 297–301). Oxford, UK: Elsevier.

Dholakia, R. R., & Dholakia, N. (2001). Social marketing and development. In P. N. Bloom & G. T. Gundlach (Eds.), *Handbook of marketing and society* (pp. 486–505). Thousand Oaks, CA: Sage.

Donovan, R., & Henley, N. (2003). *Social marketing: Principles and practice.* East Hawthorn, Victoria, Australia: IP Communications.

Evans, W. D., Renaud, J., Blitstein, J., Hersey, J., Ray, S., Schieber, B., et al. (2007). Prevention effects of an anti-tobacco brand on adolescent smoking initiation. *Social Marketing Quarterly, 13*(2), 2–20.

Fox, M., Hamilton, W., & Lin, B. (2004). *Effects of food assistance and nutrition programs and health: Vol. 3. Literature review* (Food Assistance and Nutrition Research Report No. FANRR19-3). Retrieved September 26, 2007, from www.ers.usda.gov/Publications/FANRR19-3

Grier, S., & Bryant, C. A. (2005). Social marketing in public health. *Annual Reviews in Public Health, 26,* 6.1–6.21.

Harvey, P. D. (1999). *Let every child be wanted: How social marketing is revolutionizing contraceptive use around the world.* Westport, CT: Auburn House.

Hastings, G. (2007). *The potential of social marketing: Why should the devil have all the best tunes?* Oxford, UK: Elsevier.

Hicks, J. J. (2002). The truth. In P. Kotler, N. Robert, & N. Lee (Eds.), *Social marketing: Improving the quality of life* (pp. 48–50). Thousand Oaks, CA: Sage.

John, R., Kerby, S., & Landers, P. S. (2004). A market segmentation approach to nutrition education among low-income individuals. *Social Marketing Quarterly, 10*(3–4), 24–38.

Jones, S., & Hall, D. (2007). Be well, know your BGL: Australia's diabetes awareness campaign. In G. Hastings (Ed.), *The potential of social marketing: Why should the devil have all the best tunes?* (pp. 322–328). Oxford, UK: Elsevier.

Kotler, P., & Armstrong, G. (2001). *Principles of marketing* (9th ed.). Upper Saddle River, NJ: Prentice Hall.

Kotler, P., & Lee, N. (2007). *Social marketing: Influencing behaviors for good* (3rd ed.). Thousand Oaks, CA: Sage.

Kotler, P., Roberto, N., & Lee, N. (2002). *Social marketing: Improving the quality of life* (2nd ed.). Thousand Oaks, CA: Sage.

Lavack, A. M., Watson, L., & Markwart, J. (2007). Quit and win contests: A social marketing success story. *Social Marketing Quarterly, 13*(1), 31–52.

Lee, N., Spoeth, S., Smith, K., McElroy, L., Fraze, J. L., Robinson, A., et al. (2006). Encouraging African-American women to "Take Charge. Take the Test": The audience segmentation process for CDC's HIV testing social marketing campaign. *Social Marketing Quarterly, 13*(3), 16–28.

Lefebvre, C. (2001). Theories and models in social marketing. In P. N. Bloom & G. T. Gundlach (Eds.), *Handbook of marketing and society* (pp. 506–518). Thousand Oaks, CA: Sage.

Lefebvre, C., Doner, L. Johnston, C., Loughery, K., Balch, G. I., & Sutton, S. M. (1995). Use of database marketing and consumer-based health communication in message design: An example from the Office of Cancer Communications "5 a Day for Better Health" program. In E. Maibach & R. L. Parrot (Eds.), *Designing health messages. Approaches from communication theory and public health practice* (pp. 217–246). Thousand Oaks, CA: Sage.

Lindenberger, H., & Bryant, C. A. (2000). Promoting breastfeeding in the WIC program: A social marketing case study. *American Journal of Health Behavior, 24*(1), 53–60.

McCormack Brown, K., Bryant, C. A., Forthofer, M. S., Perrin, K. M., Quinn, G. P., Wolper, B. S., et al. (2000). Florida cares for women. *American Journal of Health Behavior, 24*(1), 44–52.

McDermott, R. J. (2003). Essentials of evaluating social marketing campaigns for health behavior change. *Health Education Monograph Series, 20,* 31–38.

McDermott, R. J., Berends, K., McCormack Brown, K., Agron, P., Black, K. M., & Pitt Barnes, S. (2005). Impact of the California Project LEAN school board member social marketing campaign. *Social Marketing Quarterly, 11*(2), 18–40.

McKenzie-Mohr, D., & Smith, W. A. (1999). *Fostering sustainable behavior: An introduction to community-based social marketing.* Gabriola Island, British Columbia, Canada: New Society.

Monaghan, P., Bryant, C. A., Baldwin, J. A., Zhu, Y., Ibrahimou, B., Lind, J. D., et al. (in press). Using community-based prevention marketing to improve farm worker safety. *Social Marketing Quarterly.*

National Social Marketing Center. (2007). *NSM Center work plan.* Retrieved September 30, 2007, from www.nsms.org.uk/public/default.aspx?PageID=7

Prochaska, J. O., DiClemente, C. C., & Norcross, J. C. (1992). In search of how people change: Applications to addictive behaviors. *American Psychologist, 47*(9), 1102–1114.

Rothschild, M. L., Mastin, B., Karsten, C., & Miller, T. (2003). *The road crew final report: A demonstration of the use of social marketing to reduce alcohol-impaired driving by individuals age 21 through 34.* Retrieved August 15, 2008, from the Wisconsin Department of Transportation Web site, www.dot.wisconsin.gov/library/publications/topic/safety/roadcrew.pdf

Siegel, M., & Lotenberg, L. D. (2007). *Marketing public health: Strategies to promote social change.* Boston: Jones & Bartlett.

Wallack, L. (2002). Public health, social change, and media advocacy. *Social Marketing Quarterly, 8,* 25–31.

Wong, F., Huhman, M., Heitzler, C., Asbury, L., Bretthauer-Mueller, R., McCarthy, S., et al. (2004). *VERB™: A social marketing campaign to increase physical activity among youth. Preventing chronic disease* [Serial online]. Retrieved November 13, 2007, from www.cdc.gov/pcd/issues/2004/jul/04_0043.htm

16

Approaches to
Policy and Advocacy

Linda M. Whiteford

This chapter presents an interdisciplinary perspective on the use of social and behaviorally based research to provide the foundations for effective advocacy and resultant policy change. It is written by a medical anthropologist with master's degrees in public health and anthropology, a doctorate in cultural anthropology, and years of research in the health arena. The perspective discussed in the chapter combines the theoretical frameworks of medical ecology and the political economy of health. The three case studies that form the core of the chapter demonstrate the power of interdisciplinary research and its applicability to the world of policy and advocacy. In addition, the research illustrates the importance of multilevel frameworks that incorporate both the physical and the sociopolitical environments in public health interventions. It draws on research conducted in Latin America and the Caribbean, included to show how research can provide information for advocacy used to effect policy. At first glance, the three case studies may appear to be disparate and unconnected. The topics are varied, as are the locations. The first case study

Author's Note: This chapter includes vignettes based on research conducted with the following people and made possible by the funding and support of the following funding and academic institutions: Environmental Health Project and May Yacoob, Carmen Laspina, and Mercedes Torres; Center for Disaster Management and Humanitarian Assistance, with Graham Tobin, Carmen Laspina, and Hugo Yepes. The Cuban primary health care study was made possible by private grants and with the support of the Department of Anthropology at the University of South Florida; more details are presented in the book coauthored by Laurence Branch, *Primary Health Care in Cuba: The Other Revolution*. The vignette used here is adapted from this book. Thanks also are due to Cecilia Vindrola Padros for her help with the bibliography.

follows an attempt to curtail a cholera epidemic in northern South America. The second study follows families in Ecuador being forced to evacuate their homes and communities because of the imminent danger of a volcano exploding and killing them. The third study looks at the Cuban development of an innovative and effective primary health care (PHC) model.

What do the case studies share, and how do they help us understand how research can shape policy? What can we learn from them about the social and behavioral foundations of public health? One point each of the case studies demonstrates is that research objectives and applications need to be identified as the research is being designed, not later. Research aimed to shape policy must recognize its potential target audiences and make sure to collect data that are meaningful to those audiences, as well as data that will expand members' ways of thinking. If one is hoping to shape, for instance, disaster response policy, data must be collected about such actual occurrences, documenting both the strengths and the failures of such policy as they occur in real time, with real people, and with real options. In the second Case Study, Disaster Response in Ecuador, we followed people who had been evacuated and resettled, interviewed them, and interviewed public officials, the Civil Defense authorities, and members of the local, state, and national governments. But what we brought to the discussion that had not been provided before were the words and opinions, hopes, and losses of the people resettled, and the policymakers wanted to hear what they had to say.

Too often, policymakers are unaware of the local realities and the real-time needs of people affected by the policies they make. Moreover, policymakers rarely have the time (or the skills) to conduct the kind of fieldwork that would provide them with that information. That is why researchers who are interested in shaping policy are in an enviable position to supply policymakers and advocates with critically needed information.

Each of the three cases provides a different story, but they all share a commitment to research criteria that makes them useful for both advocacy and policymaking. They are all multidisciplinary, bilateral, and multisite. In addition, they all highlight the importance of simultaneous local and global involvement, training, and monitoring, and they all are based on a careful review of current literature in their areas and the expansion of the research questions initially derived from that review. And last, perhaps most important, they all return to their various constituencies—the community, the state, the neighborhood, the agency or organization, and the intellectual discipline—research results in usable and appropriate forms.

CASE STUDY Cholera in Ecuador

The first case shows how research that incorporates participants from various stakeholder or interest groups increases the likelihood of the results being used to shape advocacy or policy. In addition, it demonstrates the power of participatory research methods. In 1991, an epidemic of cholera began in Peru and for 2 years spread across South America. Before it was over, more than 9,000 people had died and many more had been sickened by it (Whiteford, 1993; Whiteford et al., 1999). Cholera is an acute intestinal infection with a short incubation period that produces an enterotoxin causing copious amounts of watery diarrhea. If left untreated, cholera can quickly result in severe dehydration and death. It is particularly deadly among children and the elderly, those who are immunologically compromised, or anyone who is nutritionally or otherwise physically stressed. It has been called "the blue death" because patients nearing death from cholera have been known to turn a shade of blue or gray from the loss of fluids circulating in their bodies (Kiple, 1993).

Cholera holds a significant place in the history of understanding disease transmission due to John Snow's classic 1853 study of the cholera outbreak in London (DeSalle, 1999). Snow demonstrated that cholera was a waterborne disease by removing the handle of the Broad Street water pump (and thus making access to the water in that system unavailable), thereby stopping the spread of cholera along the lines of that water system. It was not until later that it was learned how the toxin was introduced into the drinking water (it was seepage from a contaminated cesspool that leaked the cholera bacteria into the Broad Street water system), but Snow was able to show that cholera was transmitted through contaminated water.

Waterborne diseases such as cholera are intimately affected by human activities. These activities may be related to development (dam building and associated human resettlement), inadequate water and sanitation infrastructure (open or undisinfected water systems, human or animal defecation in or near water systems), or even labor migration (returning migrants can re-infect water systems). In addition, patterns of water usage are shaped by cultural beliefs, gender-based labor patterns, history, and geography. Once the cholera bacteria is introduced into the human host by the ingestion of water contaminated with human or animal feces or urine containing the pathogen, the means to disrupt transmission will depend on factors such as the location (urban or rural population), population size (concentrated or dispersed), access to resources (water and sanitation infrastructure), cultural identity (beliefs about disease transmission, animals, the environment), and power (status, agency) of the people experiencing the outbreak.

In the Ecuadorian case, the governmental and international health authorities were able to control the outbreak in the urban centers within the first 15 months of the initial epidemic through commonly understood public health measures: improved hygiene through waste disposal and hand washing. However, the rural, dispersed, and indigenous communities of the Andean highlands continued to suffer from ongoing deaths due to the disease. The Environmental Health Project (EHP), the water and health component of the Camp, Dresser, and McKee (CDM) company, agreed to work with the Ecuadorian government to study the situation and make recommendations to reduce the continuing cholera-induced suffering in those communities. Along with May Yacoob, a medical anthropologist working for EHP, a field team was put together to conduct research on five highland communities in southern Ecuador that had continuing high levels of cholera. I was the Team Leader representing EHP. We created a national team composed of a physician from the Ecuadorian Ministry of Health (Dr. Carmen Laspina) and an Ecuadorian psychologist trained in nonformal education (Dr. Mercedes Torres). With May Yacoob in the United States and the three of us working in the field, we began the project.

Ecuador is one of the smallest countries in South America, located in the northwest between its larger and more powerful neighbors, Colombia and Peru. Ecuador straddles the equator (hence, its name), situated in both the northern and the southern hemispheres. Geographically limited

(260,000 sq. km), it encompasses both an extraordinary natural biodiversity of birds and plants and a rich cultural diversity.

Indigenous cultures such as the Shuar, Chachis, and Achuar compose some of the more than 14 distinctive ethnic groups (Perrottet, 1993). Most travelers to Ecuador know the two primary cities—Quito, the Andean capital between the two cordilleras of volcanoes that create the "spine" running from the north to the south of Ecuador, and Guayaquil, the large coastal city on the Pacific side of the country. Other travelers know the Amazon in the south or the famous weaving center, Otovalo, in the north. While the cool, high mountains of the Andes attract many visitors, the lush and fascinating Amazon region draws others. Birders and hikers from around the world visit the Galapagos, Ecuador's offshore islands, with unlimited fascination.

As a secondary center of the Spanish Empire, Ecuador never experienced the degree of glory or endured the hardships that Peru and Colombia did, but its customs and architecture reflect many cultural and physical inheritances from the Spanish occupation. Along with these, Ecuador adopted beliefs about European superiority, with the result that indigenous groups are among the most economically deprived in the country. They live in the remote regions with limited access to resources, including water and sanitation. The 20 townships where the epidemic continued to rage were in five states, two along the Pacific coast and three inland, in the highlands.

The three mountain states with the highest ongoing rates of cholera were Chimborazo, Cotopaxi, and Imbabura; they also have the largest concentration of indigenous people in Ecuador. These are states rich in indigenous traditions, festivals, rituals, and cultural beliefs and practices. All five states share high levels of poverty and the structural violence maintained by distance, both geographic and social, from power. The three mountainous states suffered also because their population was predominately indigenous, rendering them targets for prejudice and further isolating them from access to resources.

The methodology we employed brought three levels of teams to work together: what we called the national team; a regional team composed of representatives from various non-governmental, governmental, and private agencies working in the region; and a local team of members of the community. The teams were selected to represent those groups that were stakeholders, with a special interest in the area. Individuals were invited to join the teams so that we could learn from them about their work, to train them in methodologies that they could later employ (such as community mapping), and to make them the repositories of the "institutional knowledge" of the project. Our goals were (1) to use local and EHP teams in order to identify cholera-related adult behaviors in high-risk communities, with the objective of isolating behaviors and beliefs associated with potential increased risk of cholera; (2) for all three teams to gather and analyze data on environmental and domestic health behaviors; (3) to develop and implement local interventions to change high-risk behaviors; (4) to establish a locally controlled monitoring system; and (5) to train people from the local and regional teams to monitor and document ongoing activities.

We developed a local health intervention model, the Community-Based Participatory Intervention (CPI) (see the References for more details on CPI.). We trained 55 individuals in community education techniques and leadership skills, conducted ethnographic and epidemiologic research, and designed and led community-based interventions (Whiteford, Laspina, & Torres, 1996).

The project successfully identified beliefs and behaviors implicated in the spread of cholera and brought about a sustained reduction of cholera in the two project states. Using a critical medical anthropology perspective, the teams identified several actions that directly and indirectly facilitated the spread of cholera: defecation in fields or other areas close to living and eating activities; substandard hygiene related to water; water insecurity; consumption of food prepared by street vendors as well as the conditions in which they served food; food preparation and distribution during religious and community festivals; and contact with migrants returning from endemically infected coastal areas. In addition, we identified contributing environmental conditions, such as the disposal of hospital waste in open canals from which downstream residents drew their drinking water.

Research that has policy as an aim must also be cognizant of the larger context in which policymakers operate. In the cholera example, neoliberal global pressures and their resultant policies shaped the larger context in which any sustained cholera control would occur. In the late 1990s, as national governments turned their attention to global trade, they further excluded the marginalized, rural, indigenous communities from basic services. The decentralization of responsibilities often associated with neoliberal reforms frequently resulted in an increased burden on local communities. Such communities found themselves responsible for the provision of clean water or sanitation—infrastructures that the central government had failed to establish. Placing the responsibility on local communities to provide the necessary resources for developing or maintaining infrastructure made adequate water and sanitation impossible for the poor.

In the case of the cholera epidemic in Ecuador, the beliefs and behaviors of individuals in the most highly affected communities were relatively easy to identify. People recognized ways to change their own behaviors in order to reduce the likelihood of cholera, provided they could pay for soap, chlorine, and household water storage tanks. With resources made available through project funds, five target communities in two states (Chimborazo and Cotopaxi) were successful in controlling cholera and sustaining the reduction. The participatory methodology and the investment of stakeholders allowed the communities to identify geophysical barriers to care, such as population dispersion, the lack of piped water or sanitary systems, distance from urban centers and their resources, and the need for labor migration because of the lack of local jobs.

In addition, the perspective incorporated the importance of local beliefs and actions that became the framework for changes identified and supported by the community, such as increased hand washing, disposal of fecal materials away from water storage, and awareness of disease transmission routes such as common bowls for food sharing either at ritual occasions or on the street.

A final, and initially unanticipated, effect of the project was the development of leadership among both young people and women—groups traditionally excluded from leadership positions in traditional Quechua societies. When I returned to these communities on another project 10 years later, I learned that two of the community leaders from our cholera-reduction project had gone on to complete college and then returned to their communities as leaders, and cholera was no longer present in any of the five research communities. The data we generated; the analysis we conducted; and, in particular, having teams drawn from the community, statewide institutions, and the Ministries of Health and Education resulted in findings that were able to inform local, regional, and national policies. The participatory methodology employed was written into education and health plans, and the participants—from all three levels—continued to employ the participatory methodologies in their work. The participants became advocates, and the research was incorporated into regional and national policy.

CASE STUDY   Disaster Research in Ecuador

The second case study demonstrates the power of local knowledge and its necessity to inform policy. Resettling populations to remove them from hazards is an oft-used strategy, preferred by policymakers and disaster managers alike. Populations often settle near rivers (that may flood), near volcanoes (that may explode), in valleys (that may experience mudslides), or near oceans (with tsunamis) for reasons related to the quality of the soil, the fish in the ocean, and the temperate climate in the valley. Since governments cannot move the ocean, the volcano, or the river, they often choose to relocate the people who have settled near the hazard. Once relocated, the resettled people are rarely queried about their experience; hence, policymakers have little or no information about what happens to people once they are moved. Without that information, policymakers only know that the people are no longer in the line of danger, but they know nothing about how the loss of home, the disruption of social networks, and the loss of employment affects the lives of those resettled.

In October 1999, government authorities in Ecuador, in consultation with the director of the Geophysical Institute (H. Yepes, personal communication, February 4, 2000) decided that the danger of an eruption from the Tungurahua volcano and the possible consequential loss of life necessitated an immediate evacuation of the communities surrounding the tourist community of Baños, Ecuador. Some residents who were being affected by ash or threatened by mudflows had already voluntarily evacuated (United Nations Office for the Coordination of Human Affairs [OCHA], 1999). The evacuation became mandatory on October 15, 1999; people residing in the hazard risk zone were given approximately 36 hours to leave the area. Because the civilian Civil Defense force was unable to force their friends and neighbors to leave, the military enforced the evacuation (Cable News Network [CNN], 1999). In the 36 hours that elapsed between the announcement of the evacuation and the closure of the community, people left, resisted, hid, were found, and were forced out. Those least able as well as those least willing to leave felt the greatest effect of the military force. An estimated 26,000 people were moved to more than 60 locations, including private homes, hostels, and government shelters in the provinces of Tungurahua and Chimborazo, where some remained for more than a year. According to the Ecuadorian Red Cross, the Civil Defense set up 125 sites as temporary shelters, and the official count of evacuees in shelters rose to 2,443 early in November (Cruz Roja Ecuatoriana, 1999a, 1999b).

The presence of a potential disaster does not necessarily imply that either the political authorities or the local populations will take the threat seriously, particularly in terms of planning to leave their homes and belongings. Therefore, when an evacuation is enforced, people are often in a state of shock, frightened, disbelieving, and ultimately unprepared to leave. During the 1999 evacuation, people first sought to find their family members so that they could evacuate together and then tried to find family or friends living outside the evacuated areas to whom they could go for shelter. They piled into cars, stuffed their belongings onto trucks, locked up their houses, and moved in with family members in Ambato, Riobamba, or even as far away as Quito. That is, if they had cars or trucks and if they had families who would let them live with them. Many of the middle- and upper-class Bañenos left in the first 24 hours of the evacuation because they could locate their family members by telephone, they could contact friends and families in other cities to ask them to take them in, and they could move their family and belongings in their own private cars and trucks.

Others were not so fortunate; their family members may have been day laborers working away from home and not accessible by telephone. Thus, to evacuate together, families had to wait until each of their members heard about the evacuation and came home. If they could find others to take them in, and public transportation to get there, then they went to stay with friends in other cities. More often than not, by the time the family was reunited, the evacuation was well under way and public transportation was not available. Private trucks rented for the trip went back and forth along the single narrow road between Baños and Ambato (an hour's journey each way) ferrying people and their few belongings. Within hours, the road was clogged with people trying to leave either on foot or in the few available vehicles. In the last hours before the military closed the road, military trucks picked up those who were still in and around Baños. Many could not find family or friends to take them in, some were evacuated to government shelters, and others were resettled. It is clear that the poorest of the poor seem to have disappeared, and many have not returned to the hazard area. Official records of the number of people relocated in shelters or resettled to other areas are unclear, but in the most rural areas it appears that the poorest went farther into the countryside. They were not found in either the government shelters or in the resettled areas.

While the government made an attempt to resettle people where their children could continue their schooling, the resettled individuals were away from the temperate and lush ecological zone of Baños. Some from Baños were relocated to the community of Quimiag, located in the high sierra, where it is cold, damp, and moist for most of the year. Local Quimiag families contributed housing to the evacuees, but the resettled families had little furniture, no heat, and few blankets. In addition, the resettled families had lost their household gardens and chickens, as well as their neighbors and extended families—traditional means of support in times of crisis. Their kids got sick more often than kids from local families, who were not resettled, and resentment gradually grew. Local Quimiag residents came to believe that the resettled families were receiving "unfair" amounts of support from international and national aid societies, while the resettled families became suspicious of their nonresettled neighbors.

Resettled families had no recourse to settle disputes, a situation epitomized by the apparent generosity of an absentee landlord who offered the resettlement group his land on a steep hillside to plant potatoes. The resettled families called for a community workgroup (*minga*), and men, women, children, pregnant women, and women with babies on their backs or at their breasts all worked the hillside. After several weeks of cultivating the mountain slope and terracing the fields, they planted the potato crop. They were successful. Their crop came in, and the families anticipated food for the winter and potatoes to sell. However, before they could harvest the crop, the landlord took back his land and the crop with it. The community had nothing to harvest, nothing to eat, and no seed potatoes for the following year. They were living on borrowed land with no rights and no official paper to support their claims. Sadly enough, the story is neither apocryphal nor unique to this resettled group.

Agricultural practices in the area were also seriously compromised by hazardous events, including volcanic ash. For example, the water supply for agriculture was usually taken from a local canal. However, in January 2000, flow of water in the canal was interrupted due to a landslide. The evacuees were told by agronomists that there would be no water from this source for at least 6 months. They then began to collect rainfall and were determined to find water from another source, by whatever means: *"Tenemos que encontrar agua de cualquier manera."*

What emerges is a picture of the poor bearing the greatest burden for a social policy that unfairly targets them because of their relative inability to resist. The effects of the resettlement policy, so favored by emergency planners, is not equally distributed among various groups within the population but rather is concentrated among the working poor. It is the poor who, because they were dependent on public transportation, had to rely on the military to move them from their homes to a government-sponsored alternative shelter. It is they who find themselves being resettled rather than staying with friends or even in shelters. And it is their children who suffered the most negative health consequences. Children whose families were relocated were sick more often than those in shelters.

Furthermore, children in the resettled communities did not have the same access to health care as did children in shelters. The Provincial Health Directorship in the two states to which families were evacuated in 1999 took active responsibility for health in the government-sponsored shelters, particularly that of children. In contrast, those families resettled in small communities scattered throughout the two states did not receive the same level of attention. They were left to visit local clinics, health posts, or other places if they were sick enough and someone could be found to take them.

Resettling families following an emergency evacuation, therefore, can have unhealthy consequences, especially for the children. They are removed from their extended kin, from schoolmates, and from their routines. They are put into situations where their families are experiencing extreme stress as they struggle to settle somewhere new, find economically productive ways to support their families, and adjust to new surroundings, people, and expectations.

The data strongly suggest that resettlement is an unhealthy policy for children in many aspects. They fall between the various systems established to protect the youngest and most vulnerable. With scarce resources available, the public health system focuses its attention on the concentration of people evacuated into shelters, leaving scattered, resettled families to fend for themselves.

Emergency evacuation and resettlement policies can have unhealthy consequences, and furthermore, they can exacerbate already existing social cleavages. Not all people are resettled; usually, only those without other resources are identified for resettlement. The Ecuadorian research also suggested that there are ways to improve the resettlement experience that are generalizable and should be of concern for public health workers.

These data can be used to provide information to advocates and to facilitate improvements in public health policies. They are aimed at improving the health of those resettled by reducing the stress associated with the experience, and rather than making resettlement a punishment for those without access to other resources, resettlement could be a positive option. To make it such an option, the following steps should be taken: (1) town meetings and discussions should be held to inform community members of hazard risks and the remedial options available, including the resettlement of families in the event of disaster; (2) resettlement strategies should be made available to all members of the community at risk, especially when confronted with the potential of catastrophic disasters; (3) resettlement sites should be found similar to the site being vacated so that lifestyle, agricultural practices, and the like are transferable; (4) resettlement policies should include specific attention to the ongoing health care of the families after they have been relocated; (5) resettled families should be provided legitimate ways to gain ownership of the land on which they are resettled; and (6) government protection should be provided to families after they have moved.

The public health lessons learned from this analysis are important for community activists and advocates, disaster mitigation planners, civil defense authorities, and governmental policymakers. The lessons are that social and behavioral research should help policymakers situate their policies in the lived realities of daily life as well as in the larger political and economic context. For the researcher, this means that we must understand the social and cultural cleavages in the fabric of the society being studied and document the distribution of power in the society. Failure to recognize and be cognizant of the constraints and possibilities imposed by these contexts limits the efficaciousness and applicability of any recommendation, whether to policymakers or advocates.

Policies that are developed without input from the affected population or uninformed by the lived realities of those affected are doomed to failure. In the case just described, the researchers worked with and shared study findings with diverse stakeholders, including local, regional, and national politicians and policymakers in Ecuador; the international community of disaster management; the authorities in the Ecuadorian Civil Defense and Geophysical Institute, the Ministry of Health; and our colleagues in our professional disciplines. As a result, the research findings have been used by advocates to help shape civil defense and evacuation policies.

CASE STUDY   Health Research in Cuba

The third case study is about a model of health care, particularly PHC. The aim of this study was not to shape Cuban health care policy but rather to provide information to policymakers in international health care agencies and national policymakers outside Cuba. To do that, data were gathered from a variety of sources, including international health agencies such as the World Health Organization (WHO), the Pan American Health Organization (PAHO), the United Nations (UN), the Population Reference Bureau (PRB), and the Population Council, because their data are generally accepted and considered reliable. Those data were then triangulated with extensive statstical reports provided by the Cuban government. In addition,

I spent periods of time in Cuba over a span of 12 years interviewing health professionals, clients, and visiting health posts in various Cuban cities. A significant component of this long-term project was working collaboratively with Cuban social scientists and medical practitioners. Because entry to Cuba is restricted for U.S. citizens, it is important to note that all this research was legally conducted with the appropriate permissions from U.S. and Cuban government officials. The research resulted in numerous academic publications and presentations at professional meetings. However, trying to reach policymakers required another form of information presentation. To address this issue, my colleague Laurence Branch and I translated our research into a book designed for policymakers.

The resultant book, *Primary Health Care in Cuba: The Other Revolution* (Whiteford & Branch, 2007), was written so that students, researchers, practitioners, and policymakers interested in public health could see how one country put into practice an effective public, PHC system. Public health researchers have long been concerned both with the Alma Ata Declaration of 1978, which set forth the PHC agenda, and with the many failures to sustain PHC effectively since then (Heggenhougen, 1984; Janes, 2004; Morgan, 1990, 2001; Walsh & Warren, 1979; Whiteford 1990). Equally significant in the current public health literature is the role of equity, both relative and absolute, as a predictor of health outcomes, as noted in Chapter 3 (Heggenhougen, 2005; Wilkerson, 1992, 1996; Wilkerson & Marmot, 2003). The Cuban experience offers important lessons regarding the reduction of socioeconomic disparities and improvements in health status (Pardo, Márquez López, & Rojas Ochoa, 2005).

The following case study highlights the Cuban PHC system as an example of a successful translation of policy into practice. How do we begin to understand Cuba and its ability to produce a PHC system that some argue is second to none in its coverage and continuity of care? The Cuban model of PHC depends on both governmental and citizen participation, an extensive network of family medicine practitioners, widespread preventive services, and epidemiologic surveillance. There have been significant and continuous improvements in mortality and morbidity rates for the Cuban population, particularly for those living in the rural areas. The most significant improvements occurred in the areas of infant, child, and maternal health and the control and eradication of some infectious and contagious diseases. To understand how Cuba was able to succeed in increased distribution and access to health care while reducing disease rates, we need to review the evolution of the Cuban PHC model.

The 1959 Revolution, the subsequent Soviet economic support, the U.S. embargo against trade with Cuba, and Castro's longevity and unflagging commitment to public health as a basic human right each separately and together have shaped the development of health policy in Cuba. As Chomsky (2000), Feinsilver (1993), and others have noted, the development of the Cuban health care system was shaped by three assumptions that were central to the Revolution: (1) Health was the responsibility of the state; (2) health was a social as well as a biological issue; and (3) health was a national priority, requiring participation from all sectors of the government and civil society. Added to this list, as Chomsky notes, is the fact that Cuba refused to accept the concept that less economically developed countries could not support primary and preventive medicine while simultaneously supporting tertiary or hospital-based care (p. 333). This refusal to concede responsibility for health care allowed Cuba to create a complex health care system comparable with those in the more developed world rather than relying exclusively on primary care and referring patients to other countries for more advanced care.

In 1962, the Cuban government introduced an innovative form of municipal polyclinic, using the multispecialty health center as the basic building block for ambulatory care. The polyclinics, staffed by a general-practice physician, a nurse, an obstetrician/gynecologist, a pediatrician, and a social worker (Feinsilver, 2002), were charged with providing health care for workplaces, child care centers, homes, and neighborhoods.

These municipal polyclinics became the core of the nascent Cuban PHC model. They were charged with providing health screening; conducting vaccination campaigns, blood drives, and neighborhood cleanup activities (especially in relation to mosquito-borne disease, since these cleanup activities were actually vector control drives); and organizing community participation through community-based social organizations. The polyclinic model that came before the family doctor program emphasized technological interventions and biomedical approaches—lifestyle issues and behavioral medicine were given a low priority, with little attention being paid to family and community life (Iatridis, 1990). While these aims and emphases may not appear unusual, as they are common practices in many places, the model did not meet the goals set by the Cuban government. The government wanted vigorous local involvement, significant attention to the social factors influencing health, and an overt and articulated focus on improving lifestyle choices for health.

Building on a series of assessments that showed dissatisfaction, in 1984, the government introduced the *family doctor model.* The assessments showed that both patients and practitioners felt that while the community medicine model was an improvement over the previous model, it provided unequal quality of care—polyclinics that served as training centers for health practitioners provided better-quality care than nonteaching polyclinics. Social factors contributing to health continued to be undervalued, while biological/technological approaches and interventions for health and illness were considered primary (Novás & Sacasas, 1989).

The family doctor program, as the name implies, put doctor and nurse teams into communities throughout Cuba, where they were responsible for the health of the families in their neighborhoods. The government placed health posts throughout the country and built above them an apartment for the doctor's family. In addition to providing housing and the health post itself, the program explicitly tied the medical team to the community. Teams were held responsible for the health outcomes of people in their catchment areas. Perhaps the most fundamental change initiated by the family doctor program was this innovation of having a doctor and nurse live in the neighborhood for which they were responsible and the identification of a geographically defined area with approximately 120 to 150 designated families (Feinsilver, 2002; Gilpin, 1991; Whiteford, 1998b, 2000). Because residential mobility is restricted in Cuba, the family doctor program personnel got to know the people in their assigned area. Unlike clinics in other parts of the world, where targeted audiences are defined by their income, age, or pathology (e.g., pediatric practices or infectious disease specialty clinics), the medical team in a family doctor program was assigned to cover the health care needs of a population by their geographic location.

Part of the program's continuous-care regimen was attention to ongoing health problems, assessment and risk evaluation, and observing people in their behaviors outside the clinical setting. Rather than seeing people only when they came into the clinic for treatment, as is commonly the case elsewhere, the doctor-nurse team observed people in their everyday lives. This allowed medical practitioners to assess behavioral risks as well as medical complaints, to observe lifestyle patterns, and to intercede before conditions required hospitalization (Whiteford, 1998a, 1998b, 2000).

While the Cuban case is clearly used to demonstrate the success of its PHC model, I am not suggesting that any policymaker simply replicate the model in another country. The Cuban model is idiosyncratically Cuban. What makes the model work in Cuba is the complex response to Cuban culture, history, and political organization, and even to the U.S. embargo against Cuba. The take-away lessons generated from this case are that expensive medical technology is not necessary for effective community-based preventive care, that contradictions within a system are inevitable and can be useful, and that the collaborative roles of the state and the community are necessary for the health of the public.

CONCLUSION

These three cases show how research employing theories, methods, and analysis from the social and behavioral sciences can be used to shape policy. Policymakers have little time to conduct research, gather data, or conduct analyses, but their policies depend on these functions. Data incorporating an understanding of how life is lived, as well as how it is measured, are critical to the design of useful policies that can be translated into effective and sustainable programs.

As the Ecuador case shows, public health practitioners were successful in stemming the cholera epidemic in the urban areas, but without information grounded in social and behavioral research, they struggled with understanding the continued emergence of the disease in the rural indigenous areas. In the second case study, Ecuadorian governmental officials and members of the Civil Defense used their knowledge of effective ways to reduce community vulnerability by evacuating communities, but they failed to account for the importance of "home" and "place" to those evacuated. In our final case, that of PHC in Cuba, public health officials did understand the significance of having a medical practitioner living in the neighborhood to whom the residents could turn in times of need or even just with questions. Having a trusted and reliable member of the community who was responsible—along with the community itself—for the health of its members resulted in improved health outcomes.

Research that incorporates historical, cultural, and environmental processes is crucial in the transformation of "fantasy" policies into real-world and applied practices. And that is, after all, an important aim of effective public health.

REFERENCES

Cable News Network. (1999). *Evacuations ordered as Ecuadorian volcano threatens* [Electronic version]. Retrieved October 17, 1999, from www.cnn.com/WORLD/americas/9910/17/ecuador.volcano/index.html

Chomsky, A. (2000). The threat of a good example: Health and revolution in Cuba. In J. Y. Kim, J. V. Miller, A. Irwin, & J. Gershman (Eds.), *Dying for growth: Global inequality and the health of the poor* (pp. 331–357). Monroe, ME: Common Courage Press.

Cruz Roja Ecuatoriana. (1999a, October). *Un nuevo volcán amenaza Ecuador* (Ecuador: Informe Especial). Quito, Republic of Ecuador: Author.

Cruz Roja Ecuatoriana. (1999b, November). *Erupciones de los volcanes Guagua Pichincha y Tungurahua* (Ecuador: Informe Especial No. 5). Quito, Republic of Ecuador: Author.

DeSalle, R. (1999). *Epidemic! The world of infectious disease.* New York: The New Press.

Feinsilver, M. (1993). *Healing the masses: Cuban health politics at home and abroad.* Berkeley: University of California Press.

Feinsilver, M. (2002). Three decades of health reform: 1960–1990. In L. Barberia, A. Castro, & D. Nemser (Eds.), *Seminar on Cuban health system: Its evolution, accomplishments and challenges—December 11, 2001* (pp. A21–A25). Cambridge, MA: David Rockefeller Center for Latin American Studies. Retrieved October 4, 2005, from www.medanthro.net/docs/castro_cuba.pdf

Gilpin, M. (1991). Update—Cuba: On the road to a family medicine nation. *Journal of Public Health Policy, Spring,* 83–103.

Heggenhougen, H. K. (1984). Will primary health care efforts be allowed to succeed? *Social Science and Medicine, 19*(3), 217–224.

Heggenhougen, H. K. (2005). The epidemiology of inequity: Will research make a difference? *Norsk Epidemiologi, 15*(2), 127–132.

Iatridis, D. (1990). Cuba's health care policy: Prevention and active community participation. *Social Work, 35*(1), 29.

Janes, C. R. (2004). Going global in century XXI: Medical anthropology and the new primary health care. *Human Organization, 63*(4), 457–472.

Kiple, K. F. (Ed.). (1993). *The Cambridge world history of human disease.* Berkeley: Cambridge University Press.

Morgan, L. M. (1990). International politics and primary health care in Costa Rica. *Social Science and Medicine, 30*(2), 211–219.

Morgan, L. M. (2001). Community participation in health: Perpetual allure, persistent challenge. *Health Policy and Planning, 16*(3), 221–230.

Novás, J. D., & Fernández Sarcasas, J. A. (1989). From municipal polyclinics to family doctor-and-nurse teams. *Revista Cubano de General Integral, 5*(4), 556–564.

Pardo, C., Márquez López, M., & Rojas Ochoa, F. (2005). Human development and equity in Latin American and the Caribbean. *MEDICC Review, 7*(9).

Perrottet, A. (1993). *Ecuador: Insight guides.* Hong Kong: Apa Publications. (Published and distributed in Ecuador by Ediciones Libri Mundi)

United Nations Office for the Coordination of Human Affairs (OCHA). (1999). *Ecuador—volcanoes Guagua Pichincha and Tungurahua: OCHA situation report No. 3* (OCHA-GENEVA-99/0182). Retrieved October 18, 1999, from UN Office for the Coordination of Humanitarian Affairs, Geneva, www.reliefweb.int/rw/rwb.nsf/db900sid/ACOS-64DBA8?OpenDocument&rc=2&emid=VO-1999-0584-ECU

Walsh, J. A., & Warren, K. S. (1979). Selective primary health care: An interim strategy for disease control in developing countries. *New England Journal of Medicine, 301*(18), 967–974.

Whiteford, L. M. (1990). A question of adequacy: Primary health care in the Dominican Republic. *Social Science & Medicine, 30*(2), 221–226.

Whiteford, L. M. (1993). International economic policies and child health. *Social Science & Medicine, 37*(11), 1391–1400.

Whiteford, L. M. (1998a). Sembrando el futuro: Globalization and the commodification of health. In M. B. Whiteford & S. Whiteford (Eds.), *Crossing currents: Continuity and change in Latin America* (pp. 264–270). Upper Saddle River, NJ: Prentice Hall.

Whiteford, L. M. (1998b). Children's health as accumulated capital: Structural adjustment in the Dominican Republic and Cuba. In N. Scheper-Hughes & C. Sargent (Eds.), *Small wars: The cultural politics of childhood* (pp. 186–203). Berkeley: University of California Press.

Whiteford, L. M. (2000). Idioms of hope and despair: Local identity, globalization and health in Cuba and the Dominican Republic. In L. M. Whiteford & L. Manderson (Eds.), *Global health policy/local realities: The fallacy of the level playing field* (pp. 57–78). Boulder, CO: Lynne Reinner Press.

Whiteford, L. M., Arata, A., Torres, M., Montaño, D., Suarez, N., Creel, E., et al. (1999). *Diarrheal disease prevention through community-based participation interventions* (Activity Report No. 61). Arlington, VA: CDM, Environmental Health Project.

Whiteford, L. M., & Branch, L. (2007). *Primary health care in Cuba: The other revolution.* New York: Rowman & Littlefield.

Whiteford, L. M., Laspina, C., & Torres, M. (1996). *Cholera control in Ecuador: Behavior-based control activities.* Arlington, VA: CDM, Environmental Health Project.

Wilkerson, R. G. (1992). National mortality rates: The impact of inequality? *American Journal of Public Health, 82*(8), 1082–1084.

Wilkerson, R. G. (1996). *Unhealthy societies: The afflictions of inequality.* London: Routledge.

Wilkerson, R. G., & Marmot, M. (Eds.). (2003). *Social determinants of health: The solid facts.* Copenhagen, Denmark: World Health Organization, Regional Office for Europe.

PART VI

Special Topics

The final section presents special topics of public health concern, focusing on social and behavior science approaches to problem analysis and design of interventions. The five areas selected represent important foci of current research and practice: childhood obesity, mental health, unintentional injuries, violence, and occupational health. Each chapter is organized by ecological-system levels for understanding the factors that influence problem parameters and for intervening at different points of influence. Together, the chapters illustrate the broad scope of socio-ecological approaches to contemporary health issues.

Chapter 17 focuses on childhood overweight and obesity, a problem of growing concern in the United States and other industrial nations because of its long-term impact on multiple chronic diseases. Multilevel influences on diet and physical activity are reviewed, including family, school, community, media, and public policy. In this area, food marketing and advertising play a particularly important role in shaping children's diet. School-based interventions, media regulation, and policy initiatives offer alternative approaches to addressing the problem.

Public mental health is a growing field of specialization, as mental health issues are increasingly recognized as important for individual, community, and societal well-being. Chapter 18 overviews research and practice in this arena, including primary and secondary prevention of mental disorders. Knowledge and practice are rapidly changing in this field as we learn more about the complexity of genetic, psychological, and sociocultural factors that influence mental health.

Unintentional injuries are a leading cause of death in the United States and are largely preventable. Chapter 19 reviews the state of knowledge in this field, with particular focus on the social and behavioral factors that contribute to the occurrence of injuries as well as the success of control measures. The case of motorcycle injuries offers an instructive example of multilevel influences and the factors that affect the shaping of policies aimed at reducing risks, such as laws requiring helmet use. Although it is a relatively new field in public health, injury prevention is likely to expand and develop in the coming years.

All types of violence, whether child abuse, sexual assault, elder mistreatment, suicide, homicide, or political conflict, have a long history in human society, but only in recent years has violence emerged as a focus of integrated public health attention. Chapter 20 overviews this interdisciplinary field, showing how violence affects all age groups in one form or another and how interventions require multisectorial collaboration in designing effective solutions.

The field of occupational health has made noteworthy advances in protecting the health of workers across diverse employment settings. Chapter 21 highlights important accomplishments and challenges in this area, with particular attention to psychosocial factors in making the workplace a safer and healthier environment. Key issues related to risk of injury, musculoskeletal problems, job stress, violence, and work-family conflict are discussed from an ecological perspective.

17

Childhood Overweight and Obesity

Rita DiGioacchino DeBate, Carol A. Bryant, and Marissa Zwald

During the past few decades, obesity has emerged as a public health priority (Stein & Colditz, 2004; Visscher & Seidell, 2001). It also has gained widespread notice in the popular press, prompting the media to create reality shows such as *The Biggest Loser, Celebrity Fit Club,* and MTV's *Real Life* documentary of overweight adolescents' experiences at a summer "fat camp." Despite widespread recognition of its importance, attempts to combat the obesity epidemic have yielded disappointing results, in part because of the complex web of contributing factors that must be addressed (Robinson & Killen, 2001). This chapter uses the socio-ecological model described in this text to explore the multifactorial nature of this health issue.

THE CURRENT STATE OF OVERWEIGHT AND OBESITY

During 2005 to 2006, more than 33% of U.S. adults, or over 72 million people, were classified as obese (i.e., having a body mass index, or BMI, $\geq$ 30), and 36.5% of U.S. adults were classified as overweight (i.e., having a BMI between 25.0 and 29.9) (Centers for Disease Control and Prevention [CDC], 2006; Ogden, Carroll, McDowell, & Flegal, 2007). In other words, over two thirds of the U.S. adult population weighs too much. Although this problem affects people of both genders and various ages, ethnic groups, socioeconomic levels, and geographic areas, obesity is disproportionately high among some groups (Baskin, Ard, Franklin, & Allison, 2005; Stein & Colditz, 2004), especially non-Hispanic black and Mexican American women who are between 40 and 59 years of age (CDC, 2006, 2007; U.S. Department of Health and Human Services [DHHS], 2001).

Overweight also has become a serious problem among children and adolescents (Stein & Colditz, 2004). In this chapter, we have considered as overweight those children who have a BMI between the 85th and 95th percentiles on age- and gender-specific BMI charts, and those with BMIs equal to or above the 95th percentile as obese. In the United States, the number of overweight children has doubled, and the number of overweight adolescents has almost tripled, during the past 20 years (Baskin et al., 2005). The prevalence of overweight reported in the 1976 to 1980 and 2003 to 2004 National Health and Nutrition Examination Survey (NHANES) increased from 5.0% to 13.9% among 2- to 5-year-olds, from 6.5% to 18.8% among 6- to 11-year-olds, and from 5.0% to 17.4% among adolescents aged 12 to 19 years (CDC, 2007). Mexican American boys and non-Hispanic black girls appear to be at special risk of overweight and obesity (DHHS, 2001). Furthermore, the increasing prevalence of obesity in many other countries suggests that obesity is now a pandemic (Egger & Swinburn, 1997).

Public health officials are concerned about the health consequences of this rapid rise in overweight and obesity. According to the CDC, more than 300,000 premature deaths each year in the United States are linked to obesity (Allison, Fontaine, Mandon, Stevens, & Vanltallie, 1999). Excess weight has been shown to increase the risk for a variety of chronic diseases, including coronary heart disease, hypertension, stroke, gallbladder disease, type 2 diabetes, osteoarthritis, and some forms of cancer.

Childhood obesity accelerates the development of these comorbidities, and some obese children and adolescents now experience medical problems previously diagnosed almost exclusively among adults (Hassink, 2006). For example, type 2 diabetes (often called adult-onset diabetes) now accounts for 29% of diabetes in children aged 12 to 19 years (Duncan, 2006). Sixty percent of overweight children have at least one risk factor (National Center for Chronic Disease Prevention and Health Promotion, 2000) and approximately 25% have two or more risk factors for cardiovascular disease (Freedman, Dietz, Srinivasan, & Berenson, 1999). Obstructive sleep apnea (OSA) is another common diagnosis associated with obesity. If left untreated, this condition can lead to pulmonary hypertension, systemic hypertension, and right-sided heart failure (Section on Pediatric Pulmonology, Subcommittee on Obstructive Sleep Apnea Syndrome, 2002). OSA also is related to the development of cardiovascular diseases, behavioral disorders, poor school performance among children, and poor quality of life among adults (Young, Skatrud, & Peppard, 2004). Almost half of severely obese 12- to 19-year-olds have metabolic syndrome, as compared with only 4.2% within the age group as a whole (Cook, Weitzman, Auinger, Nguyen, & Dietz, 2003; Wiess et al., 2004). *Metabolic syndrome* is defined as the presence of three or more abnormalities associated with atherosclerosis and diabetes.

In addition to concerns about obesity's health consequences, the epidemic's economic impact has captured the attention of many policymakers. One study estimated that $117 billion is spent each year in the United States on direct and indirect medical costs associated with obesity (Stein & Colditz, 2004). The direct medical costs considered in the study included preventive, diagnostic, and treatment services related to overweight and obesity. The indirect costs included income lost from decreased productivity, restricted activity, absenteeism, and bed days and the value of future income lost by premature death (DHHS,

2001; Stein & Colditz, 2004). This study may have actually underestimated these costs because it did not consider some of obesity's comorbidities, such as reduced physical functioning, psychological issues (i.e., depression, eating disorders, low self-esteem), sleep apnea, and cataracts (Stein & Colditz, 2004).

In an effort to reverse the rising obesity rates, the Surgeon General has declared obesity as a national epidemic, and the CDC has launched a major initiative to help states mount primary, secondary, and tertiary preventive measures (DHHS, 2001). Child and adolescent prevention programs have been especially popular because overweight children are at greatly increased risk of becoming overweight adults and the factors contributing to weight management appear more mutable during the developmental years (Dietz, 2002). Unfortunately, these efforts have not produced long-term results (Robinson & Killen, 2001), possibly because they have overrelied on education and failed to address many of the individual-, community-, and broader societal-level factors that affect weight status (Glanz & Rimer, 2005). About one third of overweight preschoolers and one half of overweight school-age children will become overweight adults, making prevention at early ages a top priority for many public health professionals (Dietz, 2002).

In this chapter, we take a broader view of the childhood obesity problem, using the social ecological model to examine factors at multiple levels of influence on weight management among youth. We recognize the important impact physical activity has on energy balance. However, this case example focuses on the factors influencing dietary intake and gives less attention to the multiple levels of influence on physical activity.

THE MULTIFACETED NATURE OF CHILDHOOD OVERWEIGHT AND OBESITY

The social ecological model provides an excellent framework for identifying the factors that influence overweight/obesity and for examining the interaction between and within the multiple levels of influence (Davison & Birch, 2001; Glanz & Rimer, 2005). As described in Figure 17.1, the social ecological model recognizes the complex interaction among intrapersonal, interpersonal, community, and broader social and cultural levels of influence on childhood overweight and obesity. For instance, policies made at the societal level affect the type and amount of foods served by schools at the community level, and national food-marketing policies influence the foods children purchase or ask their parents to purchase for them (Institute of Medicine [IOM], 2006).

Intrapersonal-Level Risk Factors

As you may recall, the intrapersonal level includes both modifiable and nonmodifiable risk factors at the individual level. Modifiable factors include behaviors (i.e., eating behaviors, physical activity, sedentary behavior) and the beliefs, attitudes, intentions, skills, and self-perceptions that affect those behaviors. This level also includes nonmodifiable factors, such as age, race/ethnicity, sex, heredity, and genetic predisposition (Davison & Birch, 2001).

Figure 17.1 Social Ecologial Model

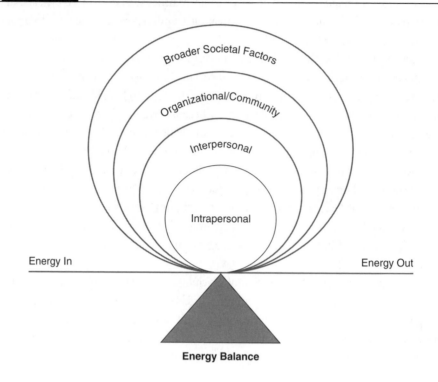

Energy Balance

Children's dietary and activity patterns play an important role in the development of overweight and obesity. Unfortunately, the methods used to assess these patterns are subject to recall error, underreporting, and misreporting, making it difficult to accurately examine their relationships with each other and with the BMI (Davis et al., 2007; IOM, 2006). Despite these challenges, current research suggests that a large number of children and adolescents eat poorly and do not get enough physical activity, creating an "energy gap" or imbalance between the number of calories consumed and the number expended (Davison & Birch, 2001; Robert Wood Johnson Foundation, 2006). Among U.S. children and adolescents, the energy gap averages 110 to 165 calories per day, while among overweight adolescents, the gap is even larger—between 700 and 1,000 calories per day, with obvious consequences for additional weight gain (Robert Wood Johnson Foundation, 2006)

Changes in children's eating behaviors are a major contributor to the energy gap. Of special concern are increased consumption of sugar-sweetened beverages and fruit drinks and fat-laden snacks such as pizza and fried potatoes during the past 30 years (IOM, 2006). According to the NHANES, one third of the calories consumed by children and adolescents now come from these sources (IOM, 2006). These findings are significant, as consumption of sugar-sweetened beverages has been linked to childhood overweight and obesity (Davis et al., 2007; Sturm, 2005).

Another trend that may be contributing to the increase in childhood overweight and obesity is decreased consumption of dairy products and fruits and vegetables. In some, but not all, studies, children who consumed more milk and/or dairy products had lower body fat percentages than those who consumed less (Davis et al., 2007). High fruit and vegetable intake may also protect children from obesity (Davis et al., 2007); however, only 20% of adolescents participating in the 2005 Youth Risk Behavior Surveillance (YRBS) consumed the recommended five or more servings of fruits and vegetables per day, and only 16% consumed three or more servings of milk per day (Eaton et al., 2006).

Three dietary practices shown to be associated with childhood obesity have also become more widespread in recent years: (1) skipping of breakfast, (2) reliance on foods purchased outside the home, and (3) increase in the portion sizes of food served both inside and outside the home (Davis et al., 2007). A review of 15 observational studies, including 2 longitudinal studies, shows that obese children and teens are more likely to skip breakfast than their leaner counterparts, most likely because those who miss breakfast have larger caloric intakes later in the day (Siega-Riz, Popkin, & Carson, 1998).

Once reserved for special occasions and travel, commercially prepared meals are now a regular part of the typical diet of U.S. citizens (Food Marketing Institute, 2000). Fast food has received considerable scrutiny because youth aged 11 to 18 years eat in quick-serve outlets on average twice a week (Paeratakul, Ferdinand, Champagne, Ryan, & Bray, 2003), and several studies suggest that fast-food consumption is associated with higher energy and higher fat intake among youth (French, Jeffery, et al., 2001; Zoumas-Morse, Rock, Sobo, & Neuhouser, 2001). Although some fast-food chains have introduced more nutritious alternatives, the extent to which children select them is not known.

The sizes of food portions served both outside and inside the home also have increased during the last few decades. A comparison of current prepared-food portion sizes with their original sizes when introduced showed that most servings are now twice the size of former standard servings, and those offered in fast-food restaurants are two to five times larger than the original sizes (Young & Nestle, 2003). As a result, a typical fast-food meal consisting of a carbonated soft drink, a cheeseburger, and fried potatoes now provides 255 calories more than it did before (IOM, 2006). Larger portion sizes are problematic because studies show that, starting as young as 5 years of age, people eat more when they are served more (Fisher, Rolls, & Birch, 2003; Rolls, Engell, & Birch, 2000).

The other major contributor to the energy gap is lowered caloric expenditure (i.e., lowered "energy out"). Higher levels of physical activity protect children from gaining excess weight (Davis et al., 2007). Unfortunately, children have become more sedentary over the past decade. Recent estimates show that nearly half the young people between the ages of 12 and 21 do not engage in regular vigorous physical activity and that approximately 10% are sedentary (Eaton et al., 2006; Shanklin, Brener, McManus, Kinchen, & Kann, 2007). These findings are especially alarming as longitudinal studies show that only 12% of youth who achieve the recommended levels of physical activity remain active as they become young adults (Davis et al., 2007).

Lack of physical activity has been linked to youth's increased reliance on television, the Internet, and electronic games for recreation. Media is a ubiquitous force in young people's lives. The typical *tween* (children from 9 to 13 years of age) lives in a house with three TVs, two VCRs, three radios, three tape players, and a computer (Siegel, Coffey, & Livingston, 2001), and 60% have a TV in their bedroom (Roberts, Foehr, Rideout, & Brodie, 1999). A recent study found that children who watched television between 2 and 4 hours per day were more likely to be overweight and 2.5 times more likely to have high blood pressure (Pardee, Worman, Lustig, Prud'homme, & Schwimmer, 2007).

A final point pertaining to intrapersonal factors: A recent review of published studies on sleep duration and childhood obesity found that children with reduced sleep had a 92% higher risk of being overweight than children who slept the recommended amount for their age (i.e., less than 5 years, 11 hours per day; 5–10 years, 10 hours per day; greater than 10 years, 9 hours per day). Interestingly, however, this association between increased sleep and lower risk for obesity was found for boys but not for girls (Johns Hopkins University Bloomberg School of Public Health, 2008).

Childhood obesity also is influenced by intrapersonal-level factors that cannot be changed, such as genetic predisposition. The human body survives in environments with fluctuating food supplies; it is equipped with efficient mechanisms for accumulating body fat and preventing the depletion of energy stores. These biological mechanisms place people with access to an abundant food supply, and without the need to work, at risk for gaining excessive amounts of weight (Brown, 2007). Some obesity researchers note that people vary genetically in ways that affect weight maintenance. Estimates of heredity's role in obesity range from 25% to over 40% (Brown, 2007). Genetic influences on obesity are still poorly understood; however, genes are believed to affect weight management by altering the metabolic rate (influencing how the body responds to excess calories—e.g., by creating heat rather than storing energy as fat), by determining the types and number of fat cells a person has, and by other mechanisms (Whitney & Rolfes, 2002).

Interpersonal-Level Factors

The interpersonal level of the ecological model refers to influence from family members, peers, and others. In the prevention of obesity, parents play a particularly important role, especially during the early years, when children depend on them for access to much of the food they eat. As the child matures, the family continues to have a major influence on children's eating behaviors and dietary intake by determining which foods are available in the home and when and where the members dine together. Parents have a long-lasting impact on their children's eating habits, even after the children move out of the house, through transmission of food attitudes, preferences, and values (IOM, 2006). Parental influence is believed to operate through several mechanisms: early infant-feeding practices and food selection (the foods parents make available to their children), parental control, modeling, and education.

Infant-Feeding Practices

Parents' influence begins at birth with their decision to breast- or bottle-feed. Breast-feeding not only protects infants from gaining too much weight while they nurse but also reduces the likelihood of their becoming obese later in life (Lindsay, Sussner, Kim, & Gortmaker, 2006). Studies estimate that children who were breast-fed are between 13% and 22% less likely to develop obesity during childhood or their adult years (Mayer-Davis et al., 2006). Breast-feeding's protective mechanisms are poorly understood but may reflect differences in how breast- and bottle-fed babies learn to regulate food intake. Those fed at the breast usually control the amount they consume based on internal satiety cues. In contrast, encouraging an infant to empty a bottle during a single feeding and use of energy-dense formulas may make it difficult for infants to respond to these internal cues (Lindsay et al., 2006). Also, breast milk's hormonal and nutritional composition may influence food intake regulation and/or protect babies in other ways from excessive adiposity (Mayer-Davis et al., 2006).

Food Availability and Accessibility

Household food availability and accessibility have a strong impact on the dietary intake of children and teens (Cullen et al., 2003; Patrick & Nicklas, 2005). For instance, the availability of carbonated soft drinks in the home has been shown to influence how much of this type of beverage 8- to 13-year-olds drink (Grimm, Harnack, & Story, 2004; Neumark-Sztainer, Wall, Perry, & Story, 2003). Studies have also shown that even when children do not like fruits and vegetables, their intake is higher when these foods are present in the household. When parents make fruits and vegetables even more accessible, for example, by making them easy to reach or cutting them into small pieces that are easy to eat, children's intake increases even more (Patrick & Nicklas, 2005).

Household food availability and children's risk for becoming overweight have been linked to parents' knowledge about nutrition and weight management (Ritchie et al., 2001). Health-conscious parents typically purchase foods that are nutritious and make them readily accessible in the home, while parents who know less about nutrition are more likely to give their children greater access to energy-dense foods and large portion sizes, thereby increasing their risk for childhood obesity (Davison & Birch, 2001).

Family meal patterns also have been linked to children's eating practices and dietary intake (Gillman, Rifas-Shiman, & Frazier, 2000). For most families, a meal is an important event, and mealtime is perhaps the only time during the day when family members have a chance to sit down and talk. A high frequency of eating meals together in families is associated with many healthful dietary intake patterns in children, including increased intake of several vitamins and minerals, fruits and vegetables, grains, and calcium-rich foods, as well as decreased soft drink consumption (Neumark-Sztainer, Hannan, Story, Croll, & Perry, 2003; Patrick & Nicklas, 2005).

Despite these benefits, the family dinner is on the decline in the United States. Many parents and children report hurried schedules, particularly in the evening, which leave little or no time for the planning, preparation, and cleanup necessary for a family meal. As the number of meals eaten together at home declines, consumption of food prepared outside the home increases, placing children and parents at increased risk of obesity (Patrick & Nicklas, 2005).

Parental Control

Parents also influence their children's eating behaviors by restricting certain foods, pressuring children to eat more, and using foods as a reward. Unfortunately, these behaviors often have the opposite effect to what was intended (Birch, 2006; Fisher & Birch, 1999). Children typically develop a preference for foods that are restricted or used as a reward while disliking foods they are forced to eat. Excessive parental control over when, what, and how much children should eat also may reduce children's regulatory ability and lead to excessive caloric intake or other types of disordered eating practices (Birch & Davison, 2001).

In addition to controlling their children's dietary behaviors, many parents help reduce children's unhealthy eating habits by setting limits on and monitoring television viewing and other forms of "screen time" that place children at risk for obesity (Ritchie et al., 2001).

Modeling and Education

Parents are powerful role models and serve as important social referents for their children's eating and physical activity practices. Children try foods they see their parents eat and, with repeated exposure, often learn to like them (Davison & Birch, 2001). In fact, parents' fruit and vegetable intake has been shown to be the best predictor of how much of these foods their children will consume between 2 and 6 years of age (Cooke et al., 2003). Studies have also shown similarities in milk and carbonated soft drink consumption habits between mothers and daughters (Grimm et al., 2004; Patrick & Nicklas, 2005).

Finally, parents are important models and sources of information and support who affect their children's physical activity levels well into adulthood (Rimal, 2003; Welk, 1999). Compared with inactive parents, physically active parents are more likely to transmit positive attitudes, beliefs, and practices about activity to their children (Davison & Birch, 2001). They also encourage their children to be active by playing with them, paying for programs that promote activity, and transporting them to locations where they can be active (Davison & Birch, 2001). Conversely, less active parents are more likely to convey negative beliefs about exercise (Skelton, DeMattia, Miller, & Olivier, 2006).

Peer, Sibling, and Adult Interactions

In addition to parents, siblings, teachers, and many other adults influence children's and teens' health behaviors (Patrick & Nicklas, 2005). Child care and school personnel have an especially important role to play because of the substantial amount of time they spend with children in these settings (IOM, 2006). Peer modeling and observational learning have been shown to affect eating behaviors, including increased intake of and preference for vegetables that were previously disliked (Patrick & Nicklas, 2005).

Activity patterns also are shaped by peers and siblings. Participation in sports, for instance, is influenced more strongly by what a child's friends do than by the family members. As children move into the teen years, the influence of peers, especially same-sex peers, increases significantly (Davison & Birch, 2001).

Organizational- and Community-Level Factors

In the following case study, the organizational and community level includes resources, norms, values, and institutional policies that affect children's energy balance and weight status. Of special importance in understanding the obesity epidemic are the school environment, community retail outlets, and certain characteristics of the physical environment, often called the "built environment."

Schools

Schools are a logical focus for understanding and reversing the childhood obesity epidemic because 95% of American youth between ages 5 and 17 spend 5 days a week there and eat between 19% and 50% of their daily intake on campus (Story, Kaphingst, & French, 2006).

The food environment in most schools includes federally regulated school food service meals and competitive foods and beverages sold à la carte, in vending machines, in school stores, or as part of fund raisers. The national school lunch and breakfast programs served over 30 million children lunch and almost 10 million children breakfast, respectively, in 2006, with the highest student participation among lower-income students, who receive meals free or at reduced price (U.S. Department of Agriculture [USDA], 2008a, 2008b). Since 1995, federally subsidized school lunches and breakfasts have had to restrict the amount of total and saturated fat in compliance with the *Dietary Guidelines for Americans,* set forth by the DHHS.

Most studies suggest that school lunches are more nutritious than other alternatives offered on campus (Davison & Birch, 2001). Students who participate in the National School Lunch Program consume more vegetables and grain foods, drink more milk and fewer sugary drinks, and eat fewer snack foods than their peers. School lunch and breakfast programs also protect some students from becoming overweight. One study shows that girls whose families participated in the Supplemental Nutrition Assistance Program and the National School Breakfast and Lunch programs had a lower risk of becoming overweight than those who did not participate in these programs (Murphy, Pagano, & Bishop, 2001; Pollitt, 1995). Although meal content has improved and students' daily fat intake has declined over the last 15 years, many nutrition experts still believe that more needs to be done to improve school lunches (Story et al., 2006).

While school breakfasts and lunches still have their critics (including many students), the greatest concern is now on "competitive foods" sold in the à la carte line, in campus vending machines and in school stores. Over half the elementary schools, 84% of middle schools, and 94% of high schools sell competitive food items on campus. The most common items are candy, soft drinks, pizza, tacos, burritos, carbonated beverages, salty snacks (e.g., chips), and high-fat baked goods (e.g., cookies) (Wechsler, McKenna, Lee, & Dietz, 2001).

Despite their abysmal nutritional content, the USDA does little to regulate competitive foods. The Department classifies items such as soft drinks, candies, and chewing gum that contain less than 5% of the recommended dietary allowance per serving for each of eight key nutrients as *foods of minimal nutritional value.* Foods in this category are not allowed to be sold in the school cafeteria during meal periods, but they can be sold in other locations on campus throughout the day. Other competitive foods, including candy bars, potato chips, cookies, and doughnuts, are not subject to federal regulation. Fortunately, many public health advocacy groups are working together to pass state and local regulations that limit or prohibit sales of some competitive foods and beverages.

Schools also provide important opportunities for children to be physically active, although many schools have reduced the amount of time devoted to physical education and recess in response to increased demands for higher academic grades and test scores (Sturm, 2005). A survey in 2000 found that only 8% of elementary schools and 6.4% of high schools provided physical education daily throughout the year for all students in each grade. As a result, recent studies estimate that only 16% of kindergartners report daily physical education in school (IOM, 2004). These findings are important because children who do not participate in physical education are less physically active overall and do less well in school than more active children (Story et al., 2006). To counter the recent decline in activity levels, many public health groups now recommend that states and local school boards adopt policies to increase physical activity requirements and standards in schools.

Community Retail Outlets

Many researchers have documented the influence that neighborhood food outlets have on local residents' dietary consumption (Wells, Ashdown, Davies, Cowett, & Yang, 2007). Availability of fruits and vegetables in local restaurants, for example, has been linked to juice and vegetable consumption patterns among African American boys (Edmonds, Baranowski, Baranowski, Cullen, & Myres, 2001), and availability of these products in local supermarkets has been shown to influence corresponding consumption patterns in neighboring households (Wrigley, Warm, & Margetts, 2003). In addition to being influenced by availability, dietary choices are also influenced by the prices of foods sold in local stores and vending machines (French, Jeffery, et al., 2001).

Unfortunately, the distribution of restaurants, supermarkets, and other food outlets place many children at risk of overweight. A recent study found that convenience stores and fast-food restaurants are now located within walking distance of at least one third of schools nationwide and over half of schools in large cities (Sturm, 2005; Zenk & Powell, 2008).

The increased availability of fast-food restaurants has received special scrutiny because of the energy-dense composition and large portion sizes of most of the menu items they sell (French, Story, & Jeffery, 2001; Grier, Mensinger, Huang, Kumanyika, & Stettler, 2007; Sturm & Datar, 2005). Although data on the relationship between fast-food restaurant proximity and patronage are mixed, many scholars are concerned about the role these restaurants play in raising the levels of obesity, especially among minority youth, because they are located in disproportionately high numbers in low-income ethnic-minority neighborhoods (Block, Scribner, & DeSalvo, 2004; Lewis et al., 2005). On the east coast of the United States, for instance, Grier and her colleagues (2007) found a threefold difference in the proportion of African American, Asian American, and Hispanic American parents who could easily walk or drive to fast-food restaurants as compared with non-Hispanic whites. Quick-serve outlets may be more popular in these neighborhoods than elsewhere because other types of food outlets are in limited supply.

Physical Features of the Community

Features of the "built environment," such as parks, sidewalks, bike trails, and gyms, also may contribute to weight management by giving local residents opportunities to be physically active (Davis et al., 2007). A recent review of studies over the last 10 years found that residents who live in low-income urban areas face greater barriers to physical activity (Black & Macinko, 2008) than other Americans. It is difficult to encourage children to walk or ride their bikes to school if the surrounding neighborhoods lack sidewalks and trails or appear unsafe. From 1977 to 2001, the percentage of children who walked to school decreased from approximately 20% to 13% (Sturm, 2005). In 2001, the average walking (6.3 minutes per day) and biking (2.1 minutes per day) travel time per day among children aged 5 to 15 years was approximately 8 minutes per day—the caloric equivalent of half a serving of a sugar-sweetened beverage (Sturm, 2005). Making the built environment more conducive to walking and biking could lead to greater use of active modes of transportation, thereby increasing physical activity among children and adolescents.

Broader Societal-Level Factors

Socioeconomic status has a powerful impact on diet and nutritional well-being. Although the relationship between income, education, and dietary patterns has not been thoroughly investigated, a variety of explanations have been given for the disproportionately high prevalence of obesity among children and teens from the lower socioeconomic brackets (IOM, 2006). Among the most likely explanations is the observation that poorer families must spend a larger proportion of their income on food expenditures, often pay higher prices for food, and, as a result, may make different food choices for their families, while diets among those in the higher social strata are more closely in line with recommended dietary guidelines.

Over a century ago, Ernst Engel demonstrated that poorer families spent a higher percentage of their income on food and often paid more for their food than those who were better off (Zimmerman, 1932). Poor people's purchasing power today tends to be diminished by their limited access to supermarkets and large grocery stores that sell healthy foods and that typically charge 10% less than convenience outlets or smaller "mom and pop" grocery stores (Black & Macinko, 2008). A 1999 survey by the USDA found that many low-income families living in rural communities have difficulty traveling to large retail outlets because they do not own a car or cannot afford to travel long distances. Because they have to rely on small grocery stores that offer fewer selections and at higher prices, they pay 2.5 times more for food than wealthier families in the rural communities and 3 times more than households in suburban neighborhoods (Kaufman, 1999).

As families' incomes rise, the demand for specific types of food also changes, with increased income accompanied by increased consumption of fruit and other expensive items. In the United States, this pattern can be seen among adolescents from lower-income families, who consume fewer fruits and vegetables than teens from more affluent homes (Lowry, Kann, Collins, & Kolbe, 1996).

Class differences in food norms and beliefs also may contribute to socioeconomic differences in food consumption and obesity rates. A study of 849 families in three European cities showed that upper-class mothers took health into account more often when purchasing foods for their families and restricted their children's intake of sweets and other nonnutritious foods more often than mothers in families with lower incomes. The mothers in poorer families considered their family's taste preferences more often and tended to agree that their children could snack as long as they ate their main meals (Hupkens, Knibbe, Otterloo, & Drop, 1998). One explanation for the difference comes from another study of mothers in the United States that showed that families on a tight budget were less likely to impose healthy foods on their children or partners because they could not afford to purchase foods that might be wasted if the family refused them (Devalt, 1991).

Food as a Symbol of Prestige

Consumption of prestige foods often is used to communicate one's social status or facilitate movement up the social ladder. While the principal sign of wealth was once the absence of work, today people must display their wealth through conspicuous consumption of commodities. Because food is such a conspicuous marker, many people adopt the dietary practices of the social group to which they aspire. Easy credit, in the form of credit cards, enables many people to consume luxury items associated with the rich.

Unfortunately, among most societal groups, foods that convey high status are also high in calories and fat. In fact, the adoption of prestigious foods is one of the first dietary changes to occur among wealthier citizens as a nation industrializes. Typically, people switch from more nutritious traditional foods to highly processed, energy-dense items, such as white flour, sugar, canned foods, candy, and soft drinks. This transitional diet results in increased consumption of fat, sugar, and calories and concomitant changes in waist circumference (Nestle, 2002).

Eating out in restaurants is another way in which people may temporarily rise above their social status (Kipke, Iverson, & Booker, 2005):

> A person does not have to belong to an exclusive club to dine on high cuisine, only have the means (cash or credit) to do so. Many exclusive restaurants restrict access, thus increasing their desirability by limiting the number of patrons they can serve. Others do so by simply elevating their prices. The diner gains both the cuisines and the elegant circumstances thought to characterize the everyday lives of those with higher social status. (McIntosh, 1996, p. 48)

Food Production and Promotion

> Food and beverage marketing to children and youth has become ubiquitous on the American landscape. Although recent public announcements by some companies suggest an interest in change, the preponderance of the foods and beverages introduced and marketed to children and youth have been high in total calories, added sugars, salt, fat, and low in nutrients. (IOM, 2006, p. 373)

In her book *Food and Politics*, Marion Nestle (2002) argues that children are an ideal market for an industry that must find ways to get consumers living in the midst of an abundant food supply to eat more. Strategies used to convince children to purchase branded products include developing new products that taste good, making eating convenient, marketing products, and supersizing products.

Many new food and beverage products are designed to appeal to children's preferences for sweets and love of novelty. Candies, snacks, cookies, cereals, and beverages lead the pack. Some companies are adding more nutritious drinks and foods, such as cheese strings, to their product lines, but these still represent a minority of new or reformulated products. Between 2000 and 2004, only 15% of the new products targeting children were low-fat, low-sugar, and/or included whole grains (Harris, 2002).

Convenience is another important attribute that the food industry uses to make its products more attractive in busy, industrialized societies. Meal replacements, easy-to-prepare meals, prepackaged school lunches, and fast-food offerings, which are high-calorie and high-fat, have replaced the more nutritious, traditional home-cooked meals, thus adding to the obesity problem (IOM, 2006).

Marketing, especially television advertising, has been shown to contribute to childhood obesity through several mechanisms. An expert panel assembled by the IOM (2006) concluded that marketing is a powerful persuader, influencing food preferences and product choices among children of ages 2 to 11 years. This finding should not be surprising; if the practice were not effective, the food industry would be unlikely to invest $10 billion annually marketing their branded food and beverages, most of which are obesogenic. In addition to television advertising, which is still the primary marketing tool used to reach youth, the food industry uses event sponsorship, outdoor media, kids' clubs, video games, music, product placement in movies and on the Internet, and cobranding with cartoon characters and other fictional or real-life spokespersons as forms of marketing. As a Kaiser Family Foundation study of food marketing showed, 85% of food companies targeting kids are now using the Internet to reach them (Moore, 2006). Among the new marketing techniques employed online are customized brand experiences, viral marketing, "advergaming," and cross-branded entertainment. Perhaps most troubling are in-school promotions such as McDonald's gift of value meal coupons to students earning good grades (York, 2007); advertising on Channel One (an in-house TV station shown in thousands of U.S. public and private schools); school contests; and contracts that give food companies exclusive rights to sell their beverages on school grounds, use their products in fund-raising drives, or incorporate their foods into the school breakfast and lunch menus (IOM, 2006; Nestle, 2002).

A second means by which food marketing influences obesity is encouraging youth to ask their parents to purchase items for them. Known as encouraging purchase requests (or the "nag factor"), this marketing strategy has been found by the IOM (2006) to be effective. In addition to spending an estimated $30 billion of their own discretionary income (Schor, 2004), children have a significant influence on the products their parents, relatives, and friends buy (McNeal, 1998). One study estimates that children from 2 to 14 years of age influence sales of more than $500 billion each year (IOM, 2006). Youth influence on food is especially powerful: 78% of youth from 8 to 17 years of age say that they influence their parents' food purchases, and 84% of their parents agreed (IOM, 2006). (While teens have greater direct and indirect purchasing power than children, the impact of advertising on their purchases and purchase requests is unclear.)

Marketing also reaches children through their parents. The fast-food industry, for instance, targets parents because they are more likely to eat in quick-serve outlets than single adults, they are gatekeepers for young children, and, as noted previously, they serve as powerful role models for children with regard to eating behaviors (Grier et al., 2007). In a study of economically disadvantaged families from diverse ethnic backgrounds, Grier and her associates (2007) found that greater exposure to fast-food promotion was associated with increased fast-food consumption. Although their study could not demonstrate cause and effect, they found an interesting relationship between parents' exposure to advertising and beliefs that fast-food dining is normative, suggesting that marketing may work by altering or reinforcing social norms.

The food industry's fourth marketing strategy is supersizing, or adding "value" to products while keeping the price low. It is unclear why supersized products are so attractive, but marketers have clearly tapped into a strong compulsion by offering consumers greatly increased quantities of food for just a few cents more. In many venues, you can purchase four times more soda, nearly three times more French fries, and two times more popcorn for less than a dollar. The impact of supersizing portions is particularly pronounced because, as we have already seen, beginning as early as 5 years of age, people appear to eat more when more is served to them (Rolls, 2003; Rolls, Roe, Kral, Meengs, & Wall, 2004).

Food Policies

The public-policy level includes local, state, and federal policies, laws, and regulations that affect food choices and people's behavior. Among those believed to affect children's obesity rates are government-sponsored dietary guidance and nutrition education programs, food labeling, regulation of children's food marketing, and food production and pricing regulations (IOM, 2006).

The USDA and the DHHS have jointly developed a set of federal dietary guidelines for the nation that reflect a new emphasis on preventing chronic disease. Graphically represented by MyPyramid (USDA, 2005c), the *Dietary Guidelines for Americans* are updated every 5 years based on the latest scientific and medical evidence (IOM, 2006; USDA, 2005a).

These guidelines serve as the basis for the nutrition education offered in all government-sponsored nutrition assistance programs and educational initiatives, including its largest social marketing project, the "5 a Day for Better Health" campaign.

Governmental policies also dictate the level of funding, the eligibility criteria, the nutritional education, the composition of food packages, and other services provided by the Supplemental Nutrition Assistance Program, the Special Supplemental Nutrition Program for Women, Infants and Children (WIC), child nutrition programs, Head Start, and school breakfast and lunch programs. These nutritional assistance programs provide an important source of food and advice for many low-income children and families, and 20% of the American population each year (USDA, 2005b). While these programs increase the quantity of food consumed by program participants, a rigorous assessment of their impact on dietary quality and weight status has not been conducted (IOM, 2006).

Governmental policies also dictate how food is labeled. Since the passage of the Nutrition Labeling and Education Act of 1990, most packaged foods are required to have labels with information regarding their caloric and fat content, which may help consumers in balancing their diet. Approximately half of American consumers read these labels when purchasing a product for the first time, usually to determine if it is high in calories or fat (IOM, 2003). At present, restaurants are exempt from posting nutrition information unless they identify an item on their menu as "healthy," making it difficult for diners to make sound nutritional choices when they eat out. However, many childhood obesity prevention advocates are promoting the display of nutrition information on menus, price lists, or packaging in fast-food and full-service chain restaurants (Center for Science in the Public Interest, 2008).

Despite the recognition of food marketing's impact on children's dietary choices, governmental policies restricting children's food advertising have been extremely controversial. In contrast to many European countries, U.S. policymakers have resisted efforts to legally regulate advertising of food and beverage, even to young children. This resistance dates back to the 1970s, when research by the Federal Trade Commission (FTC) first demonstrated that young children are unable to understand the persuasive intent of advertising and cannot distinguish ads from television programming. The FTC began to write new rules restricting children's advertising, but they were quickly stopped by Congress after the food industry complained (Elliott et al., 1981). Only recently has the subject reemerged as policymakers struggle to find ways to avoid a tidal wave of obesity-related health care costs. Recent polls suggest that the U.S. public is mixed in its views on regulation of food advertising (Evans, Finklestein, Kamerow, & Renaud, 2005; Rideout, 2004). Advocates point to the impact marketing has on children's dietary practices and their special vulnerability to advertising's persuasiveness. Opponents claim that the Constitution guarantees companies the right to advertise their products.

Food subsidies, production quotas, price supports, and tariffs also have been blamed for fueling the obesity epidemic in the United States and Europe (Elinder, 2005; Friel, Chopra, & Satcher, 2007). Corn subsidies, for example, have been shown to contribute to the consumption of soft drinks and many other products containing high-fructose corn syrup and other energy-dense products. Framed before obesity had become an issue, pricing policies offer consumers incentives for using corn, sugar, and high-fat dairy products versus less obesogenic alternatives. As a result, the IOM (1991, 2006) and other experts (Friel et al., 2007) have recommended changes in agricultural policies, to discourage production and consumption of energy-dense foods and encourage production and consumption of fruits and vegetables and low-fat dairy products, and changes in tariff regulations, to lower the prices of nutritious imported foods.

A final policy tactic, taxation, has been used in some states to make candy, soft drinks, and other high-fat, energy-dense products more expensive than healthier alternatives. Whereas taxation has proven effective in reducing tobacco sales, most efforts to tax food have been repealed before their effect on consumption patterns or dietary intake could be assessed (Jacobson & Brownell, 2000).

CONCLUSION

Our presentation of the childhood obesity epidemic has explored how various factors in each level of the socio-ecological model have an impact on childhood overweight and obesity. Although this case study is not exhaustive, we hope to have illustrated the interaction between and within multiple levels of the ecology model.

We also hope to have demonstrated the need to view obesity, like so many public health problems, as a complex web of intrapersonal, social, political, and organizational factors that will require multilevel interventions to reverse. Clearly, the challenge of arresting the obesity epidemic is daunting and will require a collaborative strategic effort on the part of elected leaders; the food and beverage industry; local and state agencies; and many community groups, including parents, teachers, and youth. Only with a shared commitment and an ecologically framed approach can we begin to gain control of this critical health problem.

REFERENCES

Allison, D., Fontaine, K., Mandon, J., Stevens, J., & Vanltallie, T. (1999). Annual deaths attributable to obesity in the United States. *Journal of the American Medical Association, 282,* 1530–1538.

Baskin, M., Ard, J., Franklin, F., & Allison, D. (2005). Prevalence of obesity in the United States. *Obesity Reviews, 6,* 5–7.

Birch, L. (2006). Child feeding practices and the etiology of obesity. *Obesity, 14*(3), 343–344.

Birch, L., & Davison, K. (2001). Family environmental factors influencing the developing behavioral controls of food intake and childhood overweight. *Pediatric Clinics of North America, 48*(4), 893–907.

Black, J., & Macinko, J. (2008). Neighborhoods and obesity. *Nutrition Reviews, 66*(1), 2–20.

Block, J., Scribner, R., & DeSalvo, K. (2004). Fast food, race/ethnicity and income: A geographic analysis. *American Journal of Preventive Medicine, 27,* 211–217.

Brown, J. (Ed.). (2007). *Nutrition now* (5th ed.). Belmont, CA: Wadsworth/Thomson Learning.

Center for Science in the Public Interest. (2008). *Nutrition policy.* Retrieved February 7, 2008, from www.cspinet.org/nutritionpolicy/index.html

Centers for Disease Control and Prevention. (2006). *Behavioral risk factor surveillance system prevalence data.* Retrieved November 30, 2007, from apps.nccd.cdc.gov/brfss/list.asp?cat=OB&yr=2006&qkey=4409&state=All

Centers for Disease Control and Prevention. (2007). *Overweight and obesity.* Retrieved November 28, 2007, from www.cdc.gov/nccdphp/dnpa/obesity/index.htm

Cook, S., Weitzman, M., Auinger, P., Nguyen, M., & Dietz, W. H. (2003). Prevalence of a metabolic syndrome phenotype in adolescents: Findings from the third national health and nutrition examination survey, 1988–1994. *Archives of Pediatric Adolescent Medicine, 157,* 821–827.

Cooke, L., Wardle, J., Gibson, E., Sapochnik, M., Sheiham, A., & Lawson, M. (2003). Demographic, familial and trait predictors of fruit and vegetable consumption by pre-school children. *Public Health Nutrition, 7*(2), 295–302.

Cullen, K., Baranowski, T., Owens, E., Marsh, T., Rittenberry, L., & de Moor, C. (2003). Availability, accessibility, and preferences for fruit, 100% fruit juice, and vegetables influence children's dietary behavior. *Health Education & Behavior, 30*(5), 615–626.

Davis, M., Gance-Cleveland, B., Hassink, S., Johnson, R., Paradis, G., & Resnicow, K. (2007). Recommendations for prevention of childhood obesity. *Pediatrics, 120*(4), S229–S253.

Davison, K., & Birch, L. (2001). Childhood overweight: A contextual model and recommendations for future research. *Obesity Reviews, 2,* 159–171.

Devalt, M. (1991). *Feeding the family in the social organization of caring as gendered work.* Chicago: University of Chicago Press.

Dietz, W. (2002). Medical consequences of obesity in children and adolescents. In C. Fairburn & K. Brownell (Eds.), *Eating disorders and obesity* (pp. 473–476). New York: Guilford Press.

Duncan, G. (2006). Prevalence of diabetes and impaired fasting glucose levels among adolescents: National Health and Nutrition Examination Survey, 1999–2002. *Archives of Pediatric Adolescent Medicine, 160,* 523–528.

Eaton, D., Kann, L., Kinchen, S., Ross, J., Hawkins, J., Harris, W., et al. (2006). Youth risk behavior surveillance—United States, 2005. *Journal of School Health, 76*(7), 353–372.

Edmonds, J., Baranowski, T., Baranowski, J., Cullen, K., & Myres, D. (2001). Ecological and socioeconomic correlates of fruit, juice, and vegetable consumption among African American boys. *Preventive Medicine, 32*(6), 476–481.

Egger, G., & Swinburn, B. (1997). An "ecological" approach to the obesity pandemic. *British Medical Journal, 315,* 477–480.

Elinder, L. (2005). Obesity, hunger, and agriculture: The damaging role of subsidies. *British Medical Journal, 331,* 1333–1336.

Elliott, S., Wilkenfeld, J., Guarino, E., Kolish, E., Jennings, C., & Siegal, D. (1981). *FTC staff report recommendation that the commission terminate proceedings for the promulgation of a trade regulation rule on children's advertising* (FTC Document TRR No. 215–60). Washington, DC: Federal Trade Commission.

Evans, W., Finklestein, E., Kamerow, D., & Renaud, J. (2005). Public perceptions of childhood obesity. *American Journal of Preventive Medicine, 28*(1), 26–32.

Fisher, J. O., & Birch, L. (1999). Restricting access to foods and children's eating. *Appetite, 32,* 405–419.

Fisher, J. O., Rolls, B., & Birch, L. (2003). Children's bite size and intake of an entree are greater with large portions than with age-appropriate or self-selected portions. *American Journal of Clinical Nutrition, 77*(5), 1164–1170.

Food Marketing Institute. (2000). *Trends in the United States: Consumer attitudes and the supermarket.* Washington, DC: Author.

Freedman, D., Dietz, W., Srinivasan, S., &, Berenson, G. S. (1999). The relation of overweight to cardiovascular risk factors among children and adolescents: The Bogalusa heart study. *Pediatrics, 103,* 1175–1182.

French, S., Jeffery, R., Story, M., Breitlow, K., Baxter, J., Hannan, P., et al. (2001). Pricing and promotion effects on low-fat vending snack purchases: The CHIPS Study. *American Journal of Public Health, 91*(1), 112–117.

French, S., Story, M., & Jeffery, R. (2001). Environmental influences on eating and physical activity. *Annual Review of Public Health, 22*, 309–335.

Friel, S., Chopra, M., & Satcher, D. (2007). Unequal weight: Equity oriented policy responses to the global obesity epidemic. *British Medical Journal, 335*, 1241–1243.

Gillman, G., Rifas-Shiman, S., & Frazier, A. (2000). Family dinner and diet quality among older children and adolescents. *Archives of Family Medicine, 9*, 235–240.

Glanz, K., & Rimer, B. (2005). *Theory at a glance: A guide for health promotion practice.* Bethesda, MD: U.S. Department of Health and Human Services, National Institutes of Health, National Cancer Institute.

Grier, S., Mensinger, J., Huang, S., Kumanyika, S., & Stettler, N. (2007). Fast-food marketing and children's fast-food consumption: Exploring parents' influences in an ethnically diverse sample. *Journal of Public Policy & Marketing, 26*(2), 221–235.

Grimm, G., Harnack, L., & Story, M. (2004). Factors associated with soft drink consumption in school-aged children. *Journal of the American Dietetic Association, 104*(8), 1244–1249.

Harris, J. (2002). Companies continue to offer new foods targeted to children [Electronic Version]. *Amber Waves, 3*, 4. Retrieved December 10, 2007, from www.ers.usda.gov/AmberWaves/June05/pdf/FindingsDHJune05.pdf

Hassink, S. (2006). *Pediatric obesity: Prevention, intervention, and treatment strategies for primary care.* Elk Grove, IL: American Academy of Pediatrics.

Hupkens, C., Knibbe, R., Otterloo, A. V., & Drop, M. (1998). Class differences in the food rules mothers impose on their children: A cross-national study. *Social Science and Medicine, 47*(9), 1331–1339.

Institute of Medicine. (2004). *Schools can play a role in preventing childhood obesity. Fact sheet.* Retrieved January 30, 2008, from www.iom.edu/Object.File/Master/22/615/0.pdf

Institute of Medicine, Committee on Dietary Guidelines Implementation. (1991). *Improving America's diet and health: From recommendations to action.* Washington, DC: National Academies Press.

Institute of Medicine, Committee on Food Marketing and the Diets of Children and Youth. (2006). *Food marketing to children and youth: Threat or opportunity.* Washington, DC: National Academies Press.

Institute of Medicine, Committee on Use of Dietary Reference Intakes in Nutrition Labeling. (2003). *Dietary reference intakes: guiding principles for nutrition labeling and fortification.* Washington, DC: National Academies Press.

Jacobson, M., & Brownell, K. (2000). Small taxes on soft drinks and snack foods to promote health. *American Journal of Public Health, 90*(6), 854–857.

Johns Hopkins University Bloomberg School of Public Health. (2008, February 8). Reduced sleep can increase childhood obesity risk. *Science Daily.* Retrieved February 16, 2008, from www.sciencedaily.com/releases/2008/02/080207104303.htm

Kaufman, P. (1999). The rural poor's access to supermarkets, large grocery stores. *Rural Development Perspectives, 13*(3), 19–25.

Kipke, M., Iverson, E., & Booker, C. (2005). Community level risks for obesity. *Obesity Research, 13*, A7.

Lewis, L., Sloane, D., Nascimento, L., Diamant, A., Guinyard, J., Yancey A., et al. (2005). African Americans' access to healthy food options in South Los Angeles restaurants. *American Journal of Public Health, 95*(4), 668–673.

Lindsay, A., Sussner, K., Kim, J., & Gortmaker, S. (2006). The role of parents in preventing childhood obesity. *The Future of Children, 16*(1), 170–186.

Lowry, R., Kann, L., Collins, J., & Kolbe, L. (1996). The effect of socioeconomic status on chronic disease risk behaviors among U.S. adolescents. *Journal of the American Medical Association, 276*(10), 792–797.

Mayer-Davis, E., Rifas-Shiman, S., Zhou, L., Hu, F., Colditz, G., & Gillman, M. (2006). Breast-feeding and risk for childhood obesity: Does maternal diabetes or obesity status matter? *Diabetes Care, 29*(10), 2231–2237.

McIntosh, W. (1996). *The sociologies of food and nutrition.* New York: Plenum Press.

McNeal, J. (1998). Tapping the three kids' markets. *American Demographics, 20*(4), 37–41.

Moore, E. (2006). *It's child's play: Online marketing of food to children.* Menlo Park, CA: Henry J. Kaiser Family Foundation.

Murphy, J., Pagano, M., & Bishop, S. (2001). *Impact of a universally-free, in-classroom school breakfast program on achievement: Results from the Abell Foundation's Baltimore Breakfast Challenge Program.* Boston: Massachusetts General Hospital.

National Center for Chronic Disease Prevention and Health Promotion. (2000). *Preventing obesity among Children.* Atlanta, GA: Centers for Disease Control and Prevention.

Nestle, M. (2002). *Food politics: How the food industry influences nutrition and health.* Berkeley: University of California Press.

Neumark-Sztainer, D., Hannan, P., Story, M., Croll, J., & Perry, C. (2003). Family meal patterns: Associations with sociodemographic characteristics and improved dietary intake among adolescents. *Journal of the American Dietetic Association, 103*(3), 317–322.

Neumark-Sztainer, D., Wall, M., Perry, C., & Story, M. (2003). Correlates of fruit and vegetable intake among adolescents. *American Journal of Preventive Medicine, 37*(3), 198–208.

Ogden, C., Carroll, M., McDowell, M., & Flegal, K. (2007). *Obesity among adults in the United States: No change since 2003–2004* (National Center for Health Statistics Data Brief). Retrieved November 8, 2007, from www.cdc.gov/nchs/data/databriefs/db01.pdf

Paeratakul, S., Ferdinand, D., Champagne, C., Ryan, D., & Bray, G. (2003). Fast-food consumption among U.S. adults and children: Dietary and nutrient intake profile. *Journal of the American Dietetic Association, 103*(10), 1332–1388.

Pardee, P., Worman, G., Lustig, R., Prud'homme, D., & Schwimmer, J. (2007). Television viewing and hypertension in obese children. *American Journal of Preventive Medicine, 33*(6), 439–443.

Patrick, H., & Nicklas, T. (2005). A review of family and social determinants of children's eating patterns and diet quality. *Journal of the American College of Nutrition, 24*(2), 83–92.

Pollitt, E. (1995). Does breakfast make a difference in school? *Journal of the American Dietetic Association, 95,* 1134–1139.

Rideout, V. (2004). *Parents, media and public policy: A Kaiser Family Foundation Survey.* Menlo Park, CA: Henry J. Kaiser Family Foundation.

Rimal, R. (2003). Intergenerational transmission of health: The role of intrapersonal, interpersonal, and communicative factors. *Health Education & Behavior, 30*(1), 10–28.

Ritchie, L., Ivey, S., Masch, M., Woodward-Lopex, G., Ikeda, J., & Crawford, P. (2001). *Pediatric overweight: A review of the literature.* Berkeley: University of California, College of Natural Resources, Center for Weight and Health.

Robert Wood Johnson Foundation. (2006, December). *Energy gap contributes to adolescent obesity* (Research Highlight, 17). Retrieved August 8, 2008, from www.rwjf.org/pr/product.jsp?id=21455

Roberts, D., Foehr, U., Rideout, V., & Brodie, M. (1999). *Kids and media at the new millennium*. Menlo Park, CA: Kaiser Family Foundation.

Robinson, T., & Killen, J. (2001). Obesity prevention for children and adolescents. In J. Thompson & L. Smolak (Eds.), *Body image, eating disorders, and obesity in youth: Assessment, prevention, and treatment* (pp. 261–292). Washington, DC: American Psychological Association.

Rolls, B. (2003). The supersizing of America: Portion size and the obesity epidemic. *Nutrition Today, 38*(2), 42–53.

Rolls, B., Engell, D., & Birch, L. (2000). Serving portion size influences 5-year-old but not 3-year-old children's food intakes. *Journal of the American Dietetic Association, 100,* 232–234.

Rolls, B., Roe, L., Kral, T., Meengs, J., & Wall, D. (2004). Increasing portion sizes of a packaged snack increases energy intake in men and women. *Appetite, 42*(1), 63–69.

Schor, J. (2004). *Born to buy: The commericialized child and the new consumer culture.* New York: Scribner.

Section on Pediatric Pulmonology, Subcommittee on Obstructive Sleep Apnea Syndrome. (2002). Clinical practice guideline: Diagnosis and management of childhood obstructive sleep apnea syndrome. *Pediatrics, 109,* 704–712.

Shanklin, S., Brener, N., McManus, T., Kinchen, S., & Kann, L. (2007). *2005 Middle school youth risk behavior survey.* Atlanta, GA: U.S. Department of Health and Human Services, Centers for Disease Control and Prevention.

Siega-Riz, A., Popkin, B., & Carson, T. (1998). Trends in breakfast consumption for children in the United States from 1965 to 1991. *American Journal of Clinical Nutrition, 67*(4), 748S–756S.

Siegel, D., Coffey, T., & Livingston, G. (2001). *The great tween buying machine: Marketing to today's tweens.* Ithaca, NY: Paramount Market.

Skelton, J., DeMattia, L., Miller, L., & Olivier, M. (2006). Obesity and its therapy: From genes to community action. *Pediatric Clinics of North America, 53,* 777–794.

Stein, C., & Colditz, G. (2004). The epidemic of obesity. *Journal of Clinical Endocrinology and Metabolism, 89*(6), 2522–2525.

Story, M., Kaphingst, M., & French, S. (2006). The role of schools in obesity prevention. *The Future of Children, 16*(1), 106–142.

Sturm, R. (2005). Childhood obesity: What we can learn from existing data on societal trends, Part 2. *Preventing Chronic Disease: Public Health Research, Practice, and Policy, 2*(2), 1–9.

Sturm, R., & Datar, A. (2005). Body mass index in elementary school children, metropolitan area food prices and food outlet density. *Public Health, 119*(12), 1059–1068.

U.S. Department of Agriculture. (2005a). *Dietary guidelines for Americans 2005: Executive summary.* Retrieved February 7, 2008, from www.health.gov/dietaryguidelines/dga2005/document/html/executivesummary.htm

U.S. Department of Agriculture. (2005b). *Food assistance and nutrition research* (Report No. 28–6). Washington, DC: Author.

U.S. Department of Agriculture. (2005c). *MyPyramid.* Retrieved February 7, 2008, from www.mypyramid.gov

U.S. Department of Agriculture. (2008a). *National food breakfast program.* Retrieved January 30, 2008, from www.fns.usda.gov/cnd/breakfast

U.S. Department of Agriculture. (2008b). *National food lunch program.* Retrieved January 30, 2008, from www.fns.usda.gov/cnd/lunch

U.S. Department of Health and Human Services, Public Health Service, Office of the Surgeon General. (2001). *The Surgeon General's call to action to prevent and decrease overweight and obesity.* Rockville, MD: Author.

Visscher, T., & Seidell, J. (2001). The public health impact of obesity. *Annual Review of Public Health, 22,* 355–360.

Wechsler, W., McKenna, M., Lee, S., & Dietz, W. (2001). Food service and foods and beverages available at school: Results from the School Health Policies and Programs Study 2000. *Journal of School Health, 71,* 313–324.

Welk, G. (1999). The youth physical activity promotion model: A conceptual bridge between theory and practice. *Quest, 51,* 5–23.

Wells, N., Ashdown, S., Davies, E., Cowett, F., & Yang, Y. (2007). Environment, design, and obesity: Opportunities for interdisciplinary collaborative research. *Environment and Behavior, 39*(1), 6–33.

Whitney, E., & Rolfes, S. (Eds.). (2002). *Understanding nutrition* (9th ed.). Belmont, CA: Wadsworth/Thomson Learning.

Wiess, R., Dziura, J., Burget, T., Tamborlane, W., Taksali, S., Yeckel, C., et al. (2004). Obesity and the metabolic syndrome in children and adolescents. *New England Journal of Medicine, 350,* 2362–2374.

Wrigley, N., Warm, D., & Margetts, B. (2003). Deprivation, diet and food retail access: Findings from the Leeds "food deserts" study. *Environment and Planning A, 35*(1), 151–188.

York, E. (2007). *McDonald's newest ad platform: Report cards.* Retrieved December 12, 2007, from http://findarticles.com/p/articles/mi_hb6398/is_200712/ai_n25582708

Young, L., & Nestle, M. (2003). Expanding portion sizes in the U.S. marketplace: Implications for nutrition counseling. *Journal of the American Dietetic Association, 103*(2), 231–234.

Young, T., Skatrud, J., & Peppard, P. (2004). Risk factors for obstructive sleep apnea in adults. *Journal of the American Medical Association, 291,* 2013–2016.

Zenk, S. N., & Powell, L. M. (2008). U.S. secondary schools and food outlets. *Health & Place, 14,* 336–346.

Zimmerman, C. (1932). Ernst Engel's law of expenditure for food. *Quarterly Journal of Economics, 47*(1), 80.

Zoumas-Morse, C., Rock, D., Sobo, E., & Neuhouser, M. (2001). Children's patterns of macronutrient intake and associations with restaurant and home eating. *Journal of the American Dietetic Association, 101*(8), 923–925.

18

Mental Health and Illness

A Public Health Perspective

Stephanie L. Marhefka

Mental health problems present an important public health issue. In 2002, the World Health Organization (WHO) identified mental illness as the second leading cause of disability worldwide, after infectious and parasitic diseases (WHO, 2002). In the United States, the National Comorbidity Study-Replication, conducted between 2001 and 2003, revealed that, at a given time, 26% of Americans have one of four types of mental health disorders, including anxiety, mood, impulse control, and substance abuse (Kessler, Chiu, Demler, Merikangas, & Walters, 2005). That study showed that 6% of Americans have what is considered a "serious" mental disorder, defined as a mental disorder that involves (a) a suicide attempt with serious lethal intent, (b) work disability or substantial limitations, or (c) being out of work or unable to perform the functions of one's typical role at least 30 days in the past year. In addition to the distress and decreased functioning caused by mental illness, people with mental disorders experience high rates of chronic health conditions (Jones et al., 2004), including the human immunodeficiency virus (HIV) as well as hepatitis B and C (Rosenburg et al., 2001). They also experience increased risk for suicide, which kills approximately 30,000 people each year in the United States alone (Centers for Disease Control and Prevention, n.d.).

In this chapter, both mental health and mental illness are discussed. For the purpose of this chapter, mental health and mental illness are defined as follows:

> *Mental health* refers to "a state of well-being in which every individual realizes his or her own potential, can cope with the normal stresses of life, can work productively and fruitfully, and is able to make a contribution to her or his community." (WHO, 2007)

Mental illness refers to any cognitive, emotional, or behavioral disorder defined in the *Diagnostic and Statistical Manual of Mental Disorders, Fourth Edition (DSM-IV)*. Mental illness includes depressive disorders, anxiety disorders, learning disorders, psychotic disorders, and many others. In this chapter, the terms *mental illness* and *mental disorders* are used synonymously.

Despite the availability of effective treatments for many mental health problems, worldwide, many people fail to receive appropriate mental health services. In developed countries, such as the United States, psychopharmacological treatment for the most prevalent disorders, such as depression and anxiety disorders, is widely accessible through primary care, and specialty mental health services, including psychological and psychiatric treatment, are available to many. Nevertheless, research suggests that less than 25% of those with mild mental disorders, less than 35% of those with moderate mental disorders, and less than 53% of those with serious mental disorders receive mental health treatment in the United States (Bijl et al., 2003; WHO World Mental Health Organization Survey Consortium, 2004). In some parts of the developing world, treatment is much less common (WHO World Mental Health Organization Survey Consortium, 2004), although treatments have been established as effective, at least for depression, schizophrenia, and substance abuse (Patel et al., 2007; Wu, Detels, Zhang, Li, & Li, 2002).

Myriad factors contribute to the high rates of mental health problems in the United States and internationally. However, it is important to note that each factor singly explains only a small proportion of mental illness. Numerous factors within various levels of influence also affect the extent to which people with mental illness receive appropriate care and treatment and experience noteworthy improvements in daily functioning.

This chapter provides an overview of some of the factors that contribute to the primary, secondary, and tertiary prevention of mental illness, using the social ecological model as a guiding framework. It should be seen as a brief tour of some of the important factors that contribute to mental illness. Moreover, readers will note that not all factors influencing mental health and illness fit clearly within one ecological level as opposed to another; this is the nature of systemic models, in which levels of influence are integrated and not always clearly differentiated. Although most influencing factors are presented at a single level, readers should note that factors at each level influence factors at other levels as well.

FACTORS INFLUENCING MENTAL HEALTH AND ILLNESS

Intrapersonal-Level Factors

At the intrapersonal level, numerous factors affect the onset of mental health problems, including age, gender, genetics, biology, and congenital conditions as well as behavior. We can look at depression for an example of how all these factors contribute to one's risks for mental illness. Worldwide, we know that the lifetime risk of depression is about twice as high in women as in men. Yet during the prepubescent period, studies show that either (a) boys and girls do not differ in rates of depression or (b) boys have higher rates of depression than girls. Between the ages of 11 and 13, the rates of depression among girls increase dramatically, and by age 15, the risk of depression is doubled for girls compared with boys. Other biological factors also contribute to risk for depression, especially genetic makeup and hormone production. It is important to note that not every person who is deemed "at risk" for depression based on these intrapersonal factors will develop a depressive disorder. Exposure to a variety of protective factors that occur across levels of the social ecological model may prevent the onset of depression.

Another illustrative example is schizophrenia. Intrapersonal risk factors for schizophrenia include genetic predisposition and exposure to psychogenic substances. Moreover, gender and age affect the manifestation of symptoms among people with schizophrenia. Among those who go on to develop schizophrenia, boys experience behavioral problems earlier than girls, and men have more social problems and work-related problems than women. Across cultures, men also tend to develop schizophrenia at younger ages. These gender differences may be explained, in part, by the protective effects of estrogen (Hafner, 2003).

A variety of intrapersonal factors also contribute to mental health care seeking, adherence to medical appointments and psychotropic medications, and recovery. Attitudes about mental illness and mental health care have been found to significantly affect care and treatment. People who are embarrassed about having a mental illness, feel that seeking mental health care is a sign of weakness, or harbor mistrust of mental health professionals are less likely to seek and adhere to mental health treatment. People who seek treatment early and adhere to appointments are more likely to recover successfully from mental health episodes and manage their mental illness over time.

Numerous studies have empirically evaluated programs for preventing mental health problems among children and adults, and yet few have directly examined the extent to which such programs are effective in preventing the onset of mental illness. Part of the problem is the difficulty of conducting a sufficiently large randomized controlled trial that has the statistical power for determining the effectiveness of prevention interventions (Cuijpers, 2003). Another limitation is our incomplete understanding of the complexity of factors that place someone at risk for mental illness and contribute to the onset of mental illness among those at risk.

The Institute of Medicine has suggested three categories of primary prevention for mental illness (Mrazek & Haggerty, 1994; Munoz, Mrazek, & Haggerty, 1996). *Universal prevention* is the most costly and is likely to be the least cost-effective, as it is designed to prevent mental illness among people with all levels of mental illness risk. However, by reaching an entire population, these programs may help reduce the stigma associated with mental illness (Bayer, Hiscock, Morton-Allen, Ukomunne, & Wake, 2007). An example of a universal prevention intervention for depression is a media campaign designed to teach people in a community how to cope with stress effectively. *Selective prevention* focuses on people with a risk factor for mental illness who have not yet experienced mental illness; this approach may be less costly than *universal prevention* but can still require reaching a large number of people with a broad array of intervention techniques to be cost-effective. A program that provides coping skills training to all children of depressed parents is a selective prevention intervention for depression. The final type, *indicated prevention*, is designed to prevent mental illness among those who have some symptoms of but have not yet developed a mental illness. This strategy may be the most cost-effective because it focuses on people at high risk for developing mental illness. A program that provides coping skills training to people who have been feeling "down in the dumps" is an example of an indicated prevention intervention for depression.

Randomized controlled trials of selective and indicated prevention interventions for mental illness are relatively few. A 2005 meta-analytic review found only 13 randomized controlled studies that examined primary prevention of mental disorders among children, adolescents, or adults (Cuijpers, Can Straten, & Smit, 2005). Results showed that interventions for preventing a depressive disorder were generally effective, while interventions for preventing posttraumatic stress disorder, which used a technique called debriefing, did not significantly reduce the risk of developing the disorder. Additionally, the review found that selective prevention interventions were not generally effective, while indicated prevention interventions generally were effective. A review of programs designed to prevent depression among children showed that educational or informational sessions alone are generally ineffective; interventions that involve psychological components, defined as skill building for reducing depression, are generally effective in the short term, although the effects are not maintained well over time (Merry, McDowell, Hetrick, Bir, & Muller, 2004).

One example of an indicated prevention intervention was tested in the Early Detection and Intervention Evaluation Trial (Morrison et al., 2004). Participants were persons aged between 17 and 35 years who were determined to be at "ultra-high risk" of developing their first episode of psychosis, based on personal and family history; 35 received the intervention, and 23 received monitoring by a case manager. The intervention involved individual cognitive therapy that was manual based yet focused on each individual's particular symptoms. As with other applications of cognitive therapy, the intervention focused on changing the way people interpreted events and experiences. Only 2 of the 35 people in the intervention group developed psychosis, while 5 in the monitoring group developed psychosis over a 12-month period. This finding suggests that cognitive therapy is an effective means of preventing the development of psychosis among those at extremely high risk.

As described in Chapter 1, early detection and treatment of a condition is considered secondary prevention in public health nomenclature. Many mental illness prevention efforts occur at this level. Two types of intrapersonal-level treatments are widely recognized for the secondary prevention of mental illness: psychotherapy and pharmacotherapy. Severe forms of acute mental illness are also treated with psychiatric hospitalization. Much has been written about the secondary prevention of mental illness using the aforementioned techniques, but a broader discussion of these interventions is beyond the scope of this chapter.

Tertiary prevention of mental illness involves a focus on a person's level of impairment, disability, and handicap, all of which relate to quality of life. Programs that incorporate exercise into care for people with mental illness have been found to benefit quality of life, perhaps through improving self-esteem and creating social interactions (Hutchinson, 2005). Other tertiary preventions for mental illness typically occur at other levels of the social ecological model.

Interpersonal-Level Factors

At the interpersonal level, social networks and social support affect the onset of mental health problems. Large social networks and high rates of perceived social support from family and friends can protect against the development of mental health problems. For example, a woman who is inclined toward depression may be less likely to experience a depressive episode if she can draw on a large social support network while she is experiencing high rates of stress (see Chapter 6 for a more thorough discussion of social networks and social support). Other interpersonal factors can contribute to the development of mental illness. For example, a man who had an insecure attachment to his mother during childhood may have difficulty forming a healthy attachment to other figures in his life. This attachment difficulty may lead to social isolation accompanied by negative thoughts about himself. His social difficulties could lead him to develop excessive anxiety in social situations, which could ultimately be so inhibiting as to make it difficult for him to leave his home, a mental health condition termed *agoraphobia*.

People are affected by the behavior of others around them in other ways, as well. For example, Alfred Bandura (1986) demonstrated how people's behavior is affected by observing others, termed *observational learning*. Observational learning can have either positive or negative impacts on the development of mental illness. A child who is living with her depressed mother may watch her mother become overwhelmed and hopeless in response to stress. Later, when the child experiences difficulties, she may adopt a similar coping style, which could result in depression. Another child may develop a more active, positive coping style from watching her mother work to solve problems in a stressful situation.

Care seeking and treatment of mental illness are also affected by interpersonal factors such as social networks, support, and integration, as well as interpersonal relationships with treatment providers. A person's social network may provide support and encouragement for mental health treatment, which could result in increased likelihood of following through with mental health care. Such support could include reminding mentally ill persons about an upcoming appointment, helping them remember to take their medication, giving them a ride to the appointment, or offering positive words about their mental health treatment, such as "It seems like you are improving since you began seeing that doctor." Less supportive people can make it more difficult for people with mental health problems to seek and adhere to care when they express negative attitudes and beliefs about mental health care or individuals with mental illness. When significant others make specific negative comments about a person's mental health problems or treatment experience, it may be especially difficult for the person to maintain involvement in mental health care. In fact, even anticipated negative reactions from significant others may impede help seeking. Studies have found that people with mental illness are more likely to avoid mental health treatment if they believe that their families would judge them negatively for identifying themselves as a person with a mental illness (Leaf, Bruce, Tischler, & Holzer, 1986), whereas they are more likely to seek mental health treatment if they perceive positive attitudes about mental health help seeking in family and friends (Greenly, Mechanic, & Cleary, 1987).

The success of mental health treatment may also depend on social integration. People with mental health problems who are well integrated into a social network have been found to recover more readily from mental illness episodes and are more likely to be employed and to maintain their own self-care (Evert, Harvey, Trauer, & Herrman, 2003).

The relationship between people with mental illness and their mental health treatment providers is another factor that can facilitate or hinder treatment adherence and success. In a recent qualitative study in Norway, some people with mental illness felt that mental health providers could not meet their interpersonal relationship needs and did not support or encourage their efforts to expand their social networks (Granerud & Severinsson, 2006). Conversely, other research has shown that when people with mental illness perceive their treatment providers as understanding and caring individuals, they are more likely to adhere to their treatment (Cameron, 1996).

A variety of interpersonal interventions have been examined for the primary prevention of mental illness. One example is the ROSE Program (Reach Out, Stand Strong, Essentials for new mothers), designed to prevent postpartum depression among high-risk mothers (Zlotnick, Miller, Pearlstein, Howard, & Sweeney, 2006). For this selective prevention intervention, expectant mothers who scored over a cutoff on a postpartum depression risk index were asked to participate if they were not currently in mental health treatment and did not have a current depressive or substance abuse disorder. Ninety-nine women were randomized into either standard care alone or standard care with the ROSE Program intervention. The ROSE Program focused on improving interpersonal relationships, building and using social support networks, and transitioning into motherhood through four prenatal group sessions and one postnatal individual session. Results suggest that the ROSE Program was effective in reducing the incidence of postpartum depression.

Interpersonal-level secondary and tertiary prevention interventions have consisted of group therapy as well as family and couples-based therapy. Multisystemic Therapy (MST) is one intervention that has been successful in the treatment of youth with antisocial behavior. MST is based on Brofenbrenner's ecological model, a systems theory much like the social ecologial model (Brofenbrenner, 1979; Curtis, Ronan, & Borduin, 2004) and targets multiple systems and levels of influence, including interpersonal relationships with peers, family, and school personnel. Therapy typically occurs in a family's home and focuses on empowering parents as the agents of change. A recent review of MST found that youth and families who received MST had greater functioning than 70% of control group participants. MST was especially effective at improving family interactions, whereas in comparison samples, intrapersonal-level interventions were associated with the worsening of family relations (Curtis et al., 2004).

Organizational-Level/Institutional-Level Factors

A variety of institutions influence the development, care, and treatment of mental illness, including the workplace, the school, and the primary-care office. One type of institution that has important implications for mental illness and care is the workplace. As discussed in Chapter 21, the workplace can affect mental health through job-related stress and job strain. People who experience large workloads and high pressures at work are at increased risk of developing depressive and anxiety disorders (Melchior et al., 2007). The workplace also affects mental health through the provision (or nonprovision) of health insurance, employee assistance programs, and sick leave benefits. Additionally, care and treatment of mental illness are affected by institutional structures including the school system, the pharmaceutical industry, and the medical system.

In recent decades, schools have been assuming a more prominent role in the secondary and tertiary prevention of mental illness (Weist, 2005). Despite challenges such as insufficient space for providing services, high turnover in school personnel, and great pressure to spend time and money on increasing test scores, many schools have been actively involved in mental health assessment and treatment. In fact, research suggests that about half the young people who receive mental health services entered care through the school system (Farmer, Burns, Phillips, Anngold, & Costello, 2003). Schools have been particularly involved in identifying children who exhibit signs of externalizing or "acting out" behavior problems, such as those with attention-deficit hyperactivity disorder (ADHD), oppositional defiant disorder (ODD), or conduct disorder (CD), as such externalizing of problems can be very disruptive in the classroom. Identification of such problems often leads to referral for a mental health evaluation and treatment as indicated. Other problems such as anxiety, depression, and suicidal ideation are detected less frequently, likely because these problems are less likely to cause disruption of an entire class or prevent a teacher from executing his or her lesson plan. School-based mental health counseling and schools' administration of psychiatric medication helps increase the likelihood that children will receive mental health treatment as indicated, although many children who receive school-based services require external mental health services as well.

At the organizational level, efforts toward primary prevention of mental disorders include wellness programs in the workplace. Programs that focus on stress reduction and health promotion, especially those that include physical exercise, may be the most effective at preventing mental illness. For example, a study conducted with casino employees in Australia tested the effects of a supervised exercise program on symptoms of depression (Atlantis, Chow, Kirby, & Singh, 2004). Employees seeking treatment for a mental health disorder were excluded from participation. Eligible participants were randomized into two conditions: (1) immediate intervention or (2) wait-list control, in which participants received no treatment for 24 weeks and then received the intervention for 24 weeks. For the intervention, participants were given instructions for getting at least 20 minutes of moderate- to high-intensity aerobic activity at least 3 days per week and doing weight training at least 2 days per week. They also received five health education seminars, 60 minutes of individual counseling per month, and weekly personalized e-mail messages with performance feedback. After 24 weeks, participants who completed the program reported significantly fewer symptoms of depression and stress than people in the wait-list control group, suggesting that this organizationally based intervention may be effective for preventing depression.

Secondary prevention, or early detection and treatment, can occur in a variety of organizational settings, including the workplace (Godard, Chevalier, Lecrubier, & Lahon, 2006), the school, and the health care delivery system (McAlpine & Wilson, 2004). It might seem intuitive for secondary prevention to occur at the primary-care office, and in fact, many people who receive mental health care are treated in nonspecialty medical clinics (Wang, Berglund, & Kessler, 2000). However, many barriers can prevent detection and treatment of mental disorders in primary care (Thielke, Vannoy, & Unutzer, 2007). Due to embarrassment or fear of stigma, patients may be reluctant to admit to experiencing mental health problems. Providers may have difficulty identifying and treating mental health problems when patients present with a variety of other health problems and providers have a limited time frame in which to address patients' needs. Primary-care providers (PCPs) are typically not well trained to diagnose and treat mental health problems, and those who are may struggle to find the time to do so during brief office visits. Moreover, the medical system, at least in the United States, is not designed to provide financial incentives for mental health diagnosis and treatment in primary care, although many providers perceive financial disincentives for referring patients to specialty mental health services (Van Voorhees, Wang, & Ford, 2003).

Efforts to improve PCPs' competencies in mental health assessment and treatment have changed service provisions but have not been effective in improving patients' mental health outcomes. Programs that aim to increase screening in primary-care settings have demonstrated increases in the rates of mental health diagnoses, although research has not found that screening alone improves mental health outcomes (Thielke et al., 2007). Similarly, training PCPs to detect and treat mental health problems has been found to increase prescriptions of psychiatric medications but has not been found to improve patient outcomes (Brown et al., 2000; Goldberg et al., 1998). Guidelines have been developed to aid PCPs in providing standard treatment for mental health problems such as major depressive disorder, anxiety disorders, and ADHD, although guidelines alone have not resulted in noteworthy improvements of mental health outcomes either (Croudace et al., 2003; Thielke et al., 2007).

A newer organizational approach to identification of mental health problems through primary care is the Behavioral Health Laboratory (Oslin et al., 2006). This strategy, implemented in the Veteran's Administration system, still depends on the PCP's recognition of possible mental health problems and referral to the program but reduces the PCP's burden by conducting a telephone assessment and providing PCPs with symptom reports and a suggested treatment plan. The Behavioral Health Laboratory was also used to monitor treatment among those prescribed antidepressants. This program is relatively inexpensive and has been found to increase the number of patients screened and identified as needing mental health care. At this time, data on mental health outcomes among participants in this program are not yet available.

For secondary and tertiary prevention, one potentially valuable strategy is to provide primary care and mental health care in the same physical location, also called centralizing or colocating care. One randomized controlled trial among a geriatric population sought to test whether it would be more helpful to provide enhanced referral to specialty mental health clinics (including scheduling, transportation, and payment) or to colocate mental health clinics with primary care (Bartels et al., 2004). They found that patients randomized to colocated services were more likely to attend mental health visits. Similarly, other studies have demonstrated the benefits of centralized care for people with substance abuse (Samet, Friedmann, & Saitz, 2001) as well as other disorders.

Another organizational approach to improving secondary and tertiary prevention is the Collaborative Care model (Katon, 2003; Thielke et al., 2007). For mental health, Collaborative Care models typically rely on a "care extender," often a nurse or a social worker, who follows the patient through problem identification to treatment planning and monitoring (Katon, 2003, p. 226). A psychiatrist often provides guidance and supervision regarding pharmacologic treatment. In this pragmatic approach, treatment is guided by outlining clear goals and tracking patient achievement through systematic assessments conducted by the care manager in the office or over the telephone. To reduce the costs of care with this model, a "stepped" approach is often implemented, in which treatment begins with low-intensity, low-cost services such as nurse management and provision of psychiatric medication by a PCP; when the care manager identifies that a more intensive approach is warranted, the treatment is intensified, and the patient is referred to a mental health specialist. Some variations of this model actively engage patients in treatment decisions, which may increase patients' motivations for following through with treatment. Studies show that the Collaborative Care model is more effective than standard care for treatment retention, mental health outcomes, and overall functioning and may be especially effective with ethnic minority group members, adolescents, and older adults who have comorbid conditions (Thielke et al., 2007; Unutzer, Katon, Callahan, et al., 2002; Unutzer, Katon, Fan, et al., 2008).

Neighborhood-Level/Community-Level Factors

Neighborhood or community conditions and norms can affect the onset as well as the care and treatment of mental illness. Using a novel approach, the Moving to Opportunity study assessed the effects of neighborhood on economic outcomes and mental health (Leventhal & Brooks-Gunn, 2003). This randomized housing mobility study provided a subset of families in high-poverty public housing the opportunity to move to low-poverty neighborhoods. Families in the experimental group were given housing vouchers and assistance with moving to low-poverty areas. Postintervention, families who moved to low-poverty neighborhoods did not differ from control participants in terms of employment or income, but parents were less likely to report psychological distress. Among children, boys in the experimental group were less likely to report symptoms of depression and anxiety, although girls did not experience these mental health benefits. The benefits of moving were experienced by children aged 8 to 13 years but not by older youth, suggesting that moving to more economically robust neighborhoods may have differential effects based on age and developmental factors.

What is it about some neighborhoods that leads to poorer mental health? Some physical characteristics of neighborhoods, such as the preponderance of buildings with lead paint, are thought to contribute directly to mental health problems. Children exposed to high levels of lead through paint or other means are at greater risk of developing cognitive or behavioral problems (Canfield et al., 2003), including ADHD (Braun, Kahn, Froehlich, Auinger, & Lanphear, 2006). Neighborhood conditions can also affect mental health indirectly by contributing to feelings of low self-worth and lack of hope for the future, which could lead to depression or other mental illnesses (Atkins, Graczyk, Frazier, & Abdul-Adil, 2003; Xue, Leventhal, Brooks-Gunn, & Earls, 2005).

Social aspects of neighborhoods can also have important effects on mental health. One might expect that greater social ties would be associated with greater mental health, regardless of the environment, although data suggest that this is not the case (Caughy, O'Campo, & Mutaner, 2003; Dupere & Perkins, 2007). In wealthier neighborhoods, socially isolated individuals tend to have worse mental health. However, in neighborhoods and communities characterized by poverty or significant fears of crime and high rates of physical and social disorder, people who are socially isolated from their neighbors have better mental health than their socially integrated peers. In such situations, social isolation is protective, perhaps because interactions with others in these disadvantaged environments can be stressful (Brodsky, 1999).

Another important factor influencing mental health care at the community level is the community's culture around mental health care. Communities of ethnic groups vary in their social norms surrounding mental health care and treatment, which could explain the differential rates of mental health service utilization across ethnic groups. For instance, research has found that mental health help seeking varies across ethnic groups. Compared with European Americans, Asian Americans—especially those who are not well acculturated into American society—have a low likelihood of seeking care for mental health problems and high rates of treatment dropout once they do seek care (Leong & Lau, 2001). Some Asian Americans are also inclined to seek medical care, rather than mental health care, for mental health problems, perhaps due to the extremely high level of stigma surrounding mental illness among the Asian American community (Leong & Lau, 2001). Cultural value orientations, especially principles of collectivism versus individualism, may also make psychotherapy difficult, if not inappropriate, for Asian Americans (Leong & Lau, 2001). African Americans may be inclined to turn to families and the clergy for help with emotional problems and to see mental health help seeking as a sign of weakness (Thompson, Bazile, & Akbar, 2004). Despite this, studies suggest that African Americans prefer counseling to antidepressant medication for the treatment of depression (Dwight-Johnson, Sherbourne, Liao, & Wells, 2000), although some African Americans may not believe that the mostly white mental health profession is truly interested in helping them (Cooper et al., 2003; Thompson et al., 2004). Thus, for African Americans, accessibility of African American mental health professionals may greatly influence their seeking care and treatment.

Even when someone is motivated to seek care, community structures may affect the ability of that person to access appropriate care. In some communities, mental health care may be difficult to access because there are few entry points into mental health care (e.g., lack of interagency linkages), because few agencies provide mental health care in the community, and because of lack of public transportation to available mental health services. Limited access to mental health services is a concern for many, especially those living in rural areas. A study of adults living with HIV in the Deep South found that over a 1-year period, rural residents were less likely than urban residents to receive mental health services. Among those with high levels of psychological distress, rural residents were also less likely to receive mental health services. Moreover, the rural residents who did receive mental health services had fewer visits than their urban peers, which may be due to the time limitations of mental health providers in rural areas (Reif, Whetten, Ostermann, & Raper, 2006).

The Positive Mental Attitudes Project (Quinn & Knifton, 2005) is a community-level intervention designed to address stigma in a community in Scotland. Community members, especially users of mental health services, youth, mental health professionals, schools, economic developers, social workers, community planners, and a local arts development team were involved in program development, including design, planning, and implementation. The resulting intervention had four components: (1) introducing antistigma curricula in secondary schools, (2) providing information and developing policies for employers, (3) training public service employees, and (4) facilitating broader social marketing efforts. Benefits were shown at multiple levels. Participating users of mental health services reported increased confidence and skills as a result of the program. Students who received the antistigma curricula reported more positive attitudes about mental health and lowered perceptions of the dangerousness of people with mental illness, a key factor associated with mental illness stigma (Link, Phelan, Bresnahan, Stueve, & Pescosolido, 1999). Public service employees who participated in the training reported improved attitudes about mental illness, and 69% of those interviewed reported that the training had changed their behavior toward people with mental illness.

Another community-level intervention that may have important implications for mental health care and treatment is linkage between mental health services and faith-based organizations. Many people turn to religious organizations or the clergy for help with mental health problems, providing a potentially important source of referral into mental health treatment. Researchers in New Haven, Connecticut, sought to better understand pastoral counseling by the African American clergy and spoke to 121 pastors about their related experiences. They found that all pastors reported that they conducted at least some counseling as part of their positions. Nearly half the pastors reported that they had referred help seekers to other services, including other clergy members, hospital emergency departments, social workers, and public mental health centers, yet only 10% to 20% of pastors reported regularly referring people to formal mental health services (Young, Griffith, & Williams, 2003). The study did not assess the willingness of pastors to work collaboratively with mental health providers, although effectively engaging pastors would be essential to such service linkages. The past decade has seen an increase in linkages between faith-based organizations and secular services, which may create a ripe environment for linking more faith-based organizations and the clergy with mental health providers.

Societal-Level Factors

The aforementioned factors influencing mental health and illness must be understood in the context of broader society. This section briefly discusses three important sources of influence at the societal level that contribute to public mental health in the United States: (1) policy, (2) the health care delivery system, and (3) the pharmaceutical industry. Before moving on, it is important to note that the impact of these societal-level factors extends beyond increased access to care. It can be argued that not only laws, policies, and programs related to mental illness prevention affect the accessibility of services but also the proliferation or amelioration of stigma related to mental health disorders. Laws and policies that provide widespread access to mental health services indirectly communicate the pervasiveness of mental health problems and the importance of care seeking, potentially decreasing beliefs that mental health problems are rare or controllable without professional assistance.

POLICY AND MENTAL HEALTH

A thorough review of policy influencing mental health in the United States or globally is well beyond the scope of this chapter; however, this section will review several key developments in public policy that have affected public mental health in the United States (Levine, 1981). In 1854, early in our nation's history, President Franklin Pierce refused to sign a bill to support state mental hospitals, arguing that the federal government should not concern itself with mental health. At that time, care of the people with serious mental health problems was generally limited to state-run institutions for "lunatics." Since then, the federal government has become increasingly involved in mental health care.

The National Institute of Mental Health was created by the National Mental Health Act in 1946 and established in 1949 to provide an infrastructure for supporting research and training initiatives aimed at promoting mental health and eliminating mental illness. In 1963, President John F. Kennedy addressed the Congress, urging change in our nation's system for preventing and treating mental illness and mental retardation. In response, Congress passed the 1963 Community Mental Health Centers Act, which allocated federal funds for the establishment of mental health care in the community, so that individuals with mental illness could be released from crowded, often underfunded institutions that did not allow for the integration of the individual with mental illness into society. This legislation required that all such centers would serve all persons in their assigned geographical "catchment" area, regardless of age, race, diagnosis, or ability to pay. The 1963 Community Mental Health Centers Act represents an important development in public mental health for its role in deinstitutionalization and, thus, reduction of mental illness stigma. Unfortunately, the legislation failed to integrate mental health services with the many ancillary services that would be required to help individuals with mental disorders live in the community, such as housing, welfare services, and medical care. As an artifact of that and other legislation, the mental health service sector is significantly fragmented, making it extremely difficult and complicated for individuals with mental disorders to access the many services they need.

In 1965, Medicare and Medicaid were established, allowing some of the poor, disabled, and elderly to obtain care in settings other than community mental health centers, including outpatient mental health clinics and psychiatric units in general hospitals (Frank & Glied, 2006). Initially, Medicare was limited in its mental health benefits, as it required high-cost sharing with states and restrictions on service utilization. In the 1980s, changes in Medicare provided greater access to psychotherapy and hospitalization and enabled reimbursement of services provided by psychologists and social workers. In contrast with Medicare, Medicaid had profound effects on mental health care. Because it did not reimburse for stays in public mental hospitals, Medicaid prompted trans-institutionalization, or transfer of many elderly people with a mental illness from state mental hospitals to nursing homes, some of which were not well equipped for mental health care. Medicaid also provided a range of outpatient mental health benefits and has become the largest payer for mental health care in the United States (Mark, Levit, Buck, Coffey, & Vandivort-Warren, 2007).

As early as 1965, efforts to establish *parity*, or equivalent insurance coverage for mental and medical care, have emerged in the U.S. House and Senate, although these efforts have not yet been successful in ensuring full mental health parity (Frank & Glied, 2006). However, since 2001, full mental health parity has been required in health care plans provided to U.S. federal employees. Evidence suggests that these federal plans reduce out-of-pocket spending for consumers of mental health care; increases in premiums and costs to providers are minimal (Goldman, 2007). As of 2007, 31 states in America have passed laws requiring mental health parity, although the laws vary in terms of which disorders are covered ("Health Care: State Laws Mandating or Regulating Mental Health Benefits," 2007). Nevertheless, many insured Americans are still without mental health coverage that is comparable with their "physical" health benefits (National Mental Health Association, 2003).

Since President Kennedy's address on mental health in the early 1960s, recent U.S. presidents have attempted to alter mental health care in this country through special investigations and reports. In 1999, during President William Clinton's administration, the Surgeon General released a report on the nation's mental health (U.S. Department of Health and Human Services, 1999). A major goal of that report was to reduce the stigma associated with mental illness. In 2002, President George W. Bush's New Freedom Commission on Mental Health was formed and charged with studying the U.S. mental health delivery system and recommending improvements. In 2003, the Commission released a report with goals and recommendations for transforming the U.S. mental health system (Druss & Goldman, 2003; Hogan, 2003). The Commission's recommendations generally involve improvements to make the mental health delivery system more accessible, less fragmented, and more effective. Other recommendations include developing programs to reduce mental illness stigma and prevent suicide, as well as increasing research focused on promoting recovery, resilience, prevention, and cures. A survey of mental health leaders a year after the release of the Commission's report suggests that the report has generated some change in the organizations related to mental health, mostly in the form of facilitating discussions, encouraging interagency linkages, and affecting organizational planning (von Esenwein et al., 2005), although the long-term mental health effects of the Commission's report remain unknown.

THE HEALTH CARE DELIVERY SYSTEM

The health care delivery system in the United States and many other countries is not always well equipped to meet the demand for mental health care. In the United States, many insurance providers using managed care consider PCPs the gatekeepers of specialty medical care (Forrest et al., 2003). Thus, many adults present to their PCP with mental health problems. Some people may visit their PCP with the stated goal of seeking mental health care. Others may not recognize their need for mental health care and may rely on their PCP to recognize the need. Yet mental health needs may go undetected by PCPs. Reasons for this include that many PCPs lack training for dealing with mental health problems and may not know how to speak with their patients about this sensitive and highly stigmatized topic, especially among cultural groups other than their own (Thielke et al., 2007). When mental health problems are detected and referrals are made, many individuals with insurance may be unable to make the copayments often required for mental health evaluation and treatment, while those without insurance who do not meet the eligibility criteria for Medicaid or Medicare experience even greater financial barriers (Safran et al., 2002).

When individuals do have insurance, their plans typically involve managed behavioral health carve-outs, meaning that behavioral health care (i.e., alcohol, drug abuse, and mental health care) is managed under a different entity than the primary insurance provider (Frank & Garfield, 2007). One encouraging trend is that behavioral health carve-outs have led to increases in mental health service use and a reduction of inpatient hospitalization for mental illness and substance abuse, which fits with nationwide efforts to treat people with mental illness in the least restrictive environment. Carve-outs have also had less positive effects on mental health care. Behavioral health care vendors do not generally reimburse PCPs for the extra time they may take to treat a person with a mental disorder, yet they often make referrals to specialty providers cumbersome. As a result, PCPs may be inclined to prescribe psychotropic medication rather than refer patients to specialty mental health services. Unfortunately, carve-outs also contribute to the fragmentation of health and mental health services, making it complex to provide adequate care to people with comorbid mental and "physical" health problems.

THE PHARMACEUTICAL INDUSTRY

In the United States, the pharmaceutical industry affects mental health care through the availability and costs of psychiatric medications. From 1991 to 2001, spending on psychotropic drugs grew 17% annually, with psychotropic drugs representing about 7% of mental health spending in 1991 to 23% of spending in 2001 (Mark et al., 2005; Mark, Levit, Coffey, et al., 2007). These increased expenditures are due to both greater utilization and rising prices (Frank, Conti, & Goldman, 2005). Since the late 1980s, new classes of drugs have been available to treat psychosis (atypical antipsychotics) and depression (selective serotonin reuptake inhibitors [SSRIs] and serotonin-norepinephrine reuptake inhibitors [SNRIs]), many of which have fewer side effects than previously available treatments. These developments have led to an increase in the use of psychotropic medication in the United

States. Studies show that patients are more likely to adhere to regimens with these newer drugs, which results in increased treatment success (Frank et al., 2005).

A major change in the past two decades is the direct marketing of psychotropic medications to consumers. Rather than relying on physicians to introduce medications to patients, people can learn about available medications simply from watching television advertisements. Research suggests that depressed people who have seen advertisements about antidepressant medication are more likely to use antidepressants than those who have not seen such advertisements, suggesting that direct marketing is effective (Donohue, Berndt, Rosenthal, Epstein, & Frank, 2004). Marketing to consumers may simplify the process of obtaining treatment for more common disorders such as depression, in that patients may be more comfortable asking their PCPs for specific medications to treat such disorders, which may make it easy for PCPs to prescribe those medications.

CONCLUSION

Mental health and illness are affected by a multitude of factors at the intrapersonal, interpersonal, organizational/institutional, neighborhood/community, and societal levels, with no factor singly explaining the development, care and treatment, or rehabilitation of mental illness. The factors influencing mental health and illness at the more microlevels of the model must be understood within the broader contexts of community and society. Our knowledge about mental health and illness is derived from the many research studies that have addressed this important topic, from epidemiological, sociological, anthropological, psychological, and political perspectives. At the same time, we are limited by the state of the science, including our incomplete understanding of the role of genetics in mental illness development and rehabilitation, as well as our insufficient knowledge of how to best support people with mental illness to help them live quality and meaningful lives. We are also limited by a fragmented health delivery system, and while we expect that defragmentation will improve the detection, care, and treatment of mental illness, the systemic changes that would be required to achieve this will become increasingly complex.

REFERENCES

Atkins, M. S., Graczyk, P. A., Frazier, S. L., & Abdul-Adil, J. (2003). Toward a new model for promoting urban children's mental health: Accessible, effective, and sustainable school-based mental health services. *School Psychology Review, 32*, 503–514.

Atlantis, E., Chow, C. M., Kirby, A., & Singh, M. F. (2004). An effective exercise-based intervention for improving mental health and quality of life measures: A randomized controlled trial. *Preventive Medicine, 39*(2), 424–434.

Bandura, A. (1986). *Social foundations of thought and action: A social cognitive theory.* Englewood Cliffs, NJ: Prentice Hall.

Bartels, S. J., Coakley, E. H., Zubritsky, C., Ware, J. H., Miles, K. M., Arean, P. A., et al. (2004). Improving access to geriatric mental health services: A randomized trial comparing treatment engagement with integrated versus enhanced referral care for depression, anxiety, and at-risk alcohol use. *American Journal of Psychiatry, 161*(8), 1455–1462.

Bayer, J. K., Hiscock, H., Morton-Allen, E., Ukomunne, O. C., & Wake, M. (2007). Prevention of mental health problems: Rationale for a universal approach. *Archives of Disease in Childhood, 92,* 34–38.

Bijl, R. V., de Graaf, R., Hiripi, E., Kessler, R. C., Kohn, R., Offord, D. R., et al. (2003). The prevalence of treated and untreated mental disorders in five countries. *Health Affairs, 22,* 122–133.

Braun, J. M., Kahn, R. S., Froehlich, T., Auinger, P., & Lanphear, B. P. (2006). Exposures to environmental toxicants and attention deficit hyperactivity disorder in U.S. children. *Environmental Health Perspectives, 114*(12), 1904–1909.

Brodsky, A. E. (1999). Making it: The components and process of resilience among urban, African-American, single mothers. *American Journal of Orthopsychiatry, 69,* 148–160.

Brofenbrenner, U. (1979). *The ecology of human development.* Cambridge, MA: Harvard University Press.

Brown, J. B., Shye, D., McFarland, B. H., Nichols, G. A., Mullooly, J. P., & Johnson, R. E. (2000). Controlled trials of CQI and academic detailing to implement a clinical practice guideline for depression. *Joint Commission Journal on Quality Improvement, 26*(1), 39–54.

Cameron, C. (1996). Patient compliance: Recognition of factors involved and suggestions for promoting compliance with therapeutic regimens. *Journal of Advanced Nursing, 24,* 244–250.

Canfield, R. L., Henderson, C. R., Jr., Cory-Slechta, D. A., Cox, C., Jusko, T. A., & Lanphear, B. P. (2003). Intellectual impairment in children with blood lead concentrations below 10 μg per deciliter. *New England Journal of Medicine, 348*(16), 1517–1526.

Caughy, M. O., O'Campo, P. J., & Mutaner, C. (2003). When being alone might be better: Neighborhood poverty, social capital, and child mental health. *Social Science & Medicine, 57,* 227–237.

Centers for Disease Control and Prevention. (n.d.). *Fast stats A to Z: Self-inflicted injury/ suicide.* Retrieved January 30, 2008, from www.cdc.gov/nchs/fastats/suicide.htm

Cooper, L. A., Gonzales, J. J., Gallo, J. J., Rost, K. M., Meredith, L. S., Rubenstein, L. V., et al. (2003). The acceptability of treatment for depression among African-American, Hispanic, and white primary care patients. *Medical Care, 41*(4), 479–489.

Croudace, T., Evans, J., Harrison, G., Sharp, D. J., Wilkinson, E., McCann, G., et al. (2003). Impact of the ICD-10 primary health care (PHC) diagnostic and management guidelines for mental disorders on detection and outcome in primary care. Cluster randomised controlled trial. *British Journal of Psychiatry, 182,* 20–30.

Cuijpers, P. (2003). Examining the effects of prevention programs on the incidence of new cases of mental disorders: The lack of statistical power. *American Journal of Psychiatry, 160*(8), 1385–1391.

Cuijpers, P., Can Straten, A., & Smit, F. (2005). Preventing the incidence of new cases of mental disorders: A meta-analytic review. *Journal of Nervous and Mental Disease, 193,* 119–125.

Curtis, N. M., Ronan, K. R., & Borduin, C. M. (2004). Multisystemic treatment: A meta-analysis of outcome studies. *Journal of Family Psychology, 18,* 411–419.

Donohue, J. M., Berndt, E. R., Rosenthal, M., Epstein, A. M., & Frank, R. G. (2004). Effects of pharmaceutical promotion on adherence to the treatment guidelines for depression. *Medical Care, 42*(12), 1176–1185.

Druss, B. G., & Goldman, H. H. (2003). New Freedom Commission Report: Introduction to the special section on the President's New Freedom Commission Report. *Psychiatric Services, 54,* 1465–1466.

Dupere, V., & Perkins, D. D. (2007). Community types and mental health: A multilevel study of local environmental stress and coping. *American Journal of Community Psychology, 39,* 107–119.

Dwight-Johnson, M., Sherbourne, C. D., Liao, D., & Wells, K. B. (2000). Treatment preferences among depressed primary care patients. *Journal of General Internal Medicine, 15*(8), 527–534.

Evert, H., Harvey, C., Trauer, T., & Herrman, H. (2003). The relationship between social networks and occupational and self-care functioning in people with psychosis. *Social Psychiatry and Psychiatric Epidemiology, 38*(4), 180–188.

Farmer, E. M. Z., Burns, B. J., Phillips, S. D., Anngold, A., & Costello, E. J. (2003). Pathways into and through mental health services for children and adolescents. *Psychiatric Services, 54,* 60–66.

Forrest, C. B., Nutting, P., Werner, J. J., Starfield, B., von Schrader, S., & Rohde, C. (2003). Managed health plan effects on the specialty referral process: Results from the Ambulatory Sentinel Practice Network referral study. *Medical Care, 41*(2), 242–253.

Frank, R. G., Conti, R. M., & Goldman, H. H. (2005). Mental health policy and psychotropic drugs. *The Milbank Quarterly, 83,* 271–298.

Frank, R. G., & Garfield, R. L. (2007). Managed behavioral health care carve-outs: Past performance and future prospects. *Annual Review of Public Health, 28,* 303–320.

Frank, R. G., & Glied, S. A. (2006). *Better but not well: Mental health policy in the United States since 1950.* Baltimore: Johns Hopkins University Press.

Godard, C., Chevalier, A., Lecrubier, Y., & Lahon, G. (2006). APRAND programme: An intervention to prevent relapses of anxiety and depressive disorders. First results of a medical health promotion intervention in a population of employees. *European Psychiatry, 21,* 451–459.

Goldberg, H. I., Wagner, E. H., Fihn, S. D., Martin, D. P., Horowitz, C. R., Christensen, D. B., et al. (1998). A randomized controlled trial of CQI teams and academic detailing: Can they alter compliance with guidelines? *Joint Commission Journal on Quality Improvement, 24*(3), 130–142.

Goldman, H. H. (2007). Considering health insurance parity for mental health and substance abuse treatment: The federal employees health benefits experience. *American Journal of Psychiatry, 164,* 1473–1474.

Granerud, A., & Severinsson, E. (2006). The struggle for social integration in the community: The experiences of people with mental health problems. *Journal of Psychiatric Mental Health Nursing, 13*(3), 288–293.

Greenly, J. R., Mechanic, D., & Cleary, P. D. (1987). Seeking help for psychological problems: A replication and extension. *Medical Care, 25,* 1113–1128.

Hafner, H. (2003). Gender differences in schizophrenia. *Psychoneuroendocrinology, 28*(Suppl. 2), 17–54.

Health care: State laws mandating or regulating mental health benefits. (2007). Retrieved February 29, 2008, from www.ncsl.org/programs/health/mentalben.htm

Hogan, M. F. (2003). The President's New Freedom Commission: Recommendations to transform mental health care in America. *Psychiatric Services, 54*(11), 1467–1474.

Hutchinson, D. S. (2005). Structured exercise for persons with serious psychiatric disabilities. *Psychiatric Services, 56*(3), 353–354.

Jones, D. R., Macias, C., Barreira, P. J., Fisher, W. H., Hargreaves, W. A., & Harding, C. M. (2004). Prevalence, severity, and co-occurrence of chronic physical health problems of persons with serious mental illness. *Psychiatric Services, 55*(11), 1250–1257.

Katon, W. J. (2003). The Institute of Medicine "Chasm" report: Implications for depression collaborative care models. *General Hospital Psychiatry, 25,* 222–229.

Kessler, R. C., Chiu, W. T., Demler, O., Merikangas, K. R., & Walters, E. E. (2005). Prevalence, severity, and comorbidity of 12-month *DSM-IV* disorders in the National Comorbidity Survey Replication. *Archives of General Psychiatry, 62*(6), 617–627.

Leaf, P. J., Bruce, M. L., Tischler, G. L., & Holzer, C. E. (1986). The relationship between demographic factors and attitudes toward mental health services. *Journal of Community Psychology, 15,* 275–284.

Leong, F. T., & Lau, A. S. (2001). Barriers to providing effective mental health services to Asian Americans. *Mental Health Services Research, 3*(4), 201–214.

Leventhal, T., & Brooks-Gunn, J. (2003). Moving to opportunity: An experimental study of neighborhood effects on mental health. *American Journal of Public Health, 93*(9), 1576–1582.

Levine, M. (1981). *The history and politics of community mental health.* New York: Oxford.

Link, B. G., Phelan, J. C., Bresnahan, M., Stueve, A., & Pescosolido, B. A. (1999). Public conceptions of mental illness: Labels, causes, dangerousness, and social distance. *American Journal of Public Health, 89*(9), 1328–1333.

Mark, T., Levit, K. R., Coffey, R. M., McKusick, D., Harwood, H., King, E. C., et al. (2007). National expenditures for mental health services and substance abuse treatment: 1993–2003. Retrieved February 17, 2008, from www.samhsa.gov/spendingestimates/SAMHSAFINAL9303.pdf

Mark, T. L., Coffey, R. M., McKusick, D., Harwood, H., King, E., Bouchery, E., et al. (2005). *National expenditures for mental health services and substance abuse treatment.* Retrieved February 17, 2008, from www.samhsa.gov/spendingestimates/SEPGenRpt013105v2BLX.pdf

Mark, T. L., Levit, K. R., Buck, J. A., Coffey, R. M., & Vandivort-Warren, R. (2007). Mental health treatment expenditure trends, 1986–2003. *Psychiatric Services 58*(8), 1041–1048.

McAlpine, D. D., & Wilson, A. R. (2004). Screening for depression in primary care: What do we still need to know? *Depression and Anxiety, 19,* 137–145.

Melchior, M., Caspi, A., Meline, B. J., Danese, A., Poulton, R., & Moffitt, T. E. (2007). Work stress precipitates depression and anxiety in young, working women and men. *Psychological Medicine, 37,* 1119–1129.

Merry, S., McDowell, H., Hetrick, S., Bir, J., & Muller, N. (2004). Psychological and/or educational interventions for the prevention of depression in children and adolescents. *Cochrane Database of Systematic Reviews, 1,* CD003380.

Morrison, A. P., French, P., Walford, L., Lewis, S. W., Kilcommons, A., Green, J., et al. (2004). Cognitive therapy for the prevention of psychosis in people at ultra-high risk: Randomised controlled trial. *British Journal of Psychiatry, 185,* 291–297.

Mrazek, P. J., & Haggerty, R. J. (1994). *Reducing risks for mental disorders: Frontiers for preventive intervention research.* Washington, DC: National Academy Press.

Munoz, R. F., Mrazek, P. J., & Haggerty, R. J. (1996). Institute of Medicine report on prevention of mental disorders summary and commentary. *American Psychologist, 51*(11), 1116–1122.

National Mental Health Association. (2003). *Can't make the grade* (NMHA State Mental Health Assessment Project). Alexandria, VA: Author.

Oslin, D. W., Ross, J., Sayers, S., Murphy, J., Kane, V., & Katz, I. R. (2006). Screening, assessment, and management of depression in VA primary care clinics. The Behavioral Health Laboratory. *Journal of General Internal Medicine, 21*(1), 46–50.

Patel, V., Araya, R., Chatterjee, S., Chisholm, D., Cohen, A., De Silva, M., et al. (2007). Treatment and prevention of mental disorders in low-income and middle-income countries. *The Lancet, 370,* 991–1005.

Quinn, N., & Knifton, L. (2005). Promoting recovery and addressing stigma: Mental health awareness through community development in a low-income area. *International Journal of Mental Health Promotion, 7,* 37–44.

Reif, S., Whetten, K., Ostermann, J., & Raper, J. L. (2006). Characteristics of HIV-infected adults in the Deep South and their utilization of mental health services: A rural vs. urban comparison. *AIDS Care, 18*, S10–S17.

Rosenberg, S. D., Goodman, L. A., Osher, F. C., Swartz, M. S., Essock, S. M., Butterfield, M. I., et al. (2001). Prevalence of HIV, hepatitis B, and hepatitis C in people with severe mental illness. *American Journal of Public Health, 91*(1), 31–37.

Safran, D. G., Neuman, P., Schoen, C., Montgomery, J. E., Li, W., Wilson, I. B., et al. (2002). Prescription drug coverage and seniors: How well are states closing the gap? [Electronic version]. *Health Affairs*, W253–W268. Retrieved February 29, 2008, from http://content.healthaffairs.org/cgi/reprint/hlthaff.w2.253v1

Samet, J. H., Friedmann, P., & Saitz, R. (2001). Benefits of linking primary medical care and substance abuse services: Patient, provider, and societal perspectives. *Archives of Internal Medicine, 161*, 85–91.

Thielke, S., Vannoy, S., & Unutzer, J. (2007). Integrating mental health and primary care. *Primary Care, 34*(3), 571–592, vii.

Thompson, V. L. S., Bazile, A., & Akbar, M. (2004). African American's perceptions of psychotherapy and psychotherapists. *Professional Psychology: Research and Practice, 35*, 19–26.

U.S. Department of Health and Human Services. (1999). *Mental health: A report of the surgeon general–executive summary.* Rockville, MD: U.S. Department of Health and Human Services, Substance Abuse and Mental Health Services Administration, National Institutes of Health, Center for Mental Health Services.

Unutzer, J., Katon, W., Callahan, C. M., Williams, J. W., Jr., Hunkeler, E., Harpole, L., et al. (2002). Collaborative care management of late-life depression in the primary care setting: A randomized controlled trial. *Journal of the American Medical Association, 288*(22), 2836–2845.

Unutzer, J., Katon, W. J., Fan, M. Y., Schoenbaum, M. C., Lin, E. H., Della Penna, R. D., et al. (2008). Long-term cost effects of collaborative care for late-life depression. *American Journal of Managed Care, 14*(2), 95–100.

Van Voorhees, B., Wang, N., & Ford, D. E. (2003). Managed care organizational complexity and access to high-quality mental health services: Perspective of U.S. primary care physicians. *General Hospital Psychiatry, 25*, 149–157.

von Esenwein, S. A., Bornemann, T., Ellingson, L., Palpant, R., Randolph, L., & Druss, B. G. (2005). A survey of mental health leaders one year after the President's New Freedom Commission report. *Psychiatric Services, 56*(5), 605–607.

Wang, P. S., Berglund, P., & Kessler, R. C. (2000). Recent care of common mental disorders in the United States: Prevalence and conformance with evidence-based recommendations. *Journal of General Internal Medicine, 15*, 284–292.

Weist, M. D. (2005). Fulfilling the promise of school-based mental health: Moving toward a public mental health promotion approach. *Journal of Abnormal Child Psychology, 33*, 735–741.

World Health Organization (WHO). (2002). *Revised Global Burden of Disease (GBD) 2002 estimates: Disability adjusted life years.* Retrieved February 5, 2008, from www.who.int/healthinfo/statistics/gbdwhoregiondaly2002.xls

World Health Organization. (2007). *What is mental health?* Retrieved February 28, 2008, from www.who.int/features/qa/62/en/index.html

WHO World Mental Health Organization Survey Consortium. (2004). Prevalence, severity, and unmet need for treatment of mental disorders in the World Health Organization World Mental Health Surveys. *Journal of the American Medical Association, 291*, 2581–2590.

Wu, Z., Detels, R., Zhang, J., Li, V., & Li, J. (2002). Community-based trial to prevent drug use among youths in Yunnan, China. *American Journal of Public Health, 92*(12), 1952–1957.

Xue, Y. P., Leventhal, T. P., Brooks-Gunn, J. P., & Earls, F. J. (2005). Neighborhood residence and mental health problems of 5- to 11-year-olds. *Archives of General Psychiatry, 62*(5), 554–563.

Young, J. L., Griffith, E. E. H., & Williams, D. R. (2003). The integral role of pastoral counseling by African-American clergy in community mental health. *Psychiatric Services, 54*, 688–692.

Zlotnick, C., Miller, I. W., Pearlstein, T., Howard, M., & Sweeney, P. (2006). A preventive intervention for pregnant women on public assistance at risk for postpartum depression. *American Journal of Psychiatry, 163*(8), 1443–1445.

19

Prevention of Unintentional Injuries

Karen Liller

njuries are the third leading cause of death in the United States, producing more than 160,000 deaths per year (National Center for Injury Prevention and Control [NCIPC], 2006). They are the leading cause of death for children, adolescents, and adults up to age 44. Since injuries greatly affect the young, their years of potential life lost (YPLLs) to injuries is quite high. Millions more individuals are injured every year, and in 2004, approximately 29.6 million were treated for an injury in a hospital emergency department (NCIPC, 2006). Injuries cost the U.S. health care system more than $400 billion dollars a year (Sattin & Corso, 2007).

While it is true that injuries directly affect the victim, there are also often profound effects on the related intrapersonal, interpersonal, organizational, community, and societal levels. For example, a person's injury will influence the role he or she plays with family or friends, as they may need to help with caretaking. Employers and workplaces are affected if the individual's work performance is affected. Also, community support may be needed, and policies at the societal level may need to be changed to better accommodate the injured individual.

Injuries have been divided into those that are *unintentional,* or done without harmful intent, and those that are considered to be *intentional.* The latter are termed *violence* and include homicide and suicide. Motor vehicle events, poisonings, falls, fires and burns, and drownings are the leading causes of deaths due to unintentional injury. In 2004, there were 112,012 unintentional injury deaths in the United States (Centers for Disease Control and Prevention [CDC], NCIPC, 2007).

Injuries are formally defined as "any unintentional or intentional damage done to the body resulting from acute exposure to thermal, mechanical or kinetic, electrical, or chemical energy or from the absence of essentials such as oxygen or heat" (National Committee for Injury Prevention and Control, 1989, p. 4). Since the agent of injury is energy and not any one particular source, energy-focused interventions have been developed. For example, in a motor vehicle crash, it is the energy of motion or the mechanical energy that must be absorbed by car seats, seat belts, and air bags, which will mitigate the effects of the crash on the individual.

This chapter focuses on unintentional injuries; related prevention efforts, including the use of the socio-ecological model; and future directions that include integrated unintentional and violence-related prevention efforts. Other chapters in the text cover the related topics of violence and occupational safety.

UNINTENTIONAL INJURIES

Unintentional injuries are the fifth leading cause of death in the United States and the leading cause of death for individuals between the ages of 1 and 44 (CDC, NCIPC, 2007; Christoffel & Gallagher, 2006). The leading cause of death due to unintentional injury across the 1 to 44 age group is motor vehicle injury. Other causes across age groups vary but largely include poisonings, falls, fires and burns, drownings, and asphyxiations. The picture for nonfatal injuries is not the same as for fatal unintentional injuries. The leading cause of nonfatal unintentional injury across the majority of age groups is falls. There were nearly 8 million unintentional falls reported in 2004, with the greatest number of these reported in the 65 years and older age group (CDC, NCIPC, 2007).

Unintentional injury rates and their causes vary according to sex, age, race, income, and setting. Falls are the most common cause of death due to fatal injury among the elderly. The very old have the highest injury death rates in general due to their fragility and comorbidity. Also, injury death rates are often higher for males than for females. This can be due to more extensive risk taking among males and more involvement in dangerous occupational tasks. Race is also important. High rates of unintentional injuries are found among minority groups, including African Americans, American Indians, and Alaska Natives (Christoffel & Gallagher, 2006). These rates in general vary inversely with income and are higher in rural areas.

The category of motor vehicle injuries encompasses several subcategories, including single-vehicle crashes, multiple-vehicle crashes, truck-automobile crashes, and so on, and can involve occupants of the vehicle, pedestrians, motorcyclists, or pedal cyclists (Christoffel & Gallagher, 2006). Most of the motor vehicle crashes involve occupants. According to the National Highway Traffic Safety Administration (NHTSA, 2007b), in 2005, there were an estimated 6,159,000 police-reported traffic crashes, in which 43,443 people were killed and 2,699,000 people were injured. Thirty-nine percent of all fatal traffic crashes involve alcohol (NHTSA, 2007b). Strategies to prevent motor vehicle injuries include seat belt and child restraint use, obeying safety laws for drivers and passengers, and avoiding substance abuse.

While motor vehicle crashes lead in terms of unintentional injury deaths across the majority of age groups, other injuries such as falls, fires and burns, poisonings, and asphyxiations are also important. Males have greater death rates from fall injuries than females, and whites have higher rates than blacks. Falls occur across the life span and in many settings, including in the home and on the job. The majority of falls leading to death occur in the home and mostly affect children and the elderly (Christoffel & Gallagher, 2006). The risk of falling increases with age, with more than one out of every three persons aged 65 or older falling each year (Christoffel & Gallagher, 2006). Preventive approaches include weight-bearing and strength-building exercises for the elderly, decreased use of psychotropic drugs, environmental modifications, adequate calcium uptake, hormone replacement for women, and education of caregivers (Christoffel & Gallagher, 2006). For injuries involving children, the use of baby gates, stationary baby walkers, appropriate window guards, straps on changing tables, and energy-absorbing surfaces on playgrounds, as well as education of parents, are important (Christoffel & Gallagher, 2006).

Fires and burns are also an important cause of death due to unintentional injury. Most of these deaths are due to house fires and occur during the winter months, when heating and lighting sources are used (Christoffel & Gallagher, 2006). Alcohol or cigarette use is an important contributor. These fires are more likely to occur in low-income areas. Important prevention efforts include the installation and maintenance of smoke detectors, having and practicing a fire-escape plan, setting hot water heaters to 120° F, and states adopting the use of fire-safe cigarettes (Christoffel & Gallagher, 2006).

Drowning is another important cause of death due to unintentional injury. Drownings in some states such as Florida are the leading cause of death for children between the ages of 1 and 4 (Christoffel & Gallagher, 2006). This is due to the large bodies of water and accessibility of swimming pools. Swimming pools are largely involved in the majority of drownings among children between the ages of 0 and 4 (Christoffel & Gallagher, 2006). Alcohol is also a major contributor in drowning. Drowning rates are high overall in minority populations and in males (Christoffel & Gallagher, 2006). Prevention efforts include four-sided fencing around pools to separate the pool from the house and the yard, supervision of children, nonuse of alcohol and other substances, never swimming alone, and use of flotation devices while boating.

There has been an increase in poisoning deaths over the last several years. In 2004, poisoning was second only to motor vehicle crashes as a cause of death from unintentional injury in the United States (CDC, 2007). Data show that poisoning mortality rates have increased each year from 1999 to 2004, rising 62.5% during this 5-year period (CDC, 2007). The largest increases were seen in females (103%), whites (75.8%), persons living in the South (113.6%), and persons aged 15 to 24 years (113.3%) (CDC, 2007). Drug poisoning deaths increased 68.3%, and the largest increases have been due to unspecified, psychotherapeutic, and narcotic drug categories (CDC, 2007). This points to the need for stronger regulatory, educational, and treatment measures to address drug overdose (CDC, 2007).

Due to the Poison Prevention Packaging Act of 1970, childhood poisoning is no longer the problem it once was. In addition, product reformulation and interventions by poison control centers have all contributed to this decline (Safe Kids, 2007). However, in 2002, there were more than 1.2 million unintentional poisonings among children aged 5 and under reported to the U.S. Poison Control Centers (Safe Kids, 2007). Although many of these poisonings are due to household cleaners, other causes include iron, alcohol, and carbon monoxide (Safe Kids, 2007). In addition, with the recent import of toys and other products with a high lead content, it is prudent that products be continually checked for children's safety. Hazardous products in the home should be stored out of the reach of children and locked in cabinets.

Unintentional asphyxiations need also to be considered. They usually involve a nonfood product such as a toy part, balloons, coins, or similar objects and the inhalation or ingestion of food (including regurgitated food) leading to obstruction of the respiratory tract (Christoffel & Gallagher, 2006). In terms of toy parts, the Consumer Product Safety Commission provides testing of small parts that might lead to choking. Also, no longer can sweatshirt hoods have dangling cords that can become caught in things such as doors of buses or playground equipment and cause suffocation. It is also important for people to learn strategies such as the Heimlich maneuver and for restaurants to have available dislodging devices for asphyxiation (Christoffel & Gallagher, 2006).

INJURY PREVENTION EFFORTS

The Socio-Ecological Model

CASE STUDY Motorcycle Injuries

The role of the socio-ecological model described in this textbook is vital to the development of unintentional injury prevention and control efforts. To illustrate the model, factors associated with motorcycle injuries and deaths are discussed here.

Nearly, 4,600 motorcyclists were killed and an additional 87,000 were injured in traffic crashes in the United States in 2005 (NHTSA, 2007a). These data represented a 13% increase in deaths and 14% increase in injuries compared with the 2004 data (NHTSA, 2007a). Motorcycle injury deaths are greater among whites and among individuals between the ages of 20 and 44 years (CDC, NCIPC, 2007). Motorcycle riding is inherently dangerous; it has been reported that per vehicle mile traveled in 2004, motorcyclists were approximately 34 times more likely than car passenger occupants to die in a crash and 6 times more likely to be injured (NHTSA, 2007a). As for the behavior of motorcyclists, 24% of motorcycle operators involved in a fatal crash in 2005 had an invalid license compared with only 12% of drivers of passenger vehicles, and motorcycle operators were 1.4 times more likely than passenger vehicle drivers to have a previous license suspension or revocation (NHTSA, 2007a). Also, in 2005, a higher percentage of motorcycle operators had blood alcohol concentrations of 0.08 grams per deciliter or higher compared with other motor vehicle drivers (NHTSA, 2007a).

Motorcycle helmet use has been a lifesaving feature for motorcycle riders. NHTSA has reported that helmets have saved the lives of 1,546 motorcyclists in 2005 and an additional 728 lives would have been saved if all motorcyclists had worn helmets. Unfortunately, motorcycle helmet use has decreased by 23 percentage points over 5 years, from 71% in 2000 to

48% in 2005 (NHTSA, 2007a). This is a very significant decline and corresponds to a 79% increase in nonuse.

In the 1970s, almost all states had universal motorcycle helmet laws or laws that cover all individuals. This was largely due to the fact that the federal government required states to enact helmet laws in order to receive certain federal safety programs and highway construction funds (Insurance Institute for Highway Safety [IIHS], 2007). However, in 1976, states lobbied Congress to stop this practice of tying funds and programs to the helmet law. That led to most states repealing these laws or greatly limiting them to cover only young riders. At the end of 2004, the number of states in which all motorcyclists were required to wear a helmet had fallen to 20 and the District of Columbia; and 26 states have laws requiring only some motorcyclists to wear a helmet (Houston & Richardson, 2007). Four states—Colorado, Illinois, Iowa, and New Hampshire—have no motorcycle helmet law. Colorado now requires motorcycle operators 17 and younger and their passengers 17 and younger to wear helmets. Research has continually shown that having universal helmet laws leads to a reduction in deaths and serious injuries and that injuries and deaths greatly increase when laws are weakened or repealed (IIHS, 2007). A recent case example of this involves the state of Florida. In 2000, Florida changed its universal motorcycle helmet law so that motorcycle and moped riders 21 years or older were exempted from wearing helmets (Muller, 2004). The exempted riders are required to have medical insurance of $10,000. A monthly time-series analysis estimated a nearly 49% increase in motorcycle occupant deaths the year after the law was changed (Muller, 2004). When controlling for travel miles and motorcycle registrations, the estimate changes to 38.2% and 21.3%, respectively (Muller, 2004). Another study has shown that in states such as Florida, in which appeals against universal coverage for the helmet law have been admitted, the motorcyclist fatality rate increased an average of 12.2% above what would have occurred had universal coverage remained (Houston & Richardson, 2007).

In terms of the socio-ecological model and motorcycle injuries and deaths, contributing factors at the intrapersonal or more proximal level include the behavior of the motorcyclist—for instance, his or her alcohol or other substance use, obeying traffic laws, and wearing a motorcycle helmet. There also may be contributing biological or psychological factors that enhance risky behaviors. Broadening the model further to include more intermediate factors is important. These include interpersonal factors such as strong peer pressure against using safety precautions. This pressure may be supported by family and home influences. Organizationally, there are clubs and associations that strongly support the repeal of the motorcycle helmet laws, along with influences at work or school that may promote this philosophy. The motorcycle groups that are against wearing helmets have been very successful in lobbying governmental bodies to repeal or weaken motorcycle helmet laws. More distal factors include those related to community and society. The community has an important role to play in the safety of motorcycle riders. In addition to providing facilities and safe roads for all motorists, safety laws need to be enforced, and there must be community support for these laws so that they become normative. As for society, government policies regarding motorcycle helmet use have been some of the most studied and debated in traffic injury prevention. The repeal and weakening of motorcycle helmet laws have led to higher injury and death rates. While injury prevention and control advocates continue to support universal helmet laws, there continues to be strong opposition from many members of Congress and the anti-helmet lobbying groups. Unfortunately, as motorcycle injuries and deaths increase, the need for expensive hospital and trauma facilities grows. These costs are passed on to society, causing great financial strain. Meeting these needs in economically distressed areas is extremely difficult (National Committee for Injury Prevention and Control, 1989).

This socio-ecological paradigm illustrates the dynamic interfaces between the individual, physical, and social environments acting on the intrapersonal, interpersonal, organizational, community, and societal levels (Hanson et al., 2005). As the lower, more intermediate, and distal factors change in a more favorable direction, the desired injury prevention outcomes should be better maintained (Hanson et al., 2005).

For example, if motorcycle injury prevention programs focused only on individual and/or behavioral changes and ignored other variables, their efficacy would be greatly reduced because of the increased inertia, especially in the lower or deeper levels of the model. The role of family and peers, the support of schools and the home, and the role of the community and society in passing proactive policies and laws such as helmet-use laws, along with financial support, are crucial to the success of prevention programs.

The use of the socio-ecological model has led to success in a variety of injury prevention areas. Other examples of road traffic injury prevention include the installation of speed cameras and primary seat belt laws, or laws that allow police to ticket a motorist solely for not wearing a seat belt. Recently, it was shown that the installation of speed cameras in an urban international setting was effective in reducing the number of road collisions, and therefore the number of people injured (Perez, Mari-Dell'Olmo, Tobias, & Borrell, 2007). This clearly points to the need for community and societal factors interfacing with behavioral factors to decrease injuries. Also, in terms of the individual level of the ecological model, it was shown that primary enforcement of seat belt laws is an effective population-based strategy to reduce sociodemographic disparities in seat belt use, and therefore in motor vehicle crashes, injuries, and deaths (Beck, Shults, Mack, & Ryan, 2007). Again, the influence of the community and society on individual and interpersonal factors can be seen.

Haddon Matrix and Countermeasures

Injury prevention researchers have for a long time used the classic Haddon Matrix and countermeasures developed by the injury pioneer William Haddon in the 1970s to guide more direct planning efforts (National Committee for Injury Prevention and Control, 1989). The understanding of energy as the agent of injury is illustrated in the Haddon Matrix. Injuries are classified by phases, or time, and factors (Christoffel & Gallagher, 2006). The phases are pre-event (before the event), event (during the event), and postevent (after the event); and the factors are host, agent (energy), more typically the vehicle or vector that carries the energy, and physical and sociocultural factors. See Table 19.1 for an illustration of the Haddon Matrix with a motor vehicle crash.

TABLE 19.1   Example of the Use of the Haddon Matrix for a Motor Vehicle Crash

Phases	Human Factors (Host)	Agent or Vector/Vehicle	Physical Environment	Sociocultural Environment
Pre-event[a]	Driver ability	Maintenance of brakes, tires, speed	Roadway markings and lighting	Attitudes about laws, alcohol, speed limits, etc.
Event[b]	Wearing seat belt, human tolerance issues	Vehicle size, load containment, etc.	Fixed objects, speed limits, recovery areas	Enforcement of mandatory traffic safety laws
Postevent[c]	Victim's overall health, age	Gas tank's ability to minimize postcrash fire	Availability of effective trauma systems	Support for trauma and EMS (emergency medical systems).

SOURCE: Adapted from Christoffel and Gallagher (2006) and the National Committee for Injury Prevention and Control (1989).

a. Pre-event: Everything that determines whether an event takes place.

b. Event: Everything that determines whether an injury results.

c. Postevent: Everything that determines whether the severity of the injury's consequences can be reduced (National Committee for Injury Prevention and Control, 1989).

Haddon also developed countermeasures that could be used more directly to develop intervention efforts. These countermeasures are largely passive in that individual behavior is not needed for many of the measures. These countermeasures are shown in Table 19.2.

For the majority of these countermeasures for a motor vehicle crash, building safer vehicles would be effective since the vehicle is the hazard. However, behaviors of individuals still come into play if you consider the need for passengers to wear seat belts; for caregivers to put children younger than 12 years in restraints in the backseat; for drivers to use airbags; and for medical professionals assisting with the transport and care of injured victims to counter the injury damage done. The Haddon Matrix and countermeasures show the important role of the socioecological model as they illustrate the intrapersonal, interpersonal, organizational, community, and societal factors that allow us to understand injury epidemiology and to develop prevention efforts more effectively.

Summary of Injury Prevention Efforts

To reinforce what has been said thus far, there have been reported to be five main elements of the ecological model in injury prevention and control (Allegrante, Marks, & Hanson, 2006, pp. 115–116): (1) Unintentional injury develops from many factors; (2) behavioral risk factors have both situational and psychological influences; (3) there are important sociological and environmental factors influencing injury; (4) prevention programs need to account for the relationships between individuals and their physical and social environments; and

TABLE 19.2	Haddon Countermeasures

1. Eliminating the production of the hazard

2. Reducing the amount of energy contained in the hazard

3. Preventing the release of the hazard

4. Modifying the rate or special distribution of the hazard

5. Separating the hazard in time or space from those to be protected

6. Separating the hazard from those to be protected by a material barrier

7. Modifying the relevant basic qualities of the hazard

8. Making individuals more resistant to the hazard

9. Countering the damage already done by the hazard

10. Stabilizing, repairing, and rehabilitating the individual changed

SOURCE: From Gielen and Sleet (2006).

(5) interventions need to consider beliefs, attitudes, behaviors, and environmental factors and involve community stakeholders when developing solutions.

Injury prevention efforts have long followed the three Es: (1) education, (2) engineering (including ergonomics and product design), and (3) enforcement (including legislation, safety policies, and regulation) (Gielen & Sleet, 2006). The earliest efforts were in automobile injury prevention and focused largely on providing education and information on the risks of injury. However, these efforts did not incorporate sophisticated theory-based approaches, access to injury prevention tools and products, or the use of social marketing and community-based participatory research (Gielen & Sleet, 2006). Consequently, their success was not great. Engineering approaches that have created safer products and environments have met with much more success, as has the enforcement of safety laws and product regulations. Even in these latter two areas, however, behavior is still important on the part of professionals and consumers alike.

FUTURE APPROACHES TO UNINTENTIONAL INJURY PREVENTION

There has been much success in unintentional injury prevention efforts over the last several years. The unintentional injury rate of today is about half of what it was in 1930—falling from 80 to 38 per 100,000 population (Baker, O'Neill, Ginsburg, & Li, 1992; CDC, NCIPC, 2007). Safer products, stronger policies, regulation, legislation, and behavior changes have all contributed to this improvement. However, injuries continue to be the leading cause of death for children and adults. As stated earlier, for the past few years, bringing about a change in behavior has become more and more important in injury prevention efforts. The majority of passive approaches need behavior change as well. The future of injury prevention clearly will involve the role of behavior, tested with sound, well-researched, behavioral theories and methods (DiClemente, Gielen, & Sleet, 2006).

In addition, sustainability of injury prevention interventions is also important for long-term success. For achieving sustainability, the following questions need to be addressed: What is the desired outcome? Are there sufficient resources? Who is responsible? (Hanson et al., 2005). The ecological system must have access to resources and must be able to mobilize them in order to maintain the outcome. In addition, sustainability needs to be built from the beginning by working with members of the community to maintain the safety outcomes using their own resources and capabilities (Hanson et al., 2005).

Finally, an exciting and promising goal to pursue is the integration of unintentional injury prevention efforts with those of violence prevention. Some of the early contributors to both unintentional and intentional injury are similar and can be studied through the use of the socio-ecological model. An example of this integrative prevention approach has been developed by Peterson and Brown (1994). They developed a working model that addresses roles for both childhood unintentional injury and childhood physical injuries due to abuse and neglect. There are background and immediate contributors to these physical injuries. They are sociocultural variables, caregiver-based variables, and child-based variables. The background contributors represent historical or continuous influences, while the immediate contributors are those specific, concrete factors that serve as discrete triggers for abuse or precipitators of injury.

In terms of background contributors, sociocultural variables include poverty, chaos, crowding, and changes in residence. Caregiver-based variables include a history of abuse or having risk-taking characteristics, emotional disturbances, substance abuse, being young and single, having unrealistic expectations of children, and supervision/discipline patterns. Child-based variables include being 0 to 4 years of age, having nonregular eating and sleeping habits, being distractible, and having high activity levels.

The immediate contributors, or triggers, also include sociocultural, caregiver-based, and child-based variables. Sociocultural factors include stress and isolation. Caregiver-based variables include the need for control and the lack of effective discipline, and child-based variables are noncompliance and impulsiveness.

The contributors clearly show the role of the socio-ecological model as they address personal and environmental factors that contribute to the risk of physical injury for a child. For example, the background sociocultural factors set the stage for lack of social supports and social isolation. Without the necessary resources, supervision may decrease, and therefore risks for unintentional injuries increase. Also, the risk now becomes greater for child abuse and neglect. This logic can be followed throughout the working model, whereby background and immediate factors related to the caregiver-based and child-based variables set the stage for both types of injuries.

However, just as the model illustrates how injuries can occur, there also is the opportunity to develop prevention programs that will address both types of injuries. Economic assistance and job training, family systems interventions, building a social service network, therapy, education for caregivers about child development, coping skills, and drop-off centers for children of parents who are stressed are just some of the ways in which coordinated interventions can be very effective (Peterson & Brown, 1994).

For integration efforts to be successful, there must be collaboration among researchers and practitioners dealing with unintentional and violence-related injury. By working together and drawing on each other's experience and knowledge, integrated interventions can be developed. Examples of opportunities for collaboration include child mortality review teams at state and county levels, development of school and community programs, and advocacy efforts (Liller, 2001). Mutual support among sectors, for example, could enhance passage of motor vehicle safety laws and policies and laws related to support for social services and prevention of abuse and neglect (Liller, 2001).

Future directions for injury prevention include the need for interdisciplinary research and practice and behavior change interventions addressing multiple levels of causality (DiClemente, Gielen, & Sleet, 2006). The use of the socio-ecological model incorporating proximal, intermediate, and distal factors will allow for the understanding of these levels. Strategies are also needed for sustaining injury prevention programs to effect behavior change, for using theoretical orientations and cost-effectiveness measures, for improving program transfer, for developing structured reporting mechanisms, and for assessing objective outcomes in research (DiClemente, Gielen, & Sleet, 2006). With these elements in place, along with the more traditional injury prevention strategies, more lives will be spared as injury morbidity and mortality decline.

REFERENCES

Allegrante, J. P., Marks, R., & Hanson, D. W. (2006). Ecological models for the prevention and control of unintentional injury. In A. C. Gielen, D. A. Sleet, & R. J. DiClemente (Eds.), *Injury and violence prevention: Behavioral science theories, methods, and applications* (pp. 105–126). San Francisco: Jossey-Bass.

Baker, S. P., O'Neill, B., Ginsburg, M. J., & Li, G. (1992). *The injury fact book* (2nd ed.). New York: Oxford University Press.

Beck, L. F., Shults, R. A., Mack, K. A., & Ryan, G. W. (2007). Associations between sociodemographics and safety belt use in states with and without primary enforcement laws. *American Journal of Public Health, 97,* 1619–1624.

Centers for Disease Control and Prevention. (2007). Unintentional poisoning deaths: United States, 1999–2004. *Morbidity and Mortality Weekly Report, 56*(5), 93–96.

Centers for Disease Control and Prevention, National Center for Injury Prevention and Control. (2007). *Injury statistics query and reporting system (WISQARS).* Retrieved July 31, 2007, from www.cdc.gov/ncipc/wisqars

Christoffel, T., & Gallagher, S. S. (2006). *Injury prevention and public health: Practical knowledge, skills, and strategies* (2nd ed.). Sudbury, MA: Jones & Bartlett.

DiClemente, R. J., Gielen, A. C., & Sleet, D. A. (2006). Behavioral sciences, injury, and violence prevention. In A. C. Gielen, D. A. Sleet, & R. J. DiClemente (Eds.), *Injury and violence prevention: Behavioral science theories, methods, and applications* (pp. 485–499). San Francisco: Jossey-Bass.

Gielen, A. C., & Sleet, D. A. (2006). Injury prevention and behavior: An evolving field. In A. C. Gielen, D. A. Sleet, & R. J. DiClemente (Eds.), *Injury and violence prevention: Behavioral science theories, methods, and applications* (pp. 1–16). San Francisco: Jossey-Bass.

Hanson, D., Hanson, J., Vardon, P., McFarlane, K., Lloyd, J., Muller, R., et al. (2005). The injury iceberg: An ecological approach to planning sustainable community safety interventions. *Health Promotion Journal of Australia, 16,* 5–10.

Houston, D. J., & Richardson, L. E. (2007). Motorcycle safety and the repeal of universal helmet laws. *American Journal of Public Health, 97,* 2063–2069.

Insurance Institute of Highway Safety. (2007). *Helmet use laws overview.* Retrieved September 29, 2007, from www.iihs.org/laws/HelmetUseOverview.aspx

Liller, K. D. (2001). The importance of integrating approaches in child abuse/neglect and unintentional injury prevention efforts: Implications for health educators. *International Electronic Journal of Health Education, 4,* 283–289.

Muller, A. (2004). Florida's motorcycle helmet law repeal and fatality rates. *American Journal of Public Health, 94,* 556–558.

National Center for Injury Prevention and Control. (2006). *Injury fact book.* Atlanta, GA: Centers for Disease Control and Prevention.

National Committee for Injury Prevention and Control. (1989). *Injury prevention: Meeting the challenge.* New York: Oxford University Press.

National Highway Traffic Safety Administration. (NHTSA). (2007a). *Traffic safety facts.* Retrieved September 29, 2007, from www-nrd.nhtsa.dot.gov/pdf/nrd-30/NCSA/TSF2005/810620.pdf

National Highway Traffic Safety Administration. (NHTSA). (2007b). *Traffic safety facts.* Retrieved November 10, 2007, from www-nrd.nhtsa.dot.gov/pdf/nrd-30/NCSA/TSF2005/810623.pdf

Perez, K., Mari-Dell'Olmo, M., Tobias, A., & Borrell, C. (2007). Reducing road traffic injuries: Effectiveness of speed cameras in an urban setting. *American Journal of Public Health, 97,* 1632–1637.

Peterson, L., & Brown, D. (1994). Integrating child injury and abuse-neglected research: Common histories, etiologies, and solutions. *Psychological Bulletin, 116,* 293–315.

Safe Kids. (2007). *Poison safety sheet.* Retrieved November 11, 2007, from www.usa.safekids.org/tier2_rl.cfm?folder_id=176

Sattin, R. W., & Corso, P. S. (2007). The epidemiology and costs of unintentional and violent injuries. In L. S. Doll, S. E. Bonzo, J. A., Mercy, & D. A. Sleet (Eds.), *Handbook of injury and violence prevention* (pp. 7–9). New York: Springer.

20

Violence and Public Health

Martha Coulter

Violence has surfaced in the United States in the past several decades as one of the most serious public health problems of our time. The impact of violence includes not only severe physical and psychological trauma but also major social and economic costs (Centers for Disease Control and Prevention [CDC], 2007b). The CDC (2007b) estimates that America has 16,800 homicides and 2.2 million medically treated injuries due to interpersonal violence annually, at a cost of $37 billion. This figure represents $33 billion in productivity losses and $4 billion in medical treatment costs. The cost of self-inflicted injuries (suicide or attempted suicide) is an additional $33 billion.

The *World Report on Violence and Health* defines violence as follows:

> The intentional use of physical force or power, threatened or actual, against oneself, another person, or against a group or community that either results in or has a high likelihood of resulting in injury, death, psychological harm, maldevelopment, or deprivation. (Krug, Dahlberg, Mercy, Zwi, & Lozano, 2002, p. 5)

Of importance in this definition is the fact that it focuses on the intentional act of violence itself and not solely on the type of outcome. Violence may result in a variety of psychological, physical, or even social problems that do not necessarily include physical injury or death (Krug et al., 2002). Traditionally, societal-level responses to violence have most frequently been from the justice system or the health care system. The attention that public health has brought to this issue has enabled a new look at the problem from an interdisciplinary, preventive, and scientific perspective (Mercy, Rosenberg, Powell, Broome, & Roper, 1993). Assessing violence from a socio-ecological perspective enables researchers to consider the multiple influences that precipitate violence and highlights the need for intervention and prevention efforts at multiple levels. Hughes, Humphrey, and Weaver (2005) stress that understanding and preventing interpersonal violence requires attention not only to the individual and the family but also to the social, cultural, community, and ethnicity factors that are implicit in the contexts in which they live. The *World Report on Violence and Health* uses the ecological model as a framework for understanding violence and considers violent outcomes to be the result of multiple levels of influence on behavior (Krug et al., 2002). Each level of influence is nested within the larger framework, from the characteristics or behavior of the individual, through the influence of relationships, to the influence of community and, finally, the influence of society. (See Figure 20.1.)

Public health attention has often been directed most specifically to issues of family violence, including child maltreatment, intimate-partner violence (IPV), and elder mistreatment. More recently, intense focus has been directed to issues of sexual violence outside the family, including dating violence; community and youth violence; suicide; and collective or political violence, such as war. The socio-ecological model is an ideal model to use in conceptualizing a field as broad as violence. This chapter will focus on four types of violence, building from the individual to the societal level:

1. *Individual level:* Self-directed violence (suicide or attempted suicide)

2. *Interpersonal level:* Interpersonal violence (family violence, sexual assault)

3. *Community level:* Community violence (homicide, youth violence)

4. *Societal violence:* Collective violence (political or ethnic violence)

FIGURE 20.1   Ecological Framework Used in the WHO *World Report on Violence and Health*

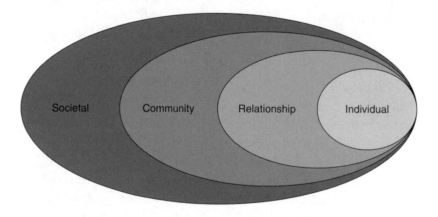

SOURCE: Krug, E. G., Dahlberg, L. L., Mercy, J. A., Zwi, A. B., and Lozano, R. (Eds.). (2002). *World Report on Violence and Health.* Geneva, Switzerland: World Health Organization. Used by permission.

While each level of the socio-ecological model will be discussed in depth later in the chapter, the following case illustration will serve to introduce a number of important issues. This illustration will demonstrate that while violence overall can be understood from the perspective of the model, each example can also be assessed using the model to explore the type of violence itself. The illustrative example that we will be examining is child sexual abuse, a type of interpersonal violence that initially seems to be limited primarily to the interpersonal level; that is, it is an act of maltreatment that an adult perpetrates on a child. We will see, however, that there are many complex issues involved. Using the socio-ecological model, we will illustrate the impact of intrapersonal, interpersonal, organizational, community, and societal influences.

Child sexual abuse is a major public health problem. In 1996, the third National Incidence Study of the U.S. Department of Health and Human Services (Sedlack & Broadhurst, 1996) reported that 300,200 children were sexually abused in 1993, a rate of 4.5 per 1,000 children. Other studies, however, that measure self-reports of childhood sexual abuse have found much higher rates, indicating that at least 20% of women and 5% to 10% of men were sexually abused as children (Barnett, Miller-Perrin, & Perrin, 2005). This wide range illustrates the difficulty of obtaining adequate information about this maltreatment problem. Causes of this difficulty include the reluctance of children to report this form of abuse and the reluctance of adults to believe it; they are complicated by the fact that there may be no physical injury and that the behavioral symptoms of sexual abuse are similar to those of other types of problems that stress children, such as parental divorce.

This illustration will explore the issue from the perspective of the child victim. Beginning with the intrapersonal (proximal) level, the individual characteristics of children that make them most vulnerable to being victimized include biological, psychological, and behavioral characteristics. From a biological perspective, gender is important—girls are more likely to be victims of sexual abuse than boys are; and age is important—rates of child sexual abuse peak at about ages 6 to 7 years and again at ages 10 to 12 (Finkelhor, 1986). From a psychological and behavioral perspective, children are often selected for victimization because the abuser can sense that they are vulnerable. The child may be passive, quiet, trusting, unhappy, or needy; she or he may be living in a divorced home. Abusers usually follow a pattern of developing the trust of and feelings of attachment in the child victim before any sexual abuse takes place (a process called "grooming"). The abuser may progress from nonsexual to sexual touching, separate the child from her or his family and friends, and condition the child through rewards or threats (Barnett et al., 2005).

The likelihood that the abuse will take place, however, does not depend solely on a child's individual characteristics but reflects also the interpersonal context of the children's lives. Their home and family are important contributors. Researchers have found that families where child sexual abuse takes place are often families where there is significant dysfunction and conflict (Finkelhor, 1988). Mothers are often out of the home, either because of employment or illness. The father may be a stepfather, or there may be no natural father in the home. The mother may have a history of being sexually abused herself and may be abused by the same person who is abusing the child. The child often has a poor relationship with his or her parents. It should be kept in mind that the abuser is usually someone in the family or someone that the child knows, not a stranger, so that the relationship of the child to other members of the family affects both the likelihood that abuse will take place and the likelihood that the child will disclose the abuse when it happens. Indeed, the relationship of the child to the mother is critical in a number of ways, as the impact of the abuse on the child is affected by the mother's response to disclosure. If she believes and supports the child, it moderates the severity of the impact (Everson, Runyan, Hunter, & Coulter, 1989).

Although disclosure of sexual abuse often depends on relationships with the other members of the child's family, it may also be influenced by the social environment outside the home. Efforts at the child's school or health care site to assist children in feeling comfortable about disclosing abuse have been helpful in reaching out to children who have been abused. The extent to which teachers and other school and community personnel are knowledgeable about the symptoms of child sexual abuse can be critical in recognition and disclosure of the problem.

The broader, more distal influences in the child's life, both in the community and in society, can also influence the likelihood that abuse will take place. Child sexual abuse takes place in all socioeconomic and ethnic groups. Finkelhor (1984) and others have discussed factors that might act as "disinhibitors" affecting the likelihood that potential abusers can maintain control over their feelings of attraction toward children. Some of those factors include the use of alcohol, attitudes toward family autonomy and secretiveness, and whether children are alone with adults, all of which are influenced by societal norms. The boundaries of what is considered appropriate behavior of adults toward children also varies a great deal, and cultural norms are powerful controls on behavior. For example, the age at which it is appropriate for a young woman to marry varies a great deal. While in one country an early marriage or an intimate relationship may be viewed positively, in other countries it may be viewed as child abuse if the girl's partner is older. Viewing a problem such as child sexual abuse from one perspective only may result in lost opportunities for understanding, prevention, and intervention.

LEVELS OF VIOLENCE FROM A SOCIO-ECOLOGICAL PERSPECTIVE

It is helpful at this point to step back and consider the different levels of violence from a socio-ecological perspective. As we take a closer look at each level of violence, the discussion will focus on which factors can be most easily identified by health systems and how that information might be used to prevent negative outcomes.

Intrapersonal Violence: Suicide

The intrapersonal level includes suicide, attempted suicide, and other self-destructive behaviors. The CDC reported that in 2004 suicide was responsible for more than 32,000 deaths in the United States alone, with males taking their own lives almost four times as often as females (Lubell, Kegler, Crosby, & Karch, 2007). Elderly males (over age 75) have the highest rates of suicide in the United States. Youth suicide, however, is a major concern as it is the third leading cause of death among youths and young adults aged 10 to 24, and there are some disturbing signs that suicide numbers may be increasing among girls aged 10 to 19 years (and especially 10–14 years) and boys aged 15 to 19 years (Lubell et al., 2007). This is a shift from an earlier pattern: The rate of suicide in this age group declined over 28% from 1990 to 2003, while from 2003 to 2004 the rate increased by 8.0% (Lubell et al., 2007). Also disturbing is the fact that among this age group there were between 100 and 200 suicide attempts for every completed suicide (as compared with 4 suicide attempts for every completed suicide among adults aged 65 or above). In fact, in 2005, almost 17% of high school students in the United States reported that they had seriously considered attempting suicide, and 8% had attempted it at least once (Eaton et al., 2006). Self-destructive behaviors that are not clearly suicidal (such as cutting oneself intentionally) but are nevertheless self-directed violence are also important issues to be studied as potential risk factors.

The factors that place individuals at risk for suicide are not well understood, but there are some indicators. About half the individuals who commit suicide have an earlier mental health diagnosis, most often depression (Patel et al., 2006). In half the cases, the family and friends of the victim describe them as being depressed at the time of their death. Family problems, school problems such as being bullied, and interpersonal problems may all contribute to this depression. Physical health problems are a major factor, especially among older adults, contributing to about 25% of suicides. Earlier suicide attempts and alcohol dependence problems are also often seen. These individual characteristics and behaviors are critical; however, interpersonal factors are also contributory, with almost 30% of suicides following problems with a current or intimate partner. A family history of suicide is a risk factor, as is suffering sexual abuse as a child. In some countries, married women are more likely to commit suicide (Krug et al., 2002).

The effect of cultural and societal factors on suicide is also important. For example, among American Indians and Alaskan Natives aged 15 to 34 years, suicide is the second leading cause of death. Krug et al. (2002) report that, internationally, the highest suicide rates are in Eastern Europe and Russia. Ethnic groups may have very distinct patterns of suicide even when they are separated by geography, and the rates of different groups within the same region vary by ethnicity.

Interpersonal Violence: Family Violence and Sexual Assault

Family Violence

In the 1960s, attention was focused most specifically on issues of child maltreatment, whereas in the past 20 years, focus has been on issues of IPV, sibling violence, and elder mistreatment. Estimates of the percentage of families in the United States in which a violent act occurs range from 20% to 55% (Barnett et al., 2005). While we will consider different forms of family violence separately to more easily describe them, it should be kept in mind that more than one of these problems frequently exist in the same family at a given time, there by increasing the likelihood of more negative outcomes. Estimates of incidence and prevalence vary widely for each type of violence, due both to variations in definitions and use of different data sources (e.g., self-reports vs. law enforcement reports or abuse reports). Underreporting is a major problem. Tjaden and Thoennes (2000) estimate that only about 20% of IPV rapes or sexual assaults, 25% of physical assaults, and 50% of stalkings of women are reported and even fewer IPV incidents against men are reported. One study found that only half of the women in a domestic violence shelter had ever called the police—and these are arguably some of the most serious cases (Coulter, Kuehnle, Byers, & Alfonso, 1999). Many experts believe that as few as 30% of child maltreatment incidents are reported, and the extent to which elder mistreatment is unreported is even less well established. What is known is that family violence is particularly serious for women and children. U.S. Department of Justice data from 1993 through 2004 revealed that 30% of all female murders (as compared with 6% of all male murders) were committed by an intimate (Catalano, 2006).

Estimates of child maltreatment, including neglect, physical abuse, sexual abuse, and psychological abuse, are based primarily on two sources: (1) cases that are reported to the child welfare agencies in the states and (2) cases that are reported to the police. The U.S. Department of Health and Human Services Administration for Children and Families reported in 2005 on data collected via the National Child Abuse and Neglect Data System, which reflects cases that were reported to state child welfare data systems. They reported that 899,000 children in the 50 states, the District of Columbia, and Puerto Rico were found to be victims of abuse and neglect in 2005, and that the number of abuse reports per year that are investigated has been increasing since 2001. The majority (62.8%) of child victims experienced neglect, followed by physical abuse (16.6%), sexual abuse (9.3%), and emotional or psychological abuse (7.1%). They also reported that an estimated rate of about 2 children per 100,000 in the national population died of abuse or neglect in 2005 (Administration for Children and Families, 2005).

Tjaden and Thoennes (2000) reported that nearly 25% of women and 7.5% of men reported being raped or physically assaulted by a current or former spouse, cohabiting partner, or date at some time in their lifetimes.

Pillemer and Finkelhor (1988), who conducted the most commonly cited population-based study, found an overall prevalence of elder mistreatment of 32 elder persons per 1,000 for an annual prevalence of 700,000 to 1.2 million cases in the United States. More recently, the U.S. Department of Health and Human Services National Elder Abuse Incidence Study (National Center on Elder Abuse & Westat, Inc., 1998) found that approximately 551,000 older adults were abused or neglected in 1996, and they acknowledge that this number may be as high as 800,000.

Understanding the causes and predictors of violence, especially family and interpersonal violence, requires careful analysis using an ecological approach. While various theoretical approaches have been explored, none have successfully explained the prevalence of violence in society. Interventions in violence prevention have usually focused on behavior change, both at the individual and the societal level. It is critical that these interventions be based on sound theoretical models and that replication be carefully conducted to provide evidence for continued use. Some of the most frequently explored theoretical approaches to the study of violence include those that try to explain patterns of family violence, such as feminist models that focus on cultural support for violence based on acceptance of patriarchal norms in the family structure, and deterrence models that focus on the low social costs of family violence. While these theories have contributed substantially to our understanding of family violence, they are nevertheless insufficient as comprehensive explanations. Theories that focus on individual behavior have also been explored in some depth. Attachment theory explores the extent to which poor attachment to parents as a child (often as a result of child neglect or physical, psychological, or sexual abuse) may result in inability to form satisfactory relationships as an adult. Social learning theory posits that patterns of behavior learned by imitating behaviors that are observed at very young ages are reinforced in the home and then repeated in adulthood. Early-childhood brain development, psychopathology, genetic influences, biochemical influences, and other individual influences are all areas that are increasingly being explored (Barnett et al., 2005) as influences and predictors of violent outcomes. An ecological model, which incorporates a variety of individual, family, societal, and cultural influences, is the most appropriate model to lend understanding to this complex problem.

Child maltreatment comprises four general areas of focus: child neglect, child physical abuse, child sexual abuse, and child psychological or emotional abuse. *Child neglect* is the most common form of child maltreatment and often the most deadly. Definitions of neglect have been varied, but the National Incidence Study (Sedlack & Broadhurst, 1996) lists a number of forms of physical neglect, including lack of supervision, abandonment, and failure to provide adequate shelter, nutrition, clothing, or hygiene. They also differentiate between situations where alternatives were available and where alternatives were not available. Physical neglect, educational neglect, developmental neglect, health care neglect, neglect of household safety, and emotional neglect are all types of neglect that have been recognized by experts in the field (Barnett et al., 2005). Most experts define neglect as acts of omission rather than commission. Neglect, unlike other forms of violence, does not always imply intentionality. Connell-Carrick and Scannapieco (2006) used an ecological model to identify the correlates of neglect. They found that children who were identified by their case managers as more vulnerable and less protected by their families were more likely to be identified as suffering from neglect. Parents who were substantiated as neglectful had poorer caretaking skills, a poorer connection with their children, attachment problems, and a lack of empathy for their children. Poor living environments (often resulting from social and economic conditions) also contribute to neglect and add stressors such as overcrowding. Differentiation between parental struggles with poverty and parental neglect has been a continually difficult task for the child welfare system and has led to substantial acrimony between parents and the child welfare system.

Exposure to parental violence has been identified as having significant negative effects on children. Some researchers argue that refusing to leave violent relationships constitutes child neglect, while others argue that parental separation may have even more detrimental effects on the children and that the impact of such family situations should be evaluated on an individual basis.

Child physical abuse is the type of abuse that has most often been studied. In 1946, the radiologist John Caffey recognized a link between a distinctive series of long-bone fractures in children and a history of battery. In 1962, Kempe, Silverman, Steele, Droegemueller, and Silver published "The Battered Child Syndrome" in the *Journal of the American Medical Association*, calling attention to the systematic, severe, intentional pattern of abuse that often results in severe neurological damage, broken bones, and injury to the skin and the skeletal system. Understanding of this problem has evolved to include current attention to other, more frequent forms of abuse, such as shaken infant syndrome. The role of cultural issues in influencing parental behavior toward children is critical to understanding the issue and to developing programs for prevention and/or intervention. There is significant controversy about issues such as corporal punishment, with some experts even recommending that corporal punishment be made illegal (Straus, 1994), as well as great variation internationally regarding the right of the state to intervene in the way parents raise their children. (Internationally, severe physical punishment of children ranges from 4% to 36% in the various countries studied [Krug et al., 2002]).

Sexual abuse of children is a frequent occurrence, most often enacted by individuals who are known to the child. While the Internet clearly adds a new element that can be exploited by abusive individuals seeking access to children, the greatest danger to children is from individuals in their immediate environment. The *emotional or psychological abuse of children* includes behaviors such as rejecting, degrading, or terrorizing children; isolating them from their family and friends, or even confining them; corrupting or exploiting them; or ignoring them to the point of severe psychological harm (Barnett et al., 2005). While this form of abuse is often accompanied by other forms of abuse as well, many experts believe that the emotional components of abuse have some of the most lasting effects. The impact of child abuse and neglect can be severe, causing both short- and long-term health and mental health problems, cognitive deficiencies, and social problems.

Intimate-partner violence, which has also been called spouse abuse and domestic violence, is a very common form of family violence, although the Bureau of Justice Statistics reports some decline in both fatal and nonfatal partner violence from 1993 to 2004 (perhaps due to increased awareness and earlier intervention; Catalano, 2006). Intimate relationships may involve current or former spouses or boyfriends or girlfriends, including homosexual partners, though there are variations in state laws that define the issue legally. Most experts believe that IPV reflects the abuser's effort to establish power and control over another person (Pence & Paymar, 1993) rather than solely his or her inability to control anger. Theories about the psychopathology of abusive individuals and about genetic influences on behavior have also been explored (see Barnett et al., 2005).

While most victims of reported IPV are women, there are significant data to support the position that men are also frequent victims of such violence. Carbone-Lopez, Kruttschnitt, and MacMillan (2006) report that while both men and women are victims of various types of domestic violence, patterns of victimization of the most serious types of systematic violence are more than two times more frequent for women than for men (3.5% vs. 1.6%). It is now recognized also that IPV is by no means limited to heterosexual couples, with gay and lesbian couples exposed to at least equal levels of violence in their relationships (Barnett et al., 2005).

The past decades have brought increased attention to the need of victims of IPV for protection, support, and advocacy. The shelter system has grown out of this recognition, as have programs that intervene with perpetrators of violence. Increasingly, there is understanding of the fact that not all abusers are the same and that intervention programs need to develop more complex models of operation if they are to be successful in preventing future recidivism. The primary response to IPV has come from the legal system; however, there is an increasing need for further development of support systems for victims, especially in the early phases of abusive relationships and when victims decide to leave the relationship. The women who are most at risk for abuse are those who are separated or divorced (Catalano, 2006), especially immediately after leaving the relationship. The health care system is also a primary participant in efforts to identify and respond to victims—research indicates that 50% of IPV victims who were murdered had sought care from their health care provider during the previous year (Sharps et al., 2001). The physical and mental health sequellae of IPV are severe and include not only repeated and chronic injury but also chronic pain syndromes; recurrent physiological symptoms such as headaches, insomnia, choking sensations, gastrointestinal symptoms, and chest, back, and pelvic pain; poor pregnancy outcomes, such as low infant birth weight, fetal death by placenta abruption, fetal fractures, rupture of the uterus, and premature labor; and other consequences such as contraction of HIV and sexually transmitted diseases, addiction, and attempted suicide (Dutton et al., 2006). Golding (1999) reports that victims are 3 to 5 times more likely to develop depression, suicidality, posttraumatic stress disorder (PTSD), and substance abuse habits than nonvictims. Individuals who are most vulnerable, such as disabled women, are at higher risk for IPV and may suffer abuse for longer periods of time—from caretakers as well as intimates. Of special concern are women who are pregnant at the time of the abuse. While being pregnant does not place women at greater risk for abuse, unplanned and unwanted pregnancies are significantly associated with violence (Jasinski, 2001). Increased attention has been given lately to assisting young women in dating relationships to recognize the signs of abusive partners, such as inappropriate jealousy or exclusive relationship requests. Vezina and Hebert (2007) find that research indicates that young women at most risk for victimization in romantic relationships include those who live in broken or dysfunctional families, are exposed to early violent episodes either as victims or as observers, are relatively uninvolved in religious activities, are suffering from depression, or are involved in high-risk behaviors. Early sexual abuse is particularly indicative of future victimization. They report also that there is some evidence that physical or sexual abuse is most often correlated with having a large number of sexual partners or relationships that are not serious, while psychological victimization is most often correlated with having a large number of serious romantic relationships.

The partners in a violent relationship are not the only victims of violence. Children who are exposed to IPV suffer a variety of negative impacts. Almost two thirds of children exposed to violence do more poorly than children who are not exposed, and their likelihood of being abusive to their own children increases from 5% to 30%. The interactions between children's development; their exposure to violence; and their family, school, and community contexts are important areas to be understood when assessing why some children are more resilient than others (Margolin, 2005).

Elder Mistreatment

Elder mistreatment refers to acts of commission or omission that result in harm or threatened harm to an older adult (Greenberg, Ramsey, Mitty, & Fulmer, 1999). It represents a serious health issue affecting the lives of thousands of older adults each year. Elder mistreatment began garnering attention in the media and among researchers in the 1980s and was initially studied in the aggregate with all forms of abuse lumped together under one heading. More recently, however, researchers have begun to refine the understanding of this phenomenon, and five categories of elder mistreatment are now generally distinguished (Comijs, Jonker, van Tilburg, & Smit, 1999; Lachs, Williams, O'Brien, Hurst, & Horwitz, 1996; National Research Council, 2003; Pillemer & Finkelhor, 1989): (1) physical abuse or aggression, (2) financial or material abuse, (3) psychological abuse or chronic verbal aggression, (4) neglect, and (5) sexual abuse.

While there is still considerable debate about what causes elder mistreatment—despite 25 years of research—there is a shared belief among experts that the consequences of elder mistreatment are severe. Elder mistreatment results in emotional difficulties such as feelings of inadequacy and self-contempt (Lewis, 1992; Metge, 1986), decreased self-esteem (Barer, 1997; Comijs, Pot, Smit, Bouter, & Jonker, 1998; Dong, 2005), and depression (Dyer, Pavlik, Pace Murphy, & Hyman, 2000; Levine, 2003). It has also been shown to result in family distress, impaired life functioning (Zarit, Todd, & Zarit, 1986), and cognitive difficulties (Barer, 1997; Dyer et al., 2000); and it has been linked to health problems such as immunologic dysfunction (Barer, 1997; Light & Lebowitz, 1994) and increased mortality (Dong, 2005; Lachs, Williams, O'Brien, Pillement, & Charlson, 1998). While typologies of victims and perpetrators are still being developed for each of the component forms of elder mistreatment, factors that place older adults at risk for elder mistreatment can be found across the individual, interpersonal, and societal levels. Factors such as a history of abuse (Kahan & Paris, 2003; Pillemer & Finkelhor, 1988; Schiamberg & Gans, 2000), dependence (Levine, 2003; Roberto, Teaster, & Duke, 2004; Schiamberg & Gans, 2000), social isolation (Litwin & Zoabi, 2004; Shugarman, Brant, Wolf, & Morris, 2003), physical or cognitive impairment (Choi & Mayer, 2000; Kahan & Paris, 2003; Roberto et al., 2004; Shugarman et al., 2003; VandeWeerd & Paveza, 2006), and depression (Flaherty & Raia, 1994; Gallagher, Wrabetz, Lovett, Del Maestro, & Rose, 1990) in older adults have been found to increase risk for varying forms of elder mistreatment. At the interpersonal level, age and gender of perpetrators (Coyne, Reichman, & Berbig, 1993), pathology of the perpetrator (Anetzberger, 1987; Bristowe & Collins, 1989), emotional problems of caregivers (Anetzberger, 1987), and depression in caregivers (VandeWeerd & Paveza, 2006) have also been found to increase risk of elder mistreatment. At the societal level, ageism and lack of training in health care professions frequently prevent recognition of mistreatment in older populations and keep many older adults from coming forward to report for fear of institutional reprisal. Research has also begun to show that many of the risk factors for elder abuse have strong interaction effects. Having a depressed person care for an elder with high levels of dementia symptoms, for example, creates a situation with higher potential risk for mistreatment than each of these risk factors taken individually (VandeWeerd & Paveza, 2006). Increased awareness of these issues is important for anyone providing services to older adults. A detailed accounting of signs and symptoms as well as screening measures for each of the component forms of abuse can be found in the *Handbook of Geriatric Assessment* (VandeWeerd, Firpro, Fulmer, & Paveza, 2005).

Sexual Assault

The BJS reported that 17.6% of all women surveyed said that they had been the victim of a completed or attempted rape at some time in their life (Catalano, 2006). Over half these women were raped while they were children or teens. Nearly 27% were younger than age 12 at the time they were raped, and over 32% were between the ages of 12 and 17. In addition, women who were raped before age 18 were twice as likely to report being raped as an adult. Sexual assault within intimate relationships is the most common form of sexual assault and the most injurious (Krug et al., 2002). If the assailant was a current or former intimate, the victim was significantly more likely to be injured than if she had been raped by other types of assailants. While reports of sexual assault against women are more common than reports of sexual assault against men, the percentage of men reporting completed or attempted rape according to the BJS was approximately 3%, a figure that represents more than 2.5 million men (Catalano, 2006).

The *World Report on Violence and Health*, which reviews all forms of sexual violence together, notes that the most important risk factor for women in terms of their vulnerability to sexual assault is being married or cohabiting with a partner (Krug et al., 2002). Other factors that raise risk, according to international studies, are being young, consuming alcohol or drugs, having been previously raped, having many sexual partners, being involved in sex work, becoming more educated and economically empowered than one's partner (where IPV is concerned), and being poor (Krug et al., 2002). Empowerment may encourage women's resistance to patriarchal norms, provoking men to resort to violence to regain control. However, the relationship between empowerment and violence is a U-shaped curve: There is a point at which greater empowerment becomes protective (Krug et al., 2002).

The factors associated internationally with sexual violence include individual factors, such as the perpetrator's attitude toward women and a history of family violence; relationship factors, such as patriarchal relationships or considerations of family honor; community factors, such as poverty and lack of employment opportunities; and societal factors, such as societal norms that are supportive of sexual violence (Krug et al., 2002).

Community Violence: Homicide and Youth Violence

Youth in our country are at particular risk of violence. Between 1981 and 2001, juveniles aged 12 to 15 were about as likely to be homicide victims as suicide victims (Snyder & Sickmund, 2006). Youth are both victims and perpetrators of crime. In a summary of several surveys, the CDC (2007a) noted that U.S adults reported approximately 1.9 million incidents of victimization by youth who were aged between 12 and 20 years, a rate of 5.1 incidents per year. Krug et al. (2002) reported that nearly 200,000 youth homicides occurred globally in

2000, with the highest rates in Latin America and Eastern Europe and the lowest rates in Western Europe. Juveniles are even more likely than adults to be victims of violence (Snyder & Sickmund, 2006). Illustrative of the utility of the socio-ecological model are several examples showing the importance of intermediate factors in assessing youth violence. Snyder and Sickmund (2006) also point out that the risk of being a violent crime victim for youth is tied more to characteristics of family and community than to individual characteristics such as race. The relationship of youth to school is an important element as well, with violent crimes against juveniles peaking at 3 p.m., when school is out; declining slightly in the early evening; and declining substantially after 9 p.m.

Juvenile offenses of some kinds have declined. The number of murders in the United States by juveniles dropped in 2002 to its lowest level since 1984 (Snyder & Sickmund, 2006) and accounted for only about 8% of all murders. Most of the murders were by male juveniles, and about half involved multiple offenders. The decline was primarily attributable to a decrease in the number of juvenile minority males using a firearm to kill male nonfamily members who were also minorities. Racial variations are apparent in the commission of various juvenile crimes. White youth are significantly more likely than black or Hispanic youth to commit vandalism, and white and Hispanic youth are more likely than black youth to report having sold drugs. At the same time, black youth report committing more assaults (Snyder & Sickmund, 2006). Snyder and Sickmund (2006) further report that youth violence is often confined to the middle teen years. Two thirds of youth who report committing lawbreaking offenses between the ages of 16 and 17 have stopped those behaviors by age 18 to 19. Family structure and connectedness to school are important factors in the likelihood that youth will be involved in crime. Membership in gangs is also an important factor. Membership in gangs is held primarily by minority youth and increases the likelihood that they will be victims of crime as well as perpetrators of crime.

The risk factors for juvenile violence have some intriguing characteristics from a prevention perspective. One study in Denmark that followed 200 children showed that complications during the mother's delivery were a predictor for the children's arrests for violence until the children were 22 years old (Krug et al., 2002). (These findings are supported by other research.) Individual personality traits such as hyperactivity and impulsiveness may further contribute to youth violence. Family dynamics are also important, with parental behaviors such as harsh discipline, abuse, and neglect increasing risk.

One facet of community violence that is receiving increasing attention is the effect on community residents of exposure to violence. Recent research indicates that negative outcomes emerge from the fear of violence that arises in a community after its exposure to violence, irrespective of the actual level of violence. The public perception that crime is increasing and the resultant fear of that crime result in poorer mental health, reduced physical functioning, and lower quality of life. Individuals who report greater fear are almost twice as likely to report depression, for example. They exercise less, see friends less often, and participate in fewer social activities than less fearful individuals (Stafford, Chandola, & Marmot, 2007).

Collective Violence: Political and Ethnic Violence

Collective violence in all its forms receives a great deal of our attention. The *World Report on Health and Violence* (Krug et al., 2002) describes collective violence as follows:

> The instrumental use of violence by people who identify themselves as members of a group—whether this group is transitory or has a more permanent identity—against another group or set of individuals, in order to achieve political, economic or social objectives. (p. 215)

We recognize various forms of collective violence, beginning with armed conflict (or war) and also including terrorism (or the intentional targeting of noncombatants for purposes of advancing a political cause), genocide (or acts committed with the intent to destroy, in whole or in part, a national, ethnic, racial, or religious group), abuses of human rights (repression, the use of torture, etc.), and organized violent crimes (such as those perpetrated in the course of gang warfare). In addition to the millions of lives lost from political violence, the impact of such violence on society is enormous. The ability of citizens to secure basic resources, such as food, water, and shelter, is often curtailed for extended periods. Some of the characteristic outcomes of these emergencies, which have profound consequences for public health, include the dislocation of populations, the destruction of social networks and ecosystems, the insecurity affecting civilians and others not engaged in fighting, and human rights abuses (Krug et al., 2002). Essential public health activities are frequently devastated in such situations, including the provision of health care and preventive services (such as the delivery of vaccinations for infants and children) for vulnerable populations.

There are severe repercussions for the population that lives in an area where collective violence takes place. Many may be forced to leave their homes and flee to other areas. Refugees suffer a wide range of physical health, mental health, and social problems. Both acculturation and acculturation stress have also been shown to be related to family violence (Caetano, Ramisetty-Mikler, Caetano-Vaeth, & Harris, 2007). Refugee children suffer tremendously from problems such as malnutrition, diarrhea, and infectious diseases (Krug et al., 2002). The direct impact of conflict on health includes the following issues:

- Increased mortality, with deaths from external causes such as weapons, from infectious diseases, and from noncommunicable disease
- Increased morbidity, due to injuries, sexual violence, infectious diseases such as HIV infection (often due to forced sexual services and rape), reproductive health problems, nutrition-related problems, and mental health problems such as anxiety, depression, posttraumatic stress disorder (PTSD), and suicidal behavior
- Increased disability, which may be physical, psychological, and/or social (Krug et al., 2002)

The combatants themselves, in addition to suffering from a variety of health, injury, and mental health problems, cause further distress in their families when they return. Recent studies have pinpointed the many secondary effects of mental health problems in returning soldiers. PTSD and depression, for example, are associated with increases in child maltreatment and IPV. Past research has established PTSD in veterans as a correlate of domestic violence and other forms of interpersonal violence (Beckham, Feldman, Kirby, Hertzberg, & Moore, 1997; Beckham, Moore, & Reynolds, 2000). In one study, family violence was significantly more prevalent among those who developed PTSD than among those who did not (Jordan et al., 1992). The increasing numbers of women in combat argues for the need for significantly increased research into the impact of deployment on their physical and mental health.

The response of states to conflict can often cause further problems for the population. Trade sanctions—a commonly used political weapon—often negatively affect the most vulnerable, such as women, children, and the elderly. One illustrative example of this is Haiti, where, following the military coup of 1991, UN economic sanctions were instituted in an effort to restore democracy and civil rights. Exports were banned to Haiti, including gasoline, food, and consumer goods. Exemptions for "humanitarian assistance" were allowed, but the impact was crippling, nevertheless. Over the next 3 years, rates of malnutrition for children under 5 increased from 27% to 50%, and thousands probably died. Deterioration of health services, power shortages, and bottlenecks in public transportation, reducing people's access to goods and services, occurred. A decline in immunization coverage caused a rise in measles and other infections. Mortality from measles increased from 1% to 14%. A country already fragile economically and socially was further endangered, with the negative impact primarily felt by the poor and vulnerable.

The World Health Assembly declared in 1981 that the role of health workers in promoting and preserving peace is a significant factor for achieving health for all (Krug et al., 2002). With the massive threats that collective violence creates, it is imperative that the health community take this charge seriously.

PREVENTION AND INTERVENTION

Interventions in family violence have traditionally been behavioral interventions. While injury researchers have focused more specific attention on understanding the immediate incident (see Chapter 19), violence researchers have given less attention to this aspect of family violence, except in the area of gun access and juvenile crime. Interventions have most often been reactive rather than preventive and have usually responded to only one type of violence at a time, such as child maltreatment or IPV, despite the high levels of co-occurrence in families. Indeed, these systems of intervention have often operated not only in parallel fashion but sometimes in conflict with each other. For example, child advocates have often held mothers to blame for not protecting their children from an abusive partner, while women's advocates have often viewed mothers as co-victims. Health professionals have not been deeply involved with these problems. Only 2% of the domestic violence victims queried in one study had ever told their health care provider about the violence (Coulter & Chez, 1997). While health care providers have been encouraged to screen for family violence, most screening has been limited to IPV screening. Fortunately, tools that screen simultaneously for a variety of types of family violence, such as child maltreatment, IPV, and elder mistreatment, are now being developed (Zink & Fisher, 2007).

The preventive services which are most often recommended focus on interpersonal and familial interventions, including support for improved parenting, with specific attention to issues of attachment and interaction, identification of early problems in intimate partner relationships, and recognition of the particular vulnerability of elders. Some of these services can be incorporated into the usual operation of primary care services providers using models that have been shown to be effective, such as home visiting models (Olds, Henderson, Tatelbaum, & Chamberlain, 1986), or models that have been developed in other countries (Coulter, 1996). Universal school-based intervention programs have shown some promise in violence prevention. The most frequent focus of these intervention programs has been on either school-based interpersonal violence, such as bullying, or on student attitudes about violence against women that could lead to dating violence and future IPV. While these programs show promise, particularly in the areas of changing attitudes and knowledge, their impact in terms of reducing the incidence of victimization are less clear (Vezina & Hebert, 2007). Murray and Graybeal (2007) conducted a methodological review of IPV prevention programs. They concluded that very little attention has been paid to empirical research in the area of IPV prevention and made a number of specific recommendations for improving future research studies. Currently few programs are designed to offer intense preventive interventions at a time when such attention might have the most effect. Increased utilization of peer support models may be a useful direction for the future. Evaluation of existing intervention programs and training of health professionals have likewise been neglected areas. The Institute of Medicine (2002) reported on the paucity of data available to help guide practice in the area of family violence. It cited reports from the U.S. Advisory Board on Child Abuse and Neglect that indicated that child maltreatment may remain the most underresearched social problem. The IOM report overall found that that while family violence is recognized as a significant social problem, its effects on society as a whole and on the health care system have not been studied adequately. It found further that the data available are inconsistent and unclear and that funding for research, educational program development, and evaluation of family violence curricula is not available.

A more global approach has been taken by those who are deeply concerned about issues of structural violence (social and economic inequities that determine who will be at risk for assaults and who will be shielded from them). Farmer (1999) recommends that healing and health be made the symbolic core of an agenda to deal with human rights; he also argues that provision of services, new research agendas, and educational mandates are critical to improving human rights and that making human rights work independent of governments and bureaucracies is critical to its success.

In summary, violence is a major health problem, and one to which we have only just begun to respond. Violence is a multifaceted problem, best understood with an ecological model that enables us to examine the linkages and connections in society that either foster or prevent its occurrence.

REFERENCES

Administration for Children and Families. (2005). *Child maltreatment 2005.* Retrieved March 14, 2008, from www.acf.hhs.gov/programs/cb/pubs/cm05/chapterthree.htm#child

Anetzberger, G. J. (1987). *The etiology of elder abuse by adult offspring.* Springfield, IL: Charles C Thomas.

Barer, B. M. (1997). The secret shame of the very old: "I've never told this to anyone else." *Journal of Mental Health and Aging, 3*(3), 365–375.

Barnett, O., Miller-Perrin, C., & Perrin, R. (2005). *Family violence across the lifespan.* Thousand Oaks, CA: Sage.

Beckham, J. C., Feldman, M. E., Kirby, A. C., Hertzberg, M. A., & Moore, S. D. (1997). Interpersonal violence and its correlates in Vietnam veterans with chronic posttraumatic stress disorder. *Journal of Clinical Psychology, 53*(8), 859–869.

Beckham, J. C., Moore, S. D., & Reynolds, V. (2000). Interpersonal hostility and violence in Vietnam combat veterans with chronic posttraumatic stress disorder: A review of theoretical models and empirical evidence. *Aggression and Violent Behavior, 5*(5), 451–466.

Bristowe, E., & Collins, J. (1989). Family mediated abuse of non-institutionalized frail elderly men and women living in British Columbia. *Journal of Elder Abuse and Neglect, 1*(1), 45–64.

Caetano, R., Ramisetty-Mikler, S., Caetano-Vaeth, P. A., & Harris, T. R. (2007). Acculturation stress, drinking, and intimate partner violence among Hispanic couples in the U.S. *Journal of Interpersonal Violence, 22*(11), 1431–1447.

Carbone-Lopez, K., Kruttschnitt, C., & MacMillan, R. (2006). Patterns of intimate partner violence and their associations with physical health, psychological distress, and substance use. *Public Health Reports, 121,* 382–392.

Catalano, S. (2006). *Intimate partner violence in the United States* (U.S. Department of Justice Bureau of Justice Statistics). Retrieved December 20, 2007, from www.ojp.usdoj.gov/bjs/intimate/ipv.htm

Centers for Disease Control and Prevention. (2007a). Effects on violence of laws and policies facilitating the transfer of youth from the juvenile to the adult justice system [Electronic version]. *Morbidity and Mortality Weekly Report.* Retrieved March 14, 2008, from www.cdc.gov/mmwr/preview/mmwrhtml/rr5609a1.htm

Centers for Disease Control and Prevention. (2007b). *Suicide.* Retrieved November 18, 2007, from www.cdc.gov/injury

Choi, N., & Mayer, J. (2000). Elder abuse, neglect and exploitation: Risk factors and prevention strategies. *Journal of Gerontological Social Work, 33*(2), 5–25.

Comijs, H. C., Jonker, C., van Tilburg, W., & Smit, J. H. (1999). Hostility and coping capacity as risk factors of elder mistreatment. *Social Psychiatry and Psychiatric Epidemiology, 34*(1), 48–52.

Comijs, H. C., Pot, A. M., Smit, J. H., Bouter, L. M., & Jonker, C. (1998). Elder abuse in the community: Prevalence and consequences. *Journal of the American Geriatrics Society, 46*(7), 885–888.

Connel-Carrick, K., & Scannapieco, M. (2006). Ecological correlates of neglect in infants and toddlers. *Journal of Interpersonal Violence, 21*(3), 306–316.

Coulter, M. (1996). Raising caring and competent children in the United States. In P. Klein (Ed.), *Early intervention: Cross cultural experiences with a mediational approach* (pp. 197–209). New York: Garland.

Coulter, M., & Chez, R. (1997). Domestic violence victims support mandatory reporting: For others. *Journal of Family Violence, 12,* 349–356.

Coulter, M., Kuehnle, K., Byers, R., & Alfonso, M. (1999). Police reporting behavior and victim-police interactions as described by women in a domestic violence shelter. *Journal of Interpersonal Violence, 14*(12), 1290–1298.

Coyne, A. C., Reichman, W. E., & Berbig, L. J. (1993). The relationship between dementia and elder abuse. *American Journal of Psychiatry, 150*(4), 643–646.

Dong, X. (2005). Medical implications of elder abuse and neglect. *Clinics in Geriatric Medicine, 21*(2), 293–313.

Dutton, M. A., Green, B. L., Kaltman, S. I., Roesch, D. M., Zeffiro, T. A., & Krause, E. D. (2006). Intimate partner violence, PTSD, and adverse health outcomes. *Journal of Interpersonal Violence, 21*(7), 955–968.

Dyer, C., Pavlik, V., Pace Murphy, K., & Hyman, D. (2000). The high prevalence of depression and dementia in elder abuse and neglect. *Journal of the American Geriatrics Society, 48*(2), 205–208.

Eaton, D. K., Kann, L., Kinchen, S. A., Ross, J. G., Hawkins. J., & Harris, W. A. (2006). Youth risk behavior surveillance: United States, 2005. *Morbidity and Mortality Weekly Report, 55*(SS-5), 1–108.

Everson, M., Runyan, D., Hunter, W., & Coulter, M. (1989). Maternal support following disclosure of incest. *Journal of Orthopsychiatry, 59,* 197–207.

Farmer, P. (1999). Pathologies of power: Rethinking health and human rights. *American Journal of Public Health, 89*(10), 1486–1496.

Finkelhor, D. (1984). *Child sexual abuse: New theory and research.* New York: Free Press.

Finkelhor, D. (1986). *A sourcebook on child sexual abuse.* Beverly Hills, CA: Sage.

Finkelhor, D. (1988). The trauma of sexual abuse. In G. E. Wyatt & G. J. Powell (Eds.), *Lasting effects of child sexual abuse* (pp. 61–82). Newbury Park, CA: Sage.

Flaherty, A., & Raia, P. (1994). Beyond risk protection and Alzheimer's disease. *Journal of Elder Abuse and Neglect, 6*(2), 75–93.

Gallagher, D., Wrabetz, A., Lovett, S., Del Maestro, S., & Rose, J. (1990). Depression and other negative affects in family caregivers. In E. Light & B. Lebowitz (Eds.), *Alzheimer's disease treatment and family stress: Directions for research* (pp. 218–244). New York: Hemisphere.

Golding, J. M. (1999). Intimate partner violence as a risk factor for mental disorders: A meta-analysis. *Journal of Family Violence, 14*(2), 99–132.

Greenberg, S. A., Ramsey, G. C., Mitty, E. L., & Fulmer, T. (1999). Elder mistreatment: Case law and ethical issues in assessment, reporting, and management. *Journal of Nursing Law, 6*(3), 1–14.

Hughes, H., Humphrey, N., & Weaver, T. (2005). Advances in violence and trauma: Toward comprehensive ecological models. *Journal of Interpersonal Violence, 20*(1), 31–38.

Institute of Medicine. (2002). *Confronting chronic neglect: The education and training of health professionals on family violence* (Report of the Committee on the Training Needs of Health Professionals to Respond to Family Violence). Washington, DC: National Academies Press.

Jasinski, J. (2001). Pregnancy and violence against women: An analysis of longitudinal data. *Journal of Interpersonal Violence, 16*(7), 712–733.

Jordan, B. K., Marmar, C. R., Fairbank, J. A., Schlenger, W. E., Kulka, R. A., Hough, R. L., et al. (1992). Problems in families of male Vietnam veterans with posttraumatic stress disorder. *Journal of Consulting and Clinical Psychology, 60*(6), 916–926.

Kahan, F., & Paris, B. (2003). Why elder abuse continues to elude the health care system. *Mount Sinai Journal of Medicine, 70*(1), 62–68.

Kempe, H., Silverman, F., Steele, B., Droegemueller, W., & Silver, H. K. (1962). The battered child syndrome. *Journal of the American Medical Association, 17,* 17–24.

Krug, E. G., Dahlberg, L. L., Mercy, J. A., Zwi, A. B., & Lozano, R. (Eds). (2002). *World report on violence and health.* Geneva, Switzerland: World Health Organization.

Lachs, M. S., Williams, C., O'Brien, S., Hurst, L., & Horwitz, R. (1996). Older adults. An 11-year longitudinal study of adult protective service use. *Archives of Internal Medicine, 156*(4), 449–453.

Lachs, M. S., Williams, C. S., O'Brien, S., Pillement, K. A., & Charlson, M. E. (1998). The mortality of elder mistreatment. *Journal of the American Medical Association, 280*(5), 428–432.

Levine, J. (2003). Elder neglect and abuse. A primer for primary care physicians. *Geriatrics, 58*(10), 37–40, 42–44.

Lewis, M. (1992). *Shame: The exposed self.* New York: Free Press.

Light, E., & Lebowitz, B. (1994). *Alzheimer's disease treatment and family stress: Directions for research.* Rockville, MD: National Institute of Mental Health.

Litwin, H., & Zoabi, S. (2004). A multivariate examination of explanations for the occurrence of elder abuse. *Social Work Research, 28*(3), 133–142.

Lubell, K. M., Kegler, S. R., Crosby, A. E., & Karch, D. (2007). Suicide trends among youths and young adults aged 10–24 years: United States, 1990–2004. *Morbidity and Mortality Weekly Report, 56*(35), 905–908. Retrieved September 30, 2007, from www.cdc.gov/mmwr/preview/mmwrhtml/mm5635a2.htm

Margolin, G. (2005). Children's exposure to violence: Exploring developmental pathways to diverse outcomes. *Journal of Interpersonal Violence, 20*(1), 72–81.

Mercy, J., Rosenberg, M., Powell, K., Broome, C., & Roper, W. (1993). Public health policy for preventing violence. *Health Affairs, Winter,* 7–29.

Metge, J. (1986). *In and out of touch: Whakamaa in cross cultural perspective.* Wellington, New Zealand: Victoria University Press.

Murray, C. E., & Graybeal, J. (2007). Methodological review of intimate partner violence prevention research. *Journal of Interpersonal Violence, 22*(10), 1250–1269.

National Center on Elder Abuse & Westat, Inc. (1998). *The national elder abuse incidence study: Final report* (Prepared for the Administration for Children and Families and the Administration on Aging, U.S. Department of Health and Human Services). Washington, DC: National Aging Information Center.

National Research Council. (2003). *Elder mistreatment: Abuse, neglect, and exploitation in an aging America* (R. J. Bonnie & R. B. Wallace, Eds.). (Report of the Panel to Review Risk and Prevalence of Elder Abuse and Neglect). Washington, DC: National Academies Press.

Olds, D. L., Henerson, C. R., Tatelbaum, R., & Chamberlain, R. (1986). Preventing child abuse and neglect: A randomized trial of nurse home visitation. *Pediatrics, 78,* 65–68.

Patel, N., Webb, K., White, D., Barker, L., Crosby, A., Deberry, M., et al. (2006). Homicides and suicides: National Violent Death Reporting System, United States, 2003–2004. *Morbidity and Mortality Weekly Report, 55*(26), 721–724.

Pence, E., & Paymar, M. (1993). *Education groups for men who batter: The Duluth model.* New York: Springer.

Pillemer, K. A., & Finkelhor, D. (1988). The prevalence of elder abuse: A random sample survey. *Gerontologist, 28*(1), 51–57.

Pillemer, K. A., & Finkelhor, D. (1989). Causes of elder abuse: Caregiver stress versus problem relatives. *American Journal of Orthopsychiatry, 59*(2), 179–187.

Roberto, K., Teaster, P., & Duke, J. (2004). Older women who experience mistreatment: Circumstances and outcomes. *Journal of Women and Aging, 16*(1–2), 3–16.

Schiamberg, L., & Gans, D. (2000). Elder abuse by adult children: An ecological framework for understanding contextual risk factors and the intergenerational character of quality of life. *International Journal of Aging and Human Development, 50*(4), 329–359.

Sedlack, A. J., & Broadhurst, D. D. (1996). *Third national incidence study on child abuse and neglect.* Washington, DC: U.S. Department of Health and Human Services.

Sharps, P., Koziol-McLain, J., Campbell, J., McFarlane, J., Sachs, C., & Xu, X. (2001). Health care providers' missed opportunities for preventing femicide. *Preventive Medicine, 33*(5), 373–380.

Shugarman, L., Brant, F., Wolf, R., & Morris, N. (2003). Identifying older people at risk of abuse during routine screening practices. *Journal of the American Geriatrics Society, 51*(1), 24–31.

Snyder, H., & Sickmund, M. (2006). *Juvenile offenders and victims: 2006 national report.* Washington, DC: U.S. Department of Justice, Office of Justice Programs. Office of Juvenile Justice and Delinquency Prevention.

Stafford, M., Chandola, T., & Marmot, M. (2007). Association between fear of crime and mental health and physical functioning. *American Journal of Public Health. 97*(11), 2076–2081.

Straus, M. (1994). *Beating the devil out of them: Corporal punishment in American families.* Lanham, MD: Lexington.

Tjaden, P., & Thoennes, N. (2000). *Extent, nature, and consequences of intimate partner violence: Findings from the National Violence Against Women Survey* (Department of Justice Publication No. NCJ 181867). Washington, DC: U.S. Department of Justice.

VandeWeerd, C., Firpro, A., Fulmer, T., & Paveza, G. (2005). Recognizing mistreatment in older adults. In J. Gallo, H. Bogner, T. Fulmer, & G. Paveza (Eds.), *Handbook of geriatric assessment* (4th ed.). Boston: Jones & Bartlett.

VandeWeerd, C., & Paveza, G. (2006) Verbal mistreatment in older adults: A look at persons with Alzheimer's disease and their caregivers in the state of Florida. *Journal of Elder Abuse and Neglect, 17*(4), 11–30.

Vezina, J., & Hebert, M. (2007). Risk factors for victimization in romantic relationships of young women. *Trauma, Violence, & Abuse, 8*(1), 33–66.

Zarit, S., Todd, P., & Zarit, J. (1986). Subjective burden of husbands and wives as caregivers: A longitudinal study. *The Gerontologist, 26,* 260–266.

Zink, T., & Fisher, B. S. (2007). Family violence quality assessment tool for primary care offices. *Quality Management in Health Care, 16*(3), 265–279.

21

Occupational Health

Paul E. Spector and Chu-Hsiang Chang

One of the major accomplishments of the 20th century was a 90% decrease in workplace fatalities in the United States, making the workplace in the United States and other Western countries the safest in history. Despite this remarkable accomplishment, there are still more than 5,000 workplace fatalities due to accidents and more than 4 million nonfatal injuries and illnesses each year in the United States alone (U.S. Department of Labor, 2007). Although much has been done to eliminate physical hazards in the workplace, far less has been done about social factors that are important to the health, safety, and well-being of people in the workplace. The new and emerging field of occupational health psychology (OHP) is dedicated to understanding how psychological and social aspects of the workplace, as well as society, contribute to the physical and psychological health of employees.

This chapter will discuss five OHP issues that affect the health, safety, and well-being of employees:

1. Injuries due to accidents on the job

2. Musculoskeletal disorders that are caused, at least in part, by carrying out job tasks

3. Job stress

4. Workplace violence, committed by coworkers and others

5. Work-family issues that arise from interference between work and nonwork demands

Each area can involve both physical and psychological health. For example, having a physical injury due to an accident can cause psychological trauma for an individual. Likewise, job stress that is primarily psychological in nature can have an impact on physical health.

A truly healthy workplace is one in which exposure to potentially unhealthy physical and social conditions is minimized. This includes the proper design of a safe physical environment, as well as the adoption of organizational policies and practices that encourage health and safety. In some cases, government legislation and oversight might be needed to encourage organizations to engage in safe practices beyond meeting standards for the physical environment.

Figure 21.1 illustrates the ecological model and displays how social influences occur at different levels. The most immediate precursor to health and well-being is the individual's own behavior. For example, failure to behave in a safe manner can lead to unnecessary exposure to workplace hazards, which can lead to accidents and violence. Such behavior occurs in a social environment that includes coworkers and supervisors who can encourage or discourage risky behavior. The immediate workgroup can have a powerful effect on behavior. A more distant influence is produced by the policies and practices of the employing organization that filter down to the immediate workgroup. Finally, at the societal level, government laws mandate policies and practices by organizations, although typically some sort of enforcement mechanism is required to ensure compliance. For example, in the United States, the Occupational Safety and Health Administration (OSHA) is a government agency that oversees compliance with government safety rules for exposure to physical hazards. Such rules have little to say about social factors in the workplace.

In the remainder of the chapter, we will discuss each of the five health and safety areas, mentioned earlier, within organizations. A great deal is known about the psychological and social factors that contribute to workplace health. Far less is known about how best to intervene in organizations to encourage safe and health-enhancing behavior by employees. The development of effective interventions remains a challenge for reducing workplace fatalities, injuries, and illness to even lower levels.

FIGURE 21.1   Ecological Model of Workplace, Health, and Safety

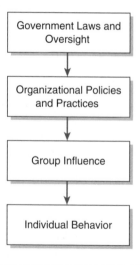

HEALTH AND SAFETY IN THE WORKPLACE

Accidents

Preventing workplace accidents is a major concern because of the associated costs for employees, organizations, and society as a whole. Nonfatal accidents and injuries resulted in an average of 6 days away from work annually for employees (National Institute for Occupational Safety and Health, 2004). Additionally, when taken together, fatal and nonfatal accidents cost an estimated $140 billion annually in the United States alone (National Safety Council, 2005–2006). Many different approaches exist to prevent accidents. Some involve designing a physically safe work environment and better equipment, while others focus on protective gear. Although these practices are helpful, they alone are not sufficient to ensure employees' safe behaviors (Zohar, 2002). Instead, employees tend to view accidents as low-probability threats and downplay the risk associated with engaging in unsafe behaviors. Moreover, because unsafe practices, such as working at a faster pace or ignoring safety procedure, tend to result in immediate payoffs or greater personal comfort, these behaviors are likely to be reinforced (Zohar & Luria, 2003). As such, researchers argue that it is essential to alter the value function associated with safe behavior through psychological and social interventions in order to prevent workplace accidents.

One psychological intervention framework that has received support is the behavioral safety approach (Alavosius, Adams, Ahern, & Follick, 2000; Geller, 1996). The behavioral safety approach emphasizes the identification of antecedents and consequences of target behaviors and changes the target behaviors by altering their antecedents or consequences, or both. Thus, a typical behavior-based intervention is likely to involve safety training and goal setting for safety performance (i.e., antecedent), followed by periodic monitoring, feedback, and rewards concerning workers' safety behaviors, which represent the consequences (Geller, 1996). Thus, the short-term benefits associated with safety behaviors are enhanced as safety performance is now associated with valued outcomes.

Research has shown that both monitoring (Sasson & Austin, 2005) and feedback (Boyce & Geller, 2001) are crucial in the initial enhancement and short- and long-term maintenance of workers' safety behaviors. Additionally, such effects appear to be augmented if coupled with positive reinforcement, such as monetary rewards or time off (e.g., Austin, Kessler, Riccobono, & Bailey, 1996; Sulzer-Azaroff, Loafman, Merante, & Hlavacek, 1990). A recent meta-analysis, which combined the results of many studies by Tuncel, Lotlikar, Salem, and Daraiseh (2006), demonstrated that interventions based on the behavioral approach significantly reduced workplace accidents and injuries, supporting the efficacy of this approach.

Another approach to promote safety performance and reduce accidents focuses on the social environment in the workplace. In particular, organizations attempt to improve employee safety performance by creating a positive safety climate (Seo, Torabi, Blair, & Ellis, 2004; Zohar & Luria, 2003; 2005). Safety climate is conceptualized as shared perceptions among members of a group or organization regarding safety policies, procedures, and practices (Ostroff, Kinicki, & Tamkins, 2003). A positive safety climate exists when organizations establish high-quality safety policies and procedures and the key personnel, including the top management and the line supervisors, encourage employees to adhere to these policies. Research indicates that safety climate can be one mechanism underlying the effects of safety training on worker compliance, such that training not only teaches workers *how* to perform their job more safely but also generates a sense of importance associated with workplace safety, which in turn results in workers performing their tasks more safely (McDiarmid & Condon, 2005).

In addition, individual perceptions of safety climate have been linked to important safety outcomes, including accidents (e.g., Hayes, Perander, Smecko, & Trask, 1998; Hofmann & Mark, 2006) and injuries (e.g., Huang, Ho, Smith, & Chen, 2006; Zacharatos, Barling, & Iverson, 2005). When measured as the shared perceptions among group members, safety climate was found to enhance employee safety performance by activating their safety motivation. For example, Neal and Griffin (2006) found that a positive safety climate resulted in employees viewing workplace safety as more important. Subsequently, they were more willing to exert effort to comply with safety standards and procedures and participate in safety-related activities. The improved safety performance was reflected in the reduced accident rates at the group level.

Finally, researchers have started to incorporate safety behaviors as part of the global employee performance and view them within an employee motivation system. For example, based on the social cognitive model of motivation (Bandura, 1991), employees self-efficacy, or their belief about their ability to successfully engage in safety performance or achieve a safety goal, should be an important factor in determining their safety performance. Indeed, studies have found that employees self-efficacy concerning safety behavior contributed positively to their utilization of protective devices (e.g., Arezes & Miguel, 2006; Lusk, Ronis, & Kerr, 1995; Melamed, Rabinowitz, Feiner, Weisberg, & Ribak, 1996). Additionally, Wallace and Chen (2006) applied human motivation theory (Higgins, 1997, 2000) to explore the motivational underpinning of employee safety behavior. They found that workplace safety climate activates employees' prevention motivation, which made them more aware of the potential threats to workplace safety and the losses associated with unsafe work behaviors. Consequently, employees engaged in more safety behaviors. Taken together, it appears that these psychological and social approaches are helpful in fostering employee cooperation to use the appropriate safety equipment and engage in safe behaviors.

Musculoskeletal Disorders

Musculoskeletal disorders (MSDs) are injuries or disorders of the muscles, nerves, tendons, joints, cartilage, and spinal disks (National Institute for Occupational Safety and Health, 2004). MSDs typically result from repetitive motion, such as bending, climbing, crawling, reaching, twisting, or overexertion and can manifest in multiple ways, including muscle strains and sprains, back pain, and carpal tunnel syndrome. Different types of jobs place different physical demands on employees, and this may result in different forms of MSDs. For example, nurses are subject to back injury from lifting patients (Rickett, Orbell, & Sheeran, 2006). Dentists tend to experience more shoulder and wrist/hand problems (Palliser, Firth, Feyer, & Paulin, 2005). Finally, because of the repeated uses of fingers and hands, workers who do a lot of typing are most likely to suffer from carpal tunnel syndrome, which is a wrist injury that causes pain, numbness, and weakness in the fingers and hands.

Because of the close connection between MSDs and the physical demands associated with the job, researchers have focused primarily on ergonomic risk factors leading to MSDs. In particular, many safety professionals have attempted to reduce MSDs by altering the environment (e.g., changing the equipment) or worker behavior (e.g., taking mandatory breaks) or a combination of both (Sasson & Austin, 2005). More recently, researchers have started to explore whether psychological and/or social (psychosocial) risk factors contribute to the development of MSDs. For example, job demands such as high time pressure and unpredictable schedules have been found to contribute to general musculoskeletal complaints (Kjellberg & Wadman, 2007; Torp, Riise, & Moen, 1999), as well as specific problems in the neck/shoulder and elbow/wrist areas (Leroyer et al., 2006; van den Heuvel, van der Beek, Blatter, Hoogendoorn, & Bongers, 2005). Negative emotions and job attitudes have been found to relate to MSDs as well. For example, work-related anxiety and low job satisfaction have been linked to lower back pain (Holmstrom, Lindell, & Moritz, 1992a) and neck/shoulder complaints (Holmstrom, Lindell, & Moritz, 1992b; Tola, Riihimaki, Videman, Viihari-Juntura, & Hanninen, 1988). Lack of social support from coworkers was found to be especially a cause for elbow/wrist problems (van den Heuvel et al., 2005), while the extent to which members of a team see themselves as a cohesive unit and the extent of management support were both negatively related to general musculoskeletal complaints (Carayon, Haims, Hoonakker, & Swanson, 2006; Torp et al., 1999).

While these studies supported the implications of psychosocial factors for MSDs above and beyond physical demands, other studies have found a more complicated interplay between physical demands and psychosocial factors in predicting MSDs. For example, in a study with German geriatric nursing home employees, musculoskeletal problems were predicted by a three-way interaction between physical job demands, psychological demands, and work control (Hollmann, Heuer, & Schmidt, 2001). In particular, having control at work appeared to alleviate the effects of psychological demands on musculoskeletal complaints. However, this effect was only present when employees had low physical job demands at work. When their job tasks were highly physical, control had minimal buffering effect on the impact of psychological demands. This complex pattern of relationship may account for other seemingly equivocal findings concerning the effects of job control on MSDs (e.g., Kjellberg & Wademan, 2007; Torp et al., 1999). Thus, while we recognize that psychosocial factors may contribute to or alleviate risks for developing MSDs, it is important to consider these factors along with the physical demands of the job in order to get a more complete picture.

Job Stress

There are many things in life that are stressful, with many of those things happening at work. Being given an unexpected assignment without needed support and training or being threatened with losing one's job would be stressful to most people. Experiencing stress in the workplace is commonplace; for example, in a British study, Warr and Payne (1983) found that 15% of the employees reported having experienced something stressful the prior day at work. Although stress is a normal part of life, excessive stress can have detrimental effects on physical and psychological health. Conversely, experiencing poor health or an injury at work can itself be stressful.

Researchers who study stress distinguish conditions or situations at work (stressors) from reactions to those conditions (strains). Stressors are things at work that require an adaptive response by the employee (Jex & Beehr, 1991) and lead to a negative emotional response, which is a form of strain. There are three categories of strain: (1) psychological (e.g., negative emotions or poor attitude about the job), (2) physical (e.g., physiological reactions such as increased blood pressure, symptoms such as headache or stomach distress, and illness), and (3) behavioral (e.g., substance use or smoking). Figure 21.2 illustrates the basic stress process. People are subjected to conditions and events at work, some of which serve as stressors. For example, an employee arrives at work 5 minutes late and is yelled at by his or her supervisor. Such events are perceived and appraised by the employee in terms of how threatening they might be to his or her personal well-being. It is likely that the employee will view being yelled at as threatening, and therefore, it will be perceived as a stressor. An immediate emotional response will occur, which might be anger at being yelled at or anxiety that the supervisor might do even worse. Those negative emotions will be associated with physiological responses, such as secretion of the stress hormone cortisol into the bloodstream. The person will engage in behavior that helps in coping with the stressful situation, and those behaviors might be constructive (e.g., the employee making sure he or she is on time the next day) or counterproductive (e.g., punching the supervisor).

Job stressors can be classified into two types: social stressors and task stressors. Social stressors arise from interactions among people in the workplace. Interpersonal conflicts and being the target of abusive behavior (being yelled at for being late) are two examples. Later in this chapter, we will discuss workplace violence, which is a form of social stressor. Task stressors involve aspects of the work itself. Common task stressors include workload (having too much to do or work tasks that are too difficult), organizational constraints (things in the workplace that interfere with doing the job, such as defective tools), role ambiguity (uncertainty about what is expected of the individual), and role conflict (conflicting demands, such as being asked to work more quickly while making fewer errors). Later in this chapter, we will discuss work-family conflict (WFC), which is a type of role conflict between work and home.

An important element in the job stress process is employee control. This refers to the ability of employees to make decisions about when, where, and how to do their jobs. Some jobs, such as that of a college professor, allow great latitude and, thus, greater control. Others,

FIGURE 21.2 The Job Stress Process

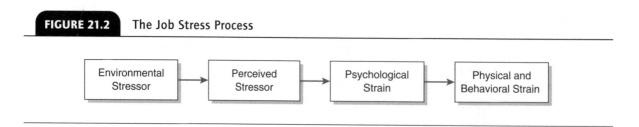

such as that of an assembly line worker, offer little control, especially if the pace of work is determined by a machine. Having control is important as it helps determine whether or not someone perceives a situation as a stressor. If an employee is working on a tight deadline, having a machine break can be a stressful event, particularly if it is important for the employee to meet the deadline. Being able to fix that machine (a form of control) will mitigate the stressfulness of the breakdown. Control too has been linked to physical and psychological health (Spector, 1986). For example, Bosma, Stansfeld, and Marmot (1998) showed that having low levels of control at work is associated with elevated risk of cardiovascular disease. The control-demand model (Karasek, 1979) suggests that control does not have a direct effect on strain but rather that it buffers the effect of stressors. As shown in Figure 21.3, when control is low, an increase in stressors is associated with an increase in strain. When control is high, however, stressors have little effect on strain levels.

The public health model of primary, secondary, and tertiary prevention is quite relevant to dealing with job stress. Primary prevention focuses on reducing job stressors in the workplace. This means the careful design of jobs to eliminate unnecessary stressors, such as balancing workloads, making sure that employees have the needed skills and tools to do the job, making sure that demands are clear and nonconflicting, and reducing conflict among employees. Secondary prevention focuses on helping employees deal with stressors that cannot be designed out of the job. This might include stress management training, which teaches employees how to cope productively with stressors, for example, by using relaxation techniques when psychological strains occur. Finally, the tertiary

FIGURE 21.3 The Control-Demand Model, Showing the Buffering Effect of Control on the Relationship Between Job Stressors and Strain

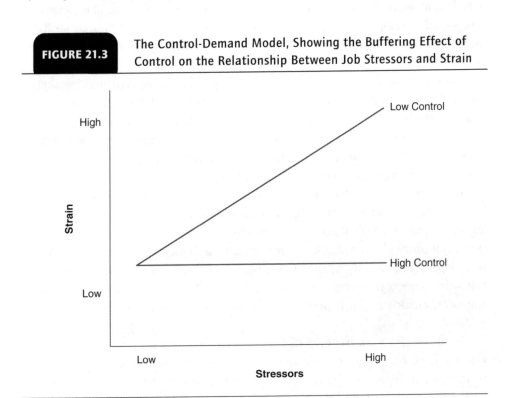

approach focuses on employees once they have experienced more than routine transient stress at work. Employee assistance programs are available to employees of most large North American organizations, providing psychological counseling services to deal with traumatic stress from work.

Violence

The U.S. Department of Labor (2007) reported that workplace violence was the fourth leading cause of workplace fatalities in 2006. Depending on the relationship between the perpetrator and the victim, workplace violence can be categorized into four types (Merchant & Lundell, 2001). Type 1 is violence by individuals with no business relationship with the organization or personal relationship with the victim, such as someone committing a robbery. This type of violence is most likely to occur to employees in jobs that involve contact with the public; exchange of money; delivery of passengers, goods, or services; and working alone (National Institute for Occupational Safety and Health, 1996). Convenience store clerks and taxicab drivers have these sorts of jobs. Type 2 violence is committed by clients, customers, or patients of the organization. For example, health care professionals can be assaulted by patients (Anderson, 2002; Lanza, 2006), whereas retail workers can be assaulted by customers (LeBlanc, Dupré, & Barling, 2006). LeBlanc and Kelloway (2002) found that employees have a higher likelihood of being assaulted when their jobs involve disciplining others and making decisions about others' lives. Type 3 is performed by the coworkers of the victim. This can occur with any kind of job in any type of organization. Type 4 is relationship violence (e.g., spouse abuse) that spills over to the workplace. Thus, the nature of the job largely determines the type of violence to which employees are most likely to be subject.

A useful model for considering the psychological and social antecedents of workplace violence has been proposed by O'Leary-Kelly, Griffin, and Glew (1996). In their model, individual employees and the organizational environment both possess characteristics that encourage violence. Often this begins with milder forms of verbal aggression, such as employees insulting one another or making nasty comments. If organizations fail to take action to discourage such acts, they may escalate into physical violence.

Based on this model, certain individuals are predisposed toward aggressive or violent behaviors. For example, trait anger and lack of self-control have been associated with higher self-reported violent acts in the workplace (Douglas & Martinko, 2001). In addition, organizational characteristics may contribute to aggressive tendencies in employees. For example, rigid and aggressive organizations may encourage their employees to behave in a more aggressive manner (Tobin, 2001). Similarly, organizations that treat their employees unfairly may also increase the chance for employee aggression (Fox, Spector, & Miles, 2001).

Finally, recent work has extended the concept of safety climate to organizational violence. In particular, violence climate refers to employees' perceptions of organizational policies, practices, and procedures regarding the control and elimination of workplace violence and verbal aggression (Spector, Coulter, Stockwell, & Matz, 2007). Violence climate predicted physical violence and verbal aggression among nurses (Spector et al., 2007). Specifically, a favorable climate was associated with low incidence of violence and aggression. Additionally, violence climate predicted physical strain, psychological strain (anxiety and depression), and perceived workplace safety. In another study, Kessler, Spector, Chang, and Parr (2008) reported similar effects of a positive violence climate and exposure to violence on employee strain, for a sample from a wide variety of jobs. Thus, it appears that aspects of the psychosocial environment in the workplace can function to either escalate or deter physical violence and verbal aggression.

The O'Leary-Kelly et al. (1996) model further suggests that the way organizations respond to aggression will alter the extent to which aggressive behaviors result in violence. In particular, organizations may deter violence if the supervisors respond quickly to employees' early aggressive acts. Indeed, previous studies have demonstrated the important role that leaders play in improving workplace safety through improvement of safety climate (e.g., Barling, Loughlin, & Kelloway, 2002; Kelloway, Mullen, & Francis, 2006). Similar effects of effective leadership on a positive violence climate may be expected, which may in turn serve to discourage aggression and violence. On the other hand, if left unnoted, organizational aggression that begins in mild and mostly verbal forms may eventually lead to physical violence, causing physical and psychological damage to employees. In this case, the proper response from supervisors may be even more crucial in discouraging future violent incidents.

For example, to deal with severe cases of violence, internal security or the police might be called. When incidents are less severe and involve employees as perpetrators, supervisors should provide employees with feedback concerning appropriate behavior, training, and, in extreme or persisting cases, disciplinary actions. When clients, customers, or patients are the perpetrators, this might involve management intervention to discuss the behavior with the perpetrator to make clear that violent acts are not permitted or tolerated. In persistent cases, management might take action to disallow the person from continued contact. These responses are aiming at not only dealing with the violent incidents but also removing the antecedents for future violence. Additionally, supervisors should be aware of and sensitive to the victims' perspectives rather than attaching blame to the victims (Hofmann & Stretzer, 1996; Kelly & Mullen, 2006). Supervisors should also be aware of the impact of a violent or aggressive incident on other bystanders, including other employees and customers. Studies have shown that vicarious experiences of workplace violence have similar effects on employee attitudes as actual exposure (Schat & Kelloway, 2000). Thus, organizations should be aware that violent incidents not only cause immediate damage to the individual but also leave a long-term negative impact on the general organizational psychosocial environment.

Work-Family Conflict

As noted earlier, WFC occurs when the demands of work interfere with the demands of home. For example, an individual might have an important work meeting on a day his or her child is sick and needs to be taken to the doctor. This is a type of stressor that arises from the interplay of work and nonwork life, leading to the sort of strains we discussed in the stress section of this chapter. There are two directions of WFC—work can interfere with family (e.g., a work emergency makes a person miss dinner with the family) or family can interfere with work (e.g., an appointment with a child's teacher makes one late for work). There are also different forms of WFC. *Time-based conflict* (as illustrated in the examples above) occurs when there are not enough hours to accomplish all work and family activities, or it can occur not because of excessive amount of time demands but because of schedule conflicts between home and work. *Strain-based conflict* occurs when exposure to stressors produces strain in one domain that spills over to the other. For example, a fight with the spouse at breakfast brings the employee to work in a bad mood. A particularly difficult day at work brings the employee home emotionally exhausted. *Behavior-based conflict* happens when behaviors in one domain are incompatible with behaviors in another and the person has trouble making the transition. For example, managers with children treat their subordinates like children and their children like employees.

There are a number of workplace factors that lead to WFC. Most notable are the number of working hours (Day & Chamberlain, 2006) and the lack of schedule flexibility, which requires the employee to be at the workplace at specified times (Major, Klein, & Ehrhart, 2002). Stressors at work can also contribute to WFC, such as role ambiguity (Ford, Heinen, & Langkamer, 2007) and workload (Spector, Allen, et al., 2007). On the other hand, family-work conflict occurs when there are high family demands, such as having children, especially when one is a single parent. Individual personality can also play a role in WFC. Emotional individuals who are high on negative affectivity (the tendency to experience negative emotions) tend to have more WFC (Bruck & Allen, 2003), as well as other job stressors.

As a type of job stressor, WFC has potential effects on a number of psychological, physical, and behavioral strains. For example, Major et al. (2002) showed that individuals reporting high levels of WFC also reported high levels of physical-health symptoms. Allen, Herst, Bruck, and Sutton (2000) showed that individuals experiencing high levels of WFC tended to be dissatisfied with their jobs. This is true for both men and women (Kossek & Ozeki, 1998), showing that the WFC is not just an issue for working women, as is sometimes assumed.

Many organizations are concerned with WFC and have taken steps to reduce it. The adoption of "family-friendly" work policies is designed to help employees balance both domains of their lives. Two of the most frequently used elements of such policies are flextime and on-site child care. There are many varieties of flextime, but all allow some degree of latitude in when the employee can work. Some forms require working a full shift within a day (usually 8 hours) but allow flexibility in the starting or stopping time. Thus, an employee has the option of beginning work anytime between 6 a.m. and 10 a.m. and leaving work between 3 p.m. and 7 p.m. (assuming an unpaid lunch hour). For a working couple, this could allow a staggering of working hours so that one spouse takes the children to school and the other picks them up after school. On-site child care is a facility that is located at the employee's place of work. This makes it easy for parents to drop their children at day care and be nearby to visit during the day, for example, at lunch time.

Although family-friendly policies seem like the ideal solution to WFC, research shows that they are not always effective (Allen, 2001). Part of the reason is that policies at the organizational level do not always translate into practices at the immediate workgroup level, so that they can have positive effects for individuals. This is a clear example of why the ecological approach is needed to link the individual with higher social levels. Allen (2001) showed that policies at the organizational level alone are not sufficient but that looking at more immediate supervisor attitudes and support for the use of such policies are required to deal with issues of WFC. They developed the concept of family-supportive organizational practices, which is the extent to which individual employees perceive their organizations to be supportive of family issues. This gets more directly at the attitudes and practices of managers and coworkers in supporting the use of family-friendly policies and the extent to which they are willing to help employees solve work-family issues. WFC can best be addressed when the organization-level policies and the immediate supervisor practices work together to help employees balance work and family demands.

CONCLUSION

Both psychological and social factors are important to the health, safety, and well-being of employees in the workplace. Whereas the 20th century saw tremendous progress in identifying and eliminating the major physical hazards in the workplace that have adverse affects on health, more recently there has been increasing awareness that a focus on the physical environment alone is insufficient. Although we now know a great deal, we need even more research to identify the psychological and social aspects of people and the workplace that are detrimental to health. Knowledge of such factors can inform the development of effective interventions to enhance employee health through a focus on employees, workgroups, and organizations.

The ecological model recognizes that there are influences on health that arise not only from the individual employee but also from larger social units ranging from the immediate work group to the employing organization, and society itself. As we discussed throughout the chapter, there are important aspects of individuals and the nature of their jobs that are important contributors to accidents, injuries, and ill health, both physical and psychological. However, a focus on the individual is incomplete, as the actions of coworkers and immediate supervisors are important. For example, coworkers and supervisors can be a major source of job stressors, and supervisor practices can contribute to unsafe work practice, violence at work, and WFC. At the organizational level, policies and practices can be implemented that facilitate health and safety for employees. There is much that top management can do to contribute to employee health, but mere writing of policy is insufficient without specific actions to make sure that those policies are enacted at the group and individual levels. Finally, government laws and regulations can do much to encourage organizations to take health and safety seriously. As with organizational policy, the writing of laws or development of regulations alone is insufficient. Government must follow up with enforcement mechanisms, as well as resources and support that assist organizations in making positive changes.

Health and safety can best be achieved when all social levels adopt compatible goals for increasing employee health and safety and they engage in cooperative action in achieving such goals. This will require a more complete understanding of workplace health and how the various social levels can best interact effectively. Imposition of policies and practices from higher (e.g., government) to lower (e.g., organization) levels is often met with resistance, so the use of effective implementation strategies is important. This begins with an understanding of how physical and social factors in the workplace combine to affect health and safety at work and the dissemination of such knowledge so that people understand how their actions affect health.

REFERENCES

Alavosius, M. P., Adams, A. E., Ahern, D. K., & Follick, M. J. (2000). Behavioral approaches to organizational safety. In J. Austin & J. E. Carr (Eds.), *Handbook of applied behavior analysis* (pp. 351–373). Reno, NV: Context Press.

Allen, T. D. (2001). Family-supportive work environments: The role of organizational perceptions. *Journal of Vocational Behavior, 58,* 414–435.

Allen, T. D., Herst, D. E. L., Bruck, C. S., & Sutton, M. (2000). Consequences associated with work-to-family conflict: A review and agenda for future research. *Journal of Occupational Health Psychology, 5,* 278–308.

Anderson, C. (2002). Workplace violence: Are some nurses more vulnerable? *Issues in Mental Health Nursing, 23,* 351–366.

Arezes, P. M., & Miguel, A. S. (2006). Does risk recognition affect workers' hearing protection utilization rate? *International Journal of Industrial Ergonomics, 36,* 1037–1043.

Austin, J., Kessler, M. L., Riccobono, J. E., & Bailey, J. (1996). Using feedback and reinforcement to improve the performance and safety of a roofing crew. *Journal of Organizational Behavior Management, 16,* 49–75.

Bandura, A. (1991). Social cognitive theory of self-regulation. *Organizational Behavior and Human Decision Processes, 50,* 248–287.

Barling, J., Loughlin, C., & Kelloway, E. K. (2002). Development and test of a model linking safety-specific transformational leadership and occupational safety. *Journal of Applied Psychology, 87,* 488–496.

Bosma, H., Stansfeld, S. A., & Marmot, M. G. (1998). Job control, personal characteristics, and heart disease. *Journal of Occupational Health Psychology, 3,* 402–409.

Boyce, T. E., & Geller, E. S. (2001). Applied behavior analysis and occupational safety: The challenge of response maintenance. *Journal of Organizational Behavior Management, 21,* 31–56.

Bruck, C. S., & Allen, T. D. (2003). The relationship between big five personality traits, negative affectivity, Type A behavior, and work-family conflict. *Journal of Vocational Behavior, 63,* 457–472.

Carayon, P., Haims, M. C., Hoonakker, P. L. T., & Swanson, N. G. (2006). Teamwork and musculoskeletal health in the context of work organization interventions in office and computer work. *Theoretical Issues in Ergonomics Science, 7,* 39–69.

Day, A. L., & Chamberlain, T. C. (2006). Committing to your work, spouse, and children: Implications for work-family conflict. *Journal of Vocational Behavior, 68,* 116–130.

Douglas, S. C., & Martinko, M. J. (2001). Exploring the role of individual differences in the prediction of workplace aggression. *Journal of Applied Psychology, 86,* 547–559.

Ford, M. T., Heinen, B. A., & Langkamer, K. L. (2007). Work and family satisfaction and conflict: A meta-analysis of cross-domain relations. *Journal of Applied Psychology, 92,* 57–80.

Fox, S., Spector, P. E., & Miles, D. (2001). Counterproductive work behavior (CWB) in response to job stressors and organizational justice: Some mediator and moderator tests for autonomy and emotions. *Journal of Vocational Behavior, 59,* 291–309.

Geller, E. S. (1996). *The psychology of safety.* Rander, PA: Chilton.

Hayes, B. E., Perander, J., Smecko, T., & Trask, J. (1998). Measuring perceptions of workplace safety: Development and validation of the Work Safety Scale. *Journal of Safety Research, 29,* 145–161.

Higgins, E. T. (1997). Beyond pleasure and pain. *American Psychologist, 52,* 1280–1300.

Higgins, E. T. (2000). Making a good decision: Value from fit. *American Psychologist, 55,* 1217–1230.

Hofmann, D. A., & Mark, B. (2006). An investigation of the relationship between safety climate and medication errors as well as other nurse and patient outcomes. *Personnel Psychology, 59,* 847–869.

Hofmann, D. A., & Stretzer, A. (1996). A cross-level investigation of factors influencing unsafe behaviors and accidents. *Personnel Psychology, 49,* 307–339.

Hollmann, S., Heuer, H., & Schmidt, K. H. (2001). Control at work: A generalized resource factor for the prevention of musculoskeletal symptoms? *Work & Stress, 15,* 29–39.

Holmstrom, E. B., Lindell, J., & Moritz, U. (1992a). Low back and neck/shoulder pain in construction workers: Occupational workload and psychosocial risk factors. Part 1: Relationship to low back pain. *Spine, 17,* 663–671.

Holmstrom, E. B., Lindell, J., & Moritz, U. (1992b). Low back and neck/shoulder pain in construction workers: Occupational workload and psychosocial risk factors. Part 2: Relationship to neck and shoulder pain. *Spine, 17,* 672–677.

Huang, Y. H., Ho, M., Smith, G. S., & Chen, P. Y. (2006). Safety climate and self-reported injury: Assessing the mediating role of employee safety control. *Accident Analysis & Prevention, 38,* 425–433.

Jex, S. M., & Beehr, T. A. (1991). Emerging theoretical and methodological issues in the study of work-related stress. *Research in Personnel and Human Resources Management, 9,* 311–365.

Karasek, R. A. (1979). Job demands, job decision latitude, and mental strain: Implications for job redesign. *Administrative Science Quarterly, 24,* 285–308.

Kelloway, E. K., Mullen, J., & Francis, L. (2006). Divergent effects of transformational and passive leadership on employee safety. *Journal of Occupational Health Psychology, 11,* 76–86.

Kelly, E., & Mullen, J. (2006). Organizational response to workplace violence. In E. K. Kelloway, J. Barling, & J. J. Hurrell Jr. (Eds.), *Handbook of workplace violence* (pp. 493–515). Thousand Oaks, CA: Sage.

Kessler, S. R., Spector, P. E., Chang, C. H., & Parr, A. D. (2008). Organizational violence climate and exposure to violence and verbal aggression. *Work & Stress, 22,* 108–124.

Kjellberg, A., & Wadman, C. (2007). The role of the affective stress response as a mediator of the effect of psychosocial risk factors on musculoskeletal complaints—Part 1: Assembly workers. *International Journal of Industrial Ergonomics, 37,* 367–374.

Kossek, E. E., & Ozeki, C. (1998). Work-family conflict, policies, and the job-life satisfaction relationship: A review and directions for organizational behavior-human resources research. *Journal of Applied Psychology, 83,* 139–149.

Lanza, M. (2006). Violence in nursing. In E. K. Kelloway, J. Barling, & J. J. Hurrell Jr. (Eds.), *Handbook of workplace violence* (pp. 147–167). Thousand Oaks, CA: Sage.

LeBlanc, M. M., Dupré, K. E., & Barling, J. (2006). Public-initiated violence. In E. K. Kelloway, J. Barling, & J. J. Hurrell Jr. (Eds.), *Handbook of workplace violence* (pp. 261–280). Thousand Oaks, CA: Sage.

LeBlanc, M. M., & Kelloway, E. K. (2002). Predictors and outcomes of workplace violence and aggression. *Journal of Applied Psychology, 87,* 444–453.

Leroyer, A., Edmé, J. L., Vaxevanoglou, X., Buisset, C., Laurent, P., Desobry, P., & Frimat, P. (2006). Neck, shoulder, and hand and wrist pain among administrative employees: Relation to work-time organization and psychosocial factors at work. *Journal of Occupational & Environmental Medicine, 48,* 326–333.

Lusk, S. L., Ronis, D. L., & Kerr, M. J. (1995). Predictors of hearing protection use among workers: Implications for training programs. *Human Factors, 37,* 635–640.

Major, V. S., Klein, K. J., & Ehrhart, M. G. (2002). Work time, work interference with family, and psychological distress. *Journal of Applied Psychology, 87,* 427–436.

McDiarmid, M. A., & Condon, M. (2005). Organizational safety culture/climate and worker compliance with hazardous drug guidelines: Lessons from the blood-borne pathogen experience. *Journal of Occupational & Environmental Medicine, 47,* 740–749.

Melamed, S., Rabinowitz, S., Feiner, M., Weisberg, E., & Ribak, J. (1996). Usefulness of the protection motivation theory in explaining hearing protection device use among male industrial workers. *Health Psychology, 15,* 209–215.

Merchant, J. A. & Lundell, J. (2001). Workplace violence intervention research workshop, April 5–7, 2000, Washington, DC: Background, rationale, and summary. *American Journal of Preventive Medicine, 20,* 135–140.

National Institute for Occupational Safety and Health. (1996). *Violence in the workplace: Risk factors and prevention strategies.* Retrieved August 13, 2008, from www.cdc.gov/niosh/violnonf.html

National Institute for Occupational Safety and Health. (2004). *Worker health chartbook.* Retrieved August 13, 2008, from www.cdc.gov/niosh/docs/chartbook

National Safety Council. (2005–2006). *Injury facts, 2005–2006 edition.* Itasca, IL: Author.

Neal, A., & Griffin, M. A. (2006). A study of the lagged relationships among safety climate, safety motivation, safety behavior, and accidents at the individual and group levels. *Journal of Applied Psychology, 91,* 946–953.

O'Leary-Kelly, A. M., Griffin, R. W., & Glew, D. J. (1996). Organization-motivated aggression: A research framework. *Academy of Management Review, 21,* 225–253.

Ostroff, C., Kinicki, A. J., & Tamkins, M. M. (2003). Organizational culture and climate. In W. C. Borman, D. R. Ilgen, & R. J. Klimoski (Eds.), *Handbook of psychology: Industrial and organizational psychology* (Vol. 12, pp. 565–593). Hoboken, NJ: Wiley.

Palliser, C. R., Firth, H. M., Feyer, A. M., & Paulin, S. M. (2005). Musculoskeletal discomfort and work-related stress in New Zealand dentists. *Work & Stress, 19,* 351–359.

Rickett, B., Orbell, S., & Sheeran, P. (2006). Social-cognitive determinants of hoist usage among health care workers. *Journal of Occupational Health Psychology, 11,* 182–196.

Sasson, J. R., & Austin, J. (2005). The effects of training, feedback, and participant involvement in behavioral safety observations on office ergonomic behavior. *Journal of Organizational Behavior Management, 24,* 1–30.

Schat, A. C. H., & Kelloway, E. K. (2000). Effects of perceived control on the outcomes of workplace aggression and violence. *Journal of Occupational Health Psychology, 5,* 386–402.

Seo, D. C., Torabi, M. R., Blair, E. H., & Ellis, N. T. (2004). A cross-validation of safety climate scale using confirmatory factor analytic approach. *Journal of Safety Research, 35,* 427–445.

Spector, P. E. (1986). Perceived control by employees: A meta-analysis of studies concerning autonomy and participation at work. *Human Relations, 39,* 1005–1016.

Spector, P. E., Allen, T. D., Poelmans, S. A. Y., Lapierre, L. M., Cooper, C. L., O'Driscoll, et al. (2007). Cross-national differences in relationships of work demands, job satisfaction and turnover intentions with work-family conflict. *Personnel Psychology, 60,* 805–835.

Spector, P. E., Coulter, M. L., Stockwell, H. G., & Matz, M. W. (2007). Relationships of workplace physical violence and verbal aggression with perceived safety, perceived violence climate, and strains in a healthcare setting. *Work & Stress, 21,* 117–130.

Sulzer-Azaroff, B., Loafman, B., Merante, R. J., & Hlavacek, A. C. (1990). Improving occupational safety in a large industrial plant: A systematic replication. *Journal of Organizational Behavior Management, 11,* 99–120.

Tobin, T. J. (2001). Organizational determinants of violence in the workplace. *Aggression and Violent Behavior, 6,* 91–102.

Tola, S., Riihimaki, H., Videman, T., Viihari-Juntura, E., & Hanninen, K. (1988). Neck and shoulder symptoms among men in machine operating, dynamic physical work and sedentary work. *Scandinavian Journal of Work Environment and Health, 14,* 299–305.

Torp, S., Riise, T., & Moen, B. E. (1999). How the psychosocial work environment of motor vehicle mechanics may influence coping with musculoskeletal symptoms. *Work & Stress, 13,* 193–203.

Tuncel, S., Lotlikar, H., Salem, S., & Daraiseh, N. (2006). Effectiveness of behavior based safety interventions to reduce accidents and injuries in workplaces: Critical appraisal and meta-analysis. *Theoretical Issues in Ergonomics Science, 7,* 191–209.

U.S. Department of Labor. (2007). *Bureau of Labor Statistics injuries, illnesses and fatalities* [Electronic version]. Retrieved September 28, 2007, from www.bls.gov/iif/home.htm#tables

van den Heuvel, S. G., van der Beek, A. J., Blatter, B. M., Hoogendoorn, W. E., & Bongers, P. M. (2005). Psychosocial work characteristics in relation to neck and upper limb symptoms. *Pain, 114,* 47–53.

Wallace, C., & Chen, G. (2006). A multilevel integration of personality, climate, self-regulation, and performance. *Personnel Psychology, 59,* 529–557.

Warr, P., & Payne, R. (1983). Affective outcomes of paid employment in a random sample of British workers. *Journal of Occupational Behavior, 4,* 91–104.

Zacharatos, A., Barling, J., & Iverson, R. D. (2005). High-performance work systems and occupational safety. *Journal of Applied Psychology, 90,* 77–93.

Zohar, D. (2002). Modifying supervisory practices to improve sub-unit safety: A leadership-based intervention model. *Journal of Applied Psychology, 87,* 156–163.

Zohar, D., & Luria, G. (2003). The use of supervisory practices as leverage to improve safety behavior: A cross-level intervention model. *Journal of Safety Research, 34,* 567–577.

Zohar, D., & Luria, G. (2005). A multilevel model of safety climate: Cross-level relationships between organization and group-level climates. *Journal of Applied Psychology, 90,* 616–628.

Afterword

New Directions

By Jeannine Coreil

The coming years will undoubtedly bring new opportunities and challenges for applying social and behavioral science perspectives to public health problems. In the preceding chapters, the authors highlighted the need for both more integrative approaches that transcend particular health issues as well as more in-depth understanding of specific problems. Research and practice will continue to develop in these two directions, although the tendency toward increasing specialization in science and technology will probably favor more narrowly focused solutions. Moreover, securing the political support and resources needed to implement integrated, comprehensive approaches will remain a major challenge.

Another challenge for social and behavioral scientists will be the need to translate the products of their research and interventions into something meaningful and usable by public health professionals. Practitioners want social scientists to produce "toolboxes" that can be transported from one setting to another, opened up when needed, and the appropriate tool applied to fix the problem (Erwin, 2008). Ideally, a user's manual should accompany the toolbox with instructions for which tools best fit different populations and situations. Toolbox thinking has undoubtedly contributed to the popularity of behavior change models that anchor determining factors within schematic assemblages, often placing them squarely within boxes or other bounded devices. In contrast, social scientists often apply abstract perspectives, theories, and concepts that are not easily converted into tools. They offer new ways of thinking about problems, rarely technologic solutions. If only someone could develop, for example, a good "culturometer," a device that could perform a complete cultural assessment of an individual in seconds, it would be an instant commercial success in the field.

The proliferation of behavior change and intervention models will surely continue in the coming years for reasons noted in Chapter 4. Studies that evaluate the advantages of one model over another are less likely to take place for philosophical and practical reasons. Researchers develop allegiance to particular approaches and tend to stick with them because they have career capital invested in them and need to demonstrate a track record in a line of research to be competitive for funding. Moreover, researchers are usually not interested in investing time and resources on alternative approaches they consider less useful. Pragmatically, it is usually prohibitive to test two different approaches, particularly intervention models, because of the complexity of design and the cost of data collection. Too often, attempts to test two or more theories or models fall short of their goals because they simply compare the predictive power of selected "measures" and not the whole theory or model (Levanthal, Musumeci, & Contrada, 2007). Consequently, "evidence-based" practice will depend on careful discernment of the kinds of problems most amenable to different approaches rather than empirical assessment of the relative effectiveness of alternative models.

Methodologic advances will continue to enhance the application of social and behavioral science perspectives in public health. For example, multilevel analytic methods such as hierarchical linear modeling (Raudenbush & Bryk, 2002) enable the differential analysis of individual and social contextual influences on health outcomes. The ability to identify causal determinants at different levels of social ecological systems will enable more precision in specifying explanatory factors and will help locate the most promising levels for intervention. The expansion of interest in qualitative research and methods development will also continue to strengthen the field as public health professionals recognize the value of insights gained through qualitative studies (Ulin, Robinson, & Tolley, 2005). Strategies for "mixed-methods" research, which integrate both quantitative and qualitative techniques, are rapidly gaining acceptance as offering the best of both worlds. The recent appearance of a new journal, the *Journal of Mixed Methods Research,* reflects the growth of interest in this interdisciplinary field.

In the decades ahead, further developments will undoubtedly unfold in the theoretical, methodologic, and practical applications of social science within public health. These will not only expand in the areas outlined in this book but will take new directions as well. One area of expected growth is the critical study of public health itself as a focus of inquiry. More than 50 years ago, the sociologist Robert Straus (1957) drew the distinction between "sociology in medicine" and "sociology of medicine." Sociology *in* medicine applies the theories and methods of sociology to understand medical problems and their management, while sociology *of* medicine studies the profession of medicine as an entity. Thus far, the social and behavioral sciences have been applied largely *in* public health, to help solve health problems. The maturation of the field calls for greater attention to the study *of* public health, including its professional organization, culture, and other collective features. To do this, social scientists will need to augment their traditional positionality within public health to adopt more outsider gazes that analyze the diverse practices of public health with the goal of highlighting the consequences of taken-for-granted approaches and perspectives. The critical approach taken in Chapter 7 to the current "diversity" enterprise in public health and the description of the "culture of public health" in Chapter 8 provide examples of this approach. In addition to elaborating the cultural background of populations served, researchers will turn their attention to the organizational culture of public health, illuminating the consequences of collective identities, value orientations, epistemologic assumptions and the social construction of problems, causality, and modes of intervention.

Another thrust will likely expand critical perspectives linking issues of social justice, ethics, and health disparities. Social scientists will move beyond measurement, description, and analysis of health inequalities to advocating agendas for directed change using social theory and methods. These actions will be directed at local, national, and global levels, drawing on strategies honed in other practice domains as well as producing innovative approaches. It is hoped that the inherent tension in negotiating a balanced interface between insider and outsider perspectives will produce a rich body of work that further enhances social and behavioral science contributions to public health.

REFERENCES

Erwin, D. (2008, February 27). *Applying anthropology in cancer prevention: Through the looking glass.* Paper presented at the University of South Florida, Tampa.

Levanthal, H., Musumeci, T., & Contrada, R. (2007). Current issues and new directions in psychology and health: Theory, translation, and evidence-based practice. *Psychology & Health, 22*(4), 381–386.

Raudenbush, S. W., & Bryk, A. S. (2002). *Hierarchical linear models: Applications and data analysis methods* (2nd ed.). Thousand Oaks, CA: Sage.

Straus, R. (1957). The nature and status of medical sociology. *American Sociological Review, 22,* 200–204.

Ulin, P., Robinson, E. T., & Tolley, E. E. (2005). *Qualitative methods in public health: A field guide for applied researchers.* San Francisco: Jossey-Bass.

Index

About the Editor

Jeannine Coreil, PhD, is a professor in the Department of Community and Family Health, College of Public Health, University of South Florida. From 1980 to 1987, she served on the faculty of the University of Texas Medical Branch at Galveston and has since held a faculty position at the University of South Florida, in Tampa. In the fall of 2008, she was a visiting faculty member at the University of Aix-Marseille, France. Her areas of research include infectious diseases, illness support groups, gender and health, and qualitative research methods. She has conducted sociomedical and ethnographic research among Haitian Americans and Hispanics, in addition to numerous studies on cultural factors and health in Haiti since 1977. Her WHO/TDR-sponsored study *Support Groups for Women With Lymphatic Filariasis in Haiti* was published as a monograph in 2003. She is the coauthor of *Anthropology and Primary Health Care* (1990), along with more than 50 journal articles and book chapters. She recently completed a 5-year study (2003–2008) of stigma and tuberculosis in Haitian populations, which was funded by the National Institutes of Health. Her current research is funded by the Susan G. Komen for the Cure Foundation and focuses on cultural diversity within breast cancer support groups in Florida. She teaches courses in social theory, social and behavioral factors in health, qualitative methods, and global health. In November 2008, she assumed the position of President-Elect of the Society for Medical Anthropology. She received a bachelor's degree in psychology from the University of Louisiana-Lafayette (1972) and a master's degree in anthropology (1976) and a doctoral degree in medical anthropology (1979) from the University of Kentucky.

About the Contributors

Carol A. Bryant, PhD, MS, is Distinguished USF Health Professor and Codirector of the Florida Prevention Research Center at the University of South Florida College of Public Health. For 20 years, she has directed social marketing research on a wide variety of public health projects. With colleagues at the Florida Prevention Research Center, she is developing and evaluating an innovative framework: community-based prevention marketing for designing and tailoring behavior change interventions. In addition to research, she teaches a variety of graduate-level social marketing courses and coordinates the National Social Marketing and Public Health Conference. She is also the founding editor of the *Social Marketing Quarterly* and senior author of *The Cultural Feast: An Introduction to Food and Society.*

Eric R. Buhi is an assistant professor and director of the Collaborative for Research Understanding Sexual Health at the University of South Florida's College of Public Health. He teaches public health graduate classes in evaluation methods and quantitative analysis. His research investigates educational programs designed to reduce adolescents' HIV/sexually transmitted infection risk and the influence of the Internet, new media, and other technologies on the sexual health of young people. He earned his PhD in health education from Texas A&M University and a Master of Public Health degree from Indiana University.

Chu-Hsiang Chang is currently an assistant professor at the Department of Environmental and Occupational Health of the University of South Florida. Her research interests focus on applying behavioral science principles to occupational health and safety. Specifically, she is interested in examining how psychosocial factors and individual differences influence employee responses to environmental stressors, as well as their impact on the effectiveness of various health and safety interventions. She received her PhD in industrial/organizational psychology from the University of Akron in 2005.

Martha Coulter is Professor of Public Health at the University of South Florida and Director of the James and Jennifer Harrell Center for the Study of Family Violence. Her research expertise is in the areas of maternal and child health and family and community violence with a particular focus on child maltreatment and intimate-partner violence. She has served as a primary investigator on numerous research projects in family violence and has authored numerous publications and made numerous presentations in this field. She is codirector of a certificate program in Violence and Injury Prevention directed at community professionals and graduate students desiring specialty training in this area. Dr. Coulter received her MSW from Tulane University, her MPH from the University of California at Berkeley, and her DrPH from the University of North Carolina at Chapel Hill.

Rita DiGioacchino DeBate, PhD, MPH, CHES, is an associate professor in the Department of Community and Family Health, College of Public Health at the University of South Florida. She has a background in health behavior/health education and public health. Her research interests include obesity and eating disorders. She has authored numerous articles on body image, physical activity, and secondary prevention of eating disorders. She is the program evaluator for Girls on the Run—a developmentally focused youth sport program. She is also the principal investigator of an NIH-funded study to develop a training program for dental professionals on secondary prevention of eating disorders.

Wendy L. Hellerstedt, MPH, PhD, is a reproductive and perinatal epidemiologist and an associate professor at the University of Minnesota, Minneapolis. Her research focuses on adolescent pregnancy and sexual health, maternal health, and unintended pregnancy. She is the principal investigator (PI) of an HRSA-funded Leadership Center in Maternal and Child Public Health and co-PI of the National Children's Study—Ramsey County. In 2006, she received the University's highest teaching honor and thus holds the title of University Distinguished Teaching Professor. She is also a recipient of the Association of Teachers of Maternal and Child Health's Loretta P. Lacey Award for national leadership in research, service, and training.

J. Neil Henderson, PhD, is Professor of Medical Anthropology at the University of Oklahoma College of Public Health and Director, American Indian Diabetes Prevention Center. He is Oklahoma Choctaw. His research uses a biocultural model to study Alzheimer's in American Indian tribes, cultural constructs of Alzheimer's and diabetes, and support group development in African American and Spanish-speaking populations. He has conducted geriatric health education for culturally diverse providers across the United States. He received the Leadership in Prevention for Native Americans (2006) award from Loma Linda University School of Public Health and the Award of Achievement from the University of Oklahoma, College of Public Health. He is a prolific author in the scientific press, coauthor of *Social and Behavioral Foundations of Public Health* (2001) and, with Maria Vesperi, editor of *The Culture of Long Term Care* (1995).

L. Carson Henderson, RN, PhD, MPH, is an assistant professor of research in the College of Public Health at the University of Oklahoma and a clinical instructor and adjunct faculty member in the Department of Geriatric Medicine. She is a biocultural gerontologist whose research foci include cross-cultural perspectives in neuro-epidemiology and diabetes. Her research has examined diverse types of disease models of diabetes among American Indian elders and health care providers, and she continues this work through a Robert Wood Johnson grant. Concurrently, she is conducting research into the cultural construction of dementia among American Indian caregivers. She is the project coordinator for the American Indian Diabetes Center, funded by the NIH Center for Minority Health and Health Disparities, and coinvestigator for research examining the cultural construction of gestational diabetes among American Indian women.

Karen Liller, PhD, is Associate Dean for Academic and Student Affairs and a tenured full professor at the University of South Florida College of Public Health. She specializes in the prevention of child and adolescent unintentional injuries and has been the recipient of several awards for her teaching and research efforts. She has published extensively in top peer-reviewed publications and was named one of the top 15 national women scholars in health education and health promotion. She is the editor of *Injury Prevention for Children and Adolescents: Research, Practice, and Advocacy,* published by the American Public Health Association.

Stephanie L. Marhefka, PhD, is Assistant Professor in the Department of Community and Family Health at the University of South Florida, where she teaches the introductory Master of Public Health course on the social and behavioral sciences in public health. She is a clinical and health psychologist with experience in a variety of health care settings. She has served as faculty for Fogarty International AIDS Training Programs serving Nigeria and India. Her research interests include HIV/AIDS, mental health and coping, adherence to medical regimens, sexual health promotion, sexual risk reduction, and pregnancy as an opportunity for health promotion and risk reduction. She has published peer-reviewed articles related to the mental health of adolescents and children living with HIV, adherence to medical regimens among children and families living with HIV, and the sexual health and development of children and youth.

Robert J. McDermott has an academic career spanning 33 years, which includes positions held at the University of Wisconsin–Madison (UW-Madison), Southern Illinois University–Carbondale, and the University of South Florida (USF) College of Public Health. He is codirector of the Florida Prevention Research Center at USF and codeveloper of the community-based prevention marketing (CBPM) framework. He has contributed to more than 300 publications and is a fellow of the American School Health Association, American Academy of Health Behavior, Royal Institute of Public Health, American Association for Health Education, and Royal Society for Health Promotion. He received his BS, MS, and PhD degrees from the UW-Madison.

Mimi Nichter, PhD, is an associate professor in the Department of Anthropology at the University of Arizona, where she also holds joint appointments in the Department of Family Studies and Human Development and the College of Public Health. Her research interests include tobacco use among adolescents and emerging adults, body image and dieting among teens, and women's health in national and global contexts. She has conducted long-term fieldwork in South and Southeast Asia on maternal and child health. She is currently working in India and Indonesia on an NIH Fogarty project in which culturally appropriate tobacco cessation programs are being developed and implemented in community and clinical settings. She is the author of numerous articles on national and global health issues and has written two books: *Fat Talk: What Girls and Their Parents Say About Dieting* (2000) and *Anthropology and International Health: Asian Case Studies* (with Mark Nichter, 2001).

Paul E. Spector is a distinguished university professor of industrial/organizational (I/O) psychology and I/O Doctoral Program Director at the University of South Florida. He is also Director of the NIOSH-funded Sunshine Education and Research Center's Occupational Health Psychology program. He is Associate Editor for Point/Counterpoint for *Journal of Organizational Behavior* and is on the editorial boards of *Journal of Applied Psychology, Journal of Occupational and Organizational Psychology, Organizational Research Methods,* and *Personnel Psychology.* In 1991, the Institute for Scientific Information listed him as one of the 50 highest-impact contemporary researchers (out of over 102,000) in psychology worldwide.

Linda M. Whiteford, Associate Vice President for Academic Affairs and Strategic Initiatives in the Office of the Provost, is Professor of Anthropology at the University of South Florida. She is a medical anthropologist who has worked in numerous international settings. Much of her work has focused on maternal/child and reproductive health, water scarcity and waterborne diseases such as cholera and dengue fever, and, most recently, human health during and following disasters such as volcanic eruptions. She has been a consultant for organizations such as the World Bank, the World Health Organization, the Pan American Health Organization, the United States Agency for International Development, and the Canadian Agency for International Development. She holds a doctorate in cultural anthropology and master's degrees in both anthropology and public health.

Marissa Zwald, BS, is an MPH student and graduate research assistant in the Department of Community and Family Health at the University of South Florida in Tampa.

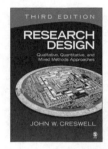
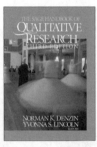
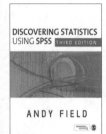
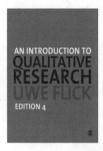
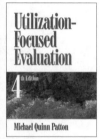
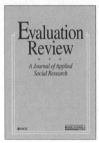
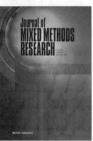
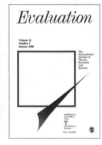
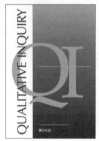
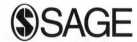